SURGERY - PROCEDURES, COMPLICATIONS, AND RESULTS

ENHANCED RECOVERY AFTER SURGERY (ERAS) IN BARIATRIC SURGERY

SURGERY - PROCEDURES, COMPLICATIONS, AND RESULTS

Additional books and e-books in this series can be found on Nova's website under the Series tab.

SURGERY - PROCEDURES, COMPLICATIONS, AND RESULTS

ENHANCED RECOVERY AFTER SURGERY (ERAS) IN BARIATRIC SURGERY

JAIME RUIZ-TOVAR
EDITOR

nova
Medicine & Health
New York

Library of Congress Cataloging-in-Publication Data

ISBN: 978-1-53619-976-5

Published by Nova Science Publishers, Inc. † New York

CONTENTS

PREFACE

Obesity is considered a pandemic in developed countries. The reality is that obesity rates are increasing in developed and developing countries and this is beginning to be a real problem.

Although we are living in a society based on the image of the person, based on the concept that a good image is associated with success (professional and personal success), obesity is not only an image problem, but it is also a health problem. Obesity is associated with many metabolic disorders, such as diabetes mellitus, dyslipidemia, hypertension, sleep apnea-hypopnea syndrome, liver steatosis etc. Far away from the psychological impact, obesity and its related comorbidities are silent diseases. These disorders are mostly asymptomatic and the patients do not complain of pain or any other symptoms for a long time. It is just when the symptoms appear that the damage is already irreversible. The objective of the fight against obesity is to prevent these permanent damages, increasing life expectancy and quality of life.

The first step in the treatment of obesity is diet and physical activity, but the main problem is that patients often tire from following both and abandon them, regaining the weight they have lost. After several attempts of diets with mild weight loss and regaining more and more weight, this situation leads to a morbidly obese status. The word "morbid" means that obesity itself represents a disease.

For morbidly obese patients, bariatric surgery is the best option to achieve a significant and maintained weight loss. Thousands of bariatric procedures are performed all around the world. Two facts have contributed to this exponential development of bariatric surgery. The first one is obviously the demand of the society. The second one is the minimally invasive approach. The first procedures performed by laparotomy were associated with incredibly high complications and mortality rates. However, with the implementation of the laparoscopic approach worldwide, these complications rates have significantly decreased, implying that bariatric surgery is actually a safe procedure, with mortality rates under 0.5% and morbidity rates under 5%. Notwithstanding, the complications following laparoscopic bariatric techniques are still life-threatening conditions.

Bariatric surgery is amenable for Enhanced Recovery After Surgery protocols. ERAS programs are a multidisciplinary approach in the perioperative care of the patient undergoing major surgery, including pre, intra and postoperative measures, based on the actual evidence published in literature (evidence-based medicine), to improve the postoperative recovery of the patient. ERAS protocols have been widely developed in colorectal surgery, but given their excellent results, new protocols and guidelines have been developed in other surgical fields, including bariatric surgery. Despite the peculiarities of the morbidly obese patient, several ERAS protocols have been implemented worldwide in bariatric surgery in the last decade, confirming their safety and advantages of ERAS approaches, even on morbidly obese patients.

Spain was the first country in developing a national ERAS protocol on bariatric surgery and different publications have demonstrated the safety of this approach and overall improvement in postoperative recovery.

I hope that this book, based on the current evidence and the experience of a group of experts in the implementation of ERAS protocols on bariatric surgery, can be helpful in clinical practices. However, we must keep always in mind that the medical field obtains new data, drugs and approaches every day, so that current evidence can be outdated in the following decade, requiring future updates.

Finally, I want to thank to all the contributing authors, all of them friends and experts in the field of bariatric surgery, for their availability, time and effort in writing the chapters.

Jaime Ruiz-Tovar, MD, PhD
Editor

In: Enhanced Recovery after Surgery ... ISBN: 978-1-53619-976-5
Editor: Jaime Ruiz-Tovar

Chapter 1

PREOPERATIVE INFORMATION OF THE PATIENT AND PSYCHOLOGICAL SUITABILITY FOR BARIATRIC SURGERY

Maria de Lourdes Bolaños Muñoz[1,*], PhD, Gilberto Gonzalez Ramirez[2], MD and Diana Laura Martínez Bolaños[3]

[1]Department of Neuropsychology and Neurolingüístic, Neuroscience Institute, Universidad de Guadalajara Jalisco, México
[2]Department of Surgery and Bariatric Surgery, Real San Jose Hospital, Guadalajara Jalisco Mexico, Universidad de Guadalajara Jalisco, México
[3]Universidad Autónoma de Guadalajara, México

ABSTRACT

Obesity is a challenge for the patient itself, the family's patients the clinical approach, and the surgery team. Also for the society economically, politically, and as a health pandemic illness.

---

* Corresponding Author's Email: mariad.bolanosm@academicos.udg.mx.

Nothing statically has been more for sure in the obesity ill than the complications related. And now in the settings of these new contexts that imply the SARS-COV 19 pandemic complications which means a new wide window that we need to close trying to avoid the fatalities that would be a high cost to pay for everyone. For these reasons and others well known the patients seeking an obesity surgery must be more than ever well informed and with a highly accurate psychological profiling looking the best treatment for each patient in their settings. And avoid cooking recipes. Now it is a challenge for everyone.

In this chapter, we are going to boarding the basic information pre-op for those patients, like expectations, possible risk, and complications, and at the same time an accurate psychologist profile for the best surgical bariatric alternatives. This is a revisional literature chapter looking for the different knowledge among the data published around the world and time.

Keywords: psychological suitability, bariatric surgery, preoperative expectations, surgical goals, weight loss

Introduction

The best surgery is for the best patient… this is not quite accurate, in the setting of the obesity world, the patients are very complex not just because they are under an obese state but because they are complex in their minds and context of life. Sometimes this context is the best predictor not always easy to be modified to achieve the goal that we are looking for. That's why we must be very careful since the beginning in the approaching of each patient in the first consultation with our bariatric team.

Background

Several reasons lead patients to choose to undergo weight loss procedures. Previous studies have demonstrated that patients have unrealistic weight loss goals. However, there is a general paucity of information on a patient's expectations in regards to comorbidity improvement and resolution [1].

In developed countries, 10–20% of the adult population is obese [2]. In the USA, over 130 million adults are overweight or obese. Indeed, obesity is now the second most common cause of death in the USA, accounting for 300,000 deaths annually or approximately 14% of all deaths [3]. Organizations such as the National Institutes of Health and the Surgeon General of the USA have acknowledged the severity of the obesity problem and have urged the development of public health strategies to curb the epidemic [4].

Bariatric surgery is the only procedure that has been consistently shown to result in sustainable long-term weight loss and significant improvement in medical comorbidity [5]. Bariatric surgery is recommended for well informed and motivated patients with a Body Mass Index (BMI) ≥40 kg/m^2 or for individuals with a BMI ≥35 kg/m^2 and one or more severe obesity-related comorbidities, such as type II diabetes, hypertension, hyperlipidemia, obstructive sleep apnea, nonalcoholic fatty liver disease, and gastroesophageal reflux disease [6].

The effectiveness of bariatric surgery (BS) is known to be superior to other dietary and medical interventions [7]. However, long-term success following BS is not guaranteed and depends greatly on patient compliance to dietary and lifestyle recommendations and nutritional counseling follow-up [8-9]. Additionally, bariatric patients who do not adhere to recommended dietary guidelines following surgery are at higher risk to develop nutrition-related complications [10]. BS candidates exhibit a high occurrence of unhealthy eating and lifestyle habits [11]. Knowledge gaps and lack of engagement in preoperative patients can result in suboptimal outcomes after surgery [8]. Expectations that are higher than realistic goals may cause disappointment with surgery outcomes [12] and therefore can negatively affect patients' motivation and adherence to long-term treatment and weight maintenance [13].

Considering that bariatric surgery leads to improvements in physical, social, and medical aspects, patients have a variety of reasons why they choose to undergo weight loss procedures. It is therefore important to examine a patient's motivation and expectations with regards to these three aspects. Previous studies examining weight loss expectations in bariatric surgery patients have demonstrated that patients have unrealistic goals [14-17].

Data on BS nutrition knowledge, weight loss expectations, and anxiety levels among BS candidates are scarce, and the optimal concept or timing for pre-surgical educational intervention remains unclear [18].

Patients with a BMI of 30–34.9 kg/m^2 with diabetes or metabolic syndrome may also be offered a bariatric procedure, although currently there is a lack of long-term data demonstrating net benefit [19].

The benefits of bariatric surgery are well documented, patients who undergo this procedure can also present with postoperative issues that need to be taken into account [20]. In fact, diverse studies have demonstrated a rise in substance use disorders [21-22], the persistence or emergence of eating disorders [23-24], and frequent body image concerns [25] after bariatric surgery. Moreover, long-term research has indicated that the psychological improvement after bariatric surgery is only temporary and not maintained in the long term [26-27].

According to the best practice update of evidence-based guidelines for psychosocial evaluation and treatment of weight-loss surgery patients, assessment should be performed by a social worker, psychologist, or psychiatrist with a background and at least some experience in the pre-and postoperative assessment of bariatric candidates [28].

Karmali et al. (2011) found that the motivating factors for the majority of patients were improvement of their medical status; however, their expectations for disease resolution or marked improvement were lower than their weight loss expectations. The reason for this discord could be related to a misconception by the patients that they have to lose an excessive amount of weight before comorbidity resolution could be achieved [1].

This knowledge gap requires further exploration, including different techniques of education and ensuring that patients have as full an understanding as possible. Before attending the educational seminar, patients generally undergo significant self-directed research into the risks and benefits of bariatric surgery. They have wide resources including hospital websites, online discussion groups, and surgical-industry-sponsored websites. Regardless of whether success rates such as % EWL are referenced from medical literature, there is usually an emphasis on success stories with results that are not necessarily typical. Combined with a patient's desire to undergo a surgical "cure" for obesity, expectations of success may be incorrect [1].

According to a recently published systematic review of patient education practices in BS, educational programs vary among centers in terms of curriculum, teaching methods, and educator and commonly use passive learning methods, primarily in classroom settings [29]. Digital communication methods such as online education programs may be utilized to increase patient engagement and minimize barriers such as time, distance, and cost [29-30].

Since several years ago, the surgical teams and medical staff related are investigating the reason of the patient´s desire to undergo bariatric surgery. Muñoz et al. published in 2007, that their patients appeared to be motivated for surgery primarily to control current medical problems. However, a significant portion of patients referred psychological and quality of life factors as important in their decision to seek weight loss surgery [31].

Unlike many other surgical and medical procedures, both short- and long-term outcomes associated with weight-loss surgery are dependent on psychological and behavioral factors present.

Patients considering bariatric surgery had a higher level of body dissatisfaction than those seeking non-surgical treatment, and this agrees with studies reporting that body image is a common motivation for bariatric surgery [32-33].

Psychological and Psychiatric Suitability

It is now clear that obese subjects more commonly report impairments in numerous psychological variables than the non-obese population. Indeed, people with obesity report high levels of depression and anxiety and a low level of self-esteem [34] that might make them psychologically more fragile [35].

High rates of psychiatric disorders among candidates for bariatric surgery seem to be the rule rather than an exception. The current and lifetime rates of psychopathology in bariatric surgery candidates are very high. About one-third of patients presenting for a preoperative evaluation have at least one current Axis I diagnosis from the DSM-V, and over two-thirds have a lifetime history of any psychiatric diagnosis [36]. The lifetime rates ranged from 36.8 to 72.6% for lifetime disorders in studies reported in USA37-39 and Europe [40-41], while in Latin America this is slightly higher (80.9%) [42].

The most frequent psychiatric disorders found in bariatric patients with morbid obesity are depression, anxiety, and eating disorders. A recent meta-analysis of 59 published papers estimated that 23% of bariatric candidates suffer from a current mood disorder and about 17% present with a current eating disorder. The most common psychiatric disorders are depression (19%), binge eating disorder (17%), and anxiety (12%). In addition, prevalence estimates are 9% for a history of suicidal ideations, 3% for substance use disorders, and 1% for Posttraumatic Stress Disorder [43].

Anxiety Disorders

Prevalence estimates for anxiety disorders (including generalized anxiety disorder and social phobia) in a bariatric population vary from 12 to 46.3% at the time of presurgical evaluation, and are even up to 37.5% for a lifetime diagnosis of anxiety disorder [44]. In addition, these rates seem to remain similarafter the surgery [45].

In patients that seek bariatric surgery, Duarte-Guerra et al. (2014) found that Anxiety disorders were the most common ones (46.3%), and generalized anxiety disorder (GAD) was the most frequent disorder (23.9%), followed by phobias; among this classification, Social Phobia showed the highest frequency (17%). Lifetime anxiety disorders were present in 54.7% of participants [42].

Affective Disorders

As outlined earlier, depression is a significant comorbidity in obese individuals.

Duarte-Guerra et al. (2014), found that the second most frequent class of disorders in patients that seek bariatric surgery were affective disorders (21.6%), bipolar disorders II (7.4%), and major depressive disorders (6.9%), being the most common disorders in this class. Affective disorders were the most frequent category of lifetime disorders (64.9%) [42].

Preoperative depression may impede postoperative weight loss, and higher depression scores after the surgery have been associated with less weight loss. However, some studies have reported that depression improves significantly after the surgery, but the improvement may begin to decline over time [5]. It is mandatory to rule out suicidal ideas, and if this is a possibility, close surveillance to any emotional change in the post-surgical period is mandatory, as existing evidence has identified an increased rate of suicide after bariatric surgery, as well as an increased rate of self-harm emergencies [46]. Unlike other psychopathologies that improve after bariatric surgery, suicide risk remains high and warrants long-term supervision [47].

Eating Disorders

Among the most common eating disorder in the presurgical candidates is binge eating disorders (BED). Their rates vary from 4 to 49% and are difficult to estimate primarily due to classification problems because the actual diagnostic criteria were not developed until the publication of DSM-V.48. The report of Duarte-Guerra et al. (2014) showed that the frequency of eating disorders was 20.1%, with binge eating disorder being 16.5% of the cases. Lifetime eating disorders were diagnosed in 35.1%, with binge eating disorders being 29.8%. Women were significantly more likely than men to meet the criteria for a lifetime for bulimia ($p = 0.02$) [42].

Substance Use Disorders

A lifetime history of substance use disorder is more likely in bariatric surgery candidates compared with the general population [28]. About one-third of patients have a lifetime history of alcohol use disorder [44]. In contrast, current rates of alcohol and substance use are only around

3% and are much lower than in the general population [19]. Duarte-Guerra et al. (2014) reported a total of 3.1% of the sample reported any SUD, with men being significantly more likely than women to meet the criteria for such disorders ($p = 0.01$) [42].

Thought Disorders

There is very limited research that has examined whether bariatric surgery can be safe and effective in patients diagnosed with thought disorders, including schizophrenia [48]. These patients are typically denied for the surgery despite an overall lack of research supports this recommendation. Patients with thought disorders exhibit deficits in memory, attention, and executive functioning, and similar cognitive deficits are associated with obesity across the lifespan and can be further exacerbated by medical comorbidities such as sleep apnea and type II diabetes [44]. It has been reported that patients with thought disorders have similar weight-loss outcomes as matched controls; however, their underlying psychopathology may worsen following the surgery [49].

Personality Disorders

Mauri et al. (2008) reported a frequency of 19.5% of patient candidates for bariatric surgery that met the criteria for at least 1 Axis II disorder. Cluster C disorders, including avoidant, dependent, and obsessive-compulsive personality disorders, comprised virtually all the disorders in the sample. Cluster C disorders were more frequent, but not significantly, in females and the severe/very severe BMI classification [50].

Cognitive Impairment

It has been reported that obese persons exhibit impairments on formal cognitive testing, including on tasks of executive function, such as inhibitory control and impulsivity [51], attention, and memory [52-53].

Bariatric surgery patients, exhibited high rates of pre-operative cognitive impairments in attention, executive function, memory, and language [54].

Lokken et al. found that obese adults seeking bariatric surgery did demonstrate specific cognitive deficits on tests of executive function (e.g., problem-solving and planning, assessed with the Rey Complex Figure Test (CFT) and cognitive flexibility using the Wisconsin Card Sorting Test (WCST) when compared with normative data. The data provided evidence for specific cognitive deficits in the area of executive functions at baseline in morbidly obese [55].

School problems and cognitive impairment are found to be associated with increased BMI among younger bariatric candidates. Therefore, improving academic support and deficiencies in educational systems for obese students is necessary to make the assessment and intervention complete [47].

Bariatric surgery is associated with improved cognition and such improvements may be found at extended follow-up in some. The impact of bariatric surgery on cognitive function may occur in the immediate months following surgical intervention, as this is the time of the most substantial weight loss and resolution of medical comorbidities that negatively affect cognitive function [56-57]. Cognitive benefits are likely sustained if weight regain is avoided or minimized, though future studies are needed to confirm this notion [58].

Psychotropic Medications Use in Bariatric Population

Almost half of the individuals seeking bariatric surgery report current use of psychotropic medications, taking antidepressants (87.7%), followed by anxiolytics (9.6%) and mood stabilizers (2.7%) [59].

MENTAL HEALTH EVALUATION

Unlike many other surgical and medical procedures, both short- and long-term outcomes associated with weight-loss surgery are dependent on psychological and behavioral factors present before and after the surgery. Successful bariatric outcomes are not only dependent on the surgical procedures but also require significant and lifelong changes in eating patterns and physical activity. At the same time, weight-loss surgery has wide-ranging and profound psychosocial effects. A thorough and specialized preoperative psychosocial assessment is an important part of a comprehensive bariatric treatment protocol [60].

Based on the survey of present practices, preoperative psychosocial assessment has become the standard of care in about 90% of centers offering weight-loss surgery, [61] and it is required for bariatric surgery centers to be nationally accredited by the American College of Surgeons and the American Society for Metabolic and Bariatric Surgery. There is a growing emphasis that the preoperative psychosocial assessment should be used to identify possible contraindications for surgery, such as uncontrolled substance abuse or poorly controlled mental illness [19].

The psychosocial evaluation of weight-loss surgery candidates should be a multifaceted process that can serve many functions. On one hand, it can help to enhance the patient's readiness for the weight-loss procedure through increasing knowledge of surgery and postoperative behavioral regimen. On the other hand, it can help to minimize the barriers to optimal weight-loss outcomes through identifying and addressing potential postoperative challenges and establishing an ongoing connection with behavioral health providers [38]. In addition, it can be an invaluable contribution to the interdisciplinary bariatric team, through reducing clinic burden, helping managing risk and liability, and providing comprehensive guidance [60].

Psychological Assessment Tools

While there is considerable variability in the content of presurgical psychosocial assessment across different bariatric centers, information is typically gathered via a comprehensive clinical interview and administration of self-report questionnaires [5]. More than half of the programs use formal psychological testing as a part of the assessment. Despite the frequency of use of psychological testing, there are few guidelines available on which tests should be utilized to assess patients´ suitability for surgery. Commonly used symptom inventories or screening instruments assess symptoms of depression, eating disorders, and anxiety disorders. They include the Beck Depression Inventory (BDI-II), which has demonstrated satisfactory internal consistency and validity in the bariatric surgery population, [39], and Minnesota Multiphasic Personality Inventory (MMPI-2) which assesses psychiatric and personality traits and has been found reliable and valid to use in this population [41]. The Symptom Checklist-90-Revised (SCL90-R) has also been validated in bariatric surgery patients and its hostility scale was predictive to the adherence to treatment plans [62].

Another frequently used tool is the Hamilton Anxiety Rating Scale (HARS) [63]. Among the scales that search the alimentary behavior are.

Eating Disorders Inventory (EDI-2) [64] and self-report questionnaire, the Bulimic Investigatory Test, Edinburgh (BITE) [65] (62) 20 (Mauri).

It is also a good recommendation to include scales that explore the patient quality of life, such as the Impact of weight on quality of life-lite (IWQOL) [66] or the short-form Quality of Life Enjoyment and Satisfaction Questionnaire (Q-LES-Q) [67].

The GRWQ was developed to address the weight loss expectations of obese patients seeking nonoperative weight loss treatment. The GRWQ is divided into two parts—the first addresses a patient's personal weight loss goals and factors that influence their selection. The second part assesses the expectations and evaluations of a variety of specifically determined weight loss outcomes [68].

Finally, the patient's capacity for regulation and self-control in their daily life can be explored using the Barrat impulsivity scale (BIS-11), [69] or the Behavior Rating Inventory of Executive Function scale-Adult Version (BRIEF-A) [70]. The latter has the advantage that it can be administered in self-report or informant format, allowing us to obtain more objective and ecological information on the patient's functioning.

Contraindications

To summarize, the most common reasons for deferring bariatric surgery are significant psychopathology such as active psychosis (including thought disorder symptoms), current substance dependence, untreated eating disorders (specifically anorexia nervosa or bulimia nervosa), untreated depression, or patients in a situation of current emotional crisis (emotional breakdown, recent grief, etc.) and/ or active suicidal ideation [5]. In addition, intellectual disability, inadequate knowledge about the surgery resulting in the inability to provide informed consent, unrealistic expectations for weight loss, and lack of social support have been most frequently reported as nonpsychiatric contraindications [5, 40, 61, 71-73].

Discussion

Bariatric surgery has been consistently shown to be effective in long-term marked weight loss and in bringing significant improvement to medical comorbidities. We have found a substantially high prevalence of psychiatric disorders among bariatric surgery candidates. Depressive disorders, anxiety disorders, and binge eating disorders are the most common diagnoses. Part of the psychopathologies before surgery may be attenuated after surgery, though the mechanism is not clarified [47].

A substantial proportion of bariatric candidates present themselves in an overly favorable light during the psychological evaluation, and there is low congruence between clinically derived and research-based diagnoses, which may impact accurate assessment [48]. Carrying out a careful exploration of the patient's psychopathology history, and when possible to consider the report of an informant, will allow us to have a clearer and more objective impression of the patient, that helps us to identify those personality traits, as well as the presence of psychopathology that may hinder the success of the bariatric patient's treatment, and their achievement of both physical and emotional well-being. In case of not identifying any absolute contraindication, it will be possible to propose a psychological and/or psychiatric intervention program that allows us to achieve the best physical and psychosocial results.

REFERENCES

[1] Karmali S, Kadikoy H, Brandt ML, Sherman V. What is my goal? Expected weight loss and comorbidity outcomes among bariatric surgery patients. *Obes Surg.* 2011;21(5):595–603.

[2] World Health Organization. *Obesity: preventing and managing the global epidemic.* Geneva: The Organization; 2004. Report No.: Technical report series 894.

[3] Wang Y, Beydoun MA, Liang L, Caballero B, Kumanyika SK. Will all Americans become overweight or obese? Estimating the progression and cost of the US obesity epidemic. *Obesity* (Silver Spring). 2008;16(10):2323–30.

[4] National Institutes of Health. *Clinical guidelines on the identification, evaluation and treatment of overweight and obesity in adults.* Bethesda: National Institutes of Health; 1998.

[5] Müller A, Mitchell JE, Sondag C, de Zwaan M. Psychiatric aspects of bariatric surgery. *Curr Psychiatry Rep.* 2013;15(10):397.

[6] NIH conference. Gastrointestinal surgery for severe obesity. Consensus Development Conference Panel. *Ann Intern Med.* 1991;115(12):956–61.

[7] Colquitt JL, Pickett K, Loveman E, Frampton GK. Surgery for weight loss in adults. *Cochrane Libr* [Internet]. 2014; Available from: http://dx.doi.org/10.1002/14651858.cd003641.pub4

[8] Mundi MS, Lorentz PA, Grothe K, Kellogg TA, Collazo-Clavell ML. Feasibility of smartphone-based education modules and ecological momentary assessment/intervention in pre-bariatric surgery patients. *Obes Surg.* 2015;25(10):1875–81.

[9] Freire RH, Borges MC, Alvarez-Leite JI, Toulson Davisson Correia MI. Food quality, physical activity, and nutritional follow-up as determinant of weight regain after Roux-en-Y gastric bypass. *Nutrition.* 2012;28(1):53–8.

[10] Taube-Schiff M, Chaparro M, Gougeon L, Shakory S, Weiland M, Warwick K, et al. Examining nutrition knowledge of bariatric surgery patients: What happens to dietary knowledge over time? *Obes Surg.* 2016;26(5):972–82.

[11] Oved I, Vaiman IM, Hod K, Mardy-Tilbor L, Torban Y, Dagan SS. Poor health behaviors prior to laparoscopic sleeve gastrectomy surgery. *Obes Surg.* 2017;27(2):469–75.

[12] Heinberg LJ, Keating K, Simonelli L. Discrepancy between ideal and realistic goal weights in three bariatric procedures: who is likely to be unrealistic? *Obes Surg.* 2010;20(2):148–53.

[13] Sherf-Dagan S, Hod K, Mardy-Tilbor L, Gliksman S, Ben-Porat T, Sakran N, et al. The effect of pre-surgery information online lecture on nutrition knowledge and anxiety among bariatric surgery candidates. *Obes Surg.* 2018;28(7):1876–85.

[14] White MA, Masheb RM, Burke-Martindale C, Rothschild B, Grilo CM. Accuracy of self-reported weight among bariatric surgery candidates: the influence of race and weight cycling. *Obesity* (Silver Spring). 2007;15(11):2761–8.

[15] Wadden TA, Butryn ML, Sarwer DB, Fabricatore AN, Crerand CE, Lipschutz PE, et al. Comparison of psychosocial status in treatment-seeking women with class III vs. class I-II obesity. *Surg Obes Relat Dis.* 2006;2(2):138–45.

[16] Wolfe BL, Terry ML. Expectations and outcomes with gastric bypass surgery. *Obes Surg.* 2006;16(12):1622–9.

[17] Wee CC, Jones DB, Davis RB, Bourland AC, Hamel MB. Understanding patients' value of weight loss and expectations for bariatric surgery. *Obes Surg.* 2006;16(4):496–500.

[18] Groller KD. Systematic review of patient education practices in weight loss surgery. *Surg Obes Relat Dis.* 2017;13(6):1072–85.

[19] Mechanick JI, Youdim A, Jones DB, Garvey WT, Hurley DL, McMahon MM, et al. Clinical practice guidelines for the perioperative nutritional, metabolic, and nonsurgical support of the bariatric surgery patient--2013 update: cosponsored by American Association of Clinical Endocrinologists, The Obesity Society, and American Society for Metabolic & Bariatric Surgery: AACE/TOS/ASMBS Guidelines. *Obesity* (Silver Spring). 2013;21 Suppl 1(S1):S1-27.

[20] Adams TD, Gress RE, Smith SC, Halverson RC, Simper SC, Rosamond WD, et al. Long-term mortality after gastric bypass surgery. *N Engl J Med.* 2007;357(8):753–61.

[21] Svensson P-A, Anveden Å, Romeo S, Peltonen M, Ahlin S, Burza MA, et al. Alcohol consumption and alcohol problems after bariatric surgery in the Swedish obese subjects study: Alcohol Consumption and Alcohol Problems After Bariatric Surgery. *Obesity* (Silver Spring). 2013;21(12):2444–51.

[22] Conason A, Teixeira J, Hsu CH, Puma L, Knafo D, Geliebter A. Substance use following bariatric weight loss surgery. *JAMA Surg.* 2013;148(2):145–50.

[23] Colles SL, Dixon JB, O'Brien PE. Grazing and loss of control related to eating: two high-risk factors following bariatric surgery. *Obesity* (Silver Spring). 2008;16(3):615–22.

[24] Wood KV, Ogden J. Explaining the role of binge eating behaviour in weight loss post bariatric surgery. *Appetite.* 2012;59(1):177–80.

[25] Ivezaj V, Grilo CM. The complexity of body image following bariatric surgery: a systematic review of the literature. *Obes Rev.* 2018;19(8):1116–40.

[26] Herpertz S, Müller A, Burgmer R, Crosby RD, de Zwaan M, Legenbauer T. Health-related quality of life and psychological functioning 9 years after restrictive surgical treatment for obesity. *Surg Obes Relat Dis.* 2015;11(6):1361–70.

[27] Booth H, Khan O, Prevost AT, Reddy M, Charlton J, Gulliford MC, et al. Impact of bariatric surgery on clinical depression. Interrupted time series study with matched controls. *J Affect Disord.* 2015;174:644–9.

[28] Greenberg I, Sogg S, M Perna F. Behavioral and psychological care in weight loss surgery: best practice update. *Obesity* (Silver Spring). 2009;17(5):880–4.

[29] Groller KD. Systematic review of patient education practices in weight loss surgery. *Surg Obes Relat Dis.* 2017;13(6):1072–85.

[30] McGrice M, Don Paul K. Interventions to improve long-term weight loss in patients following bariatric surgery: challenges and solutions. *Diabetes Metab Syndr Obes.* 2015;8:263–74.

[31] Munoz DJ, Lal M, Chen EY, Mansour M, Fischer S, Roehrig M, et al. Why patients seek bariatric surgery: a qualitative and quantitative analysis of patient motivation. *Obes Surg.* 2007;17(11):1487–91.

[32] Libeton M, Dixon JB, Laurie C, O'Brien PE. Patient motivation for bariatric surgery: characteristics and impact on outcomes. *Obes Surg*. 2004;14(3):392–8.

[33] Wee CC, Hamel MB, Apovian CM, Blackburn GL, Bolcic-Jankovic D, Colten ME, et al. Expectations for weight loss and willingness to accept risk among patients seeking weight loss surgery. *JAMA* Surg. 2013;148(3):264–71.

[34] van Hout GCM, van Oudheusden I, van Heck GL. Psychological profile of the morbidly obese. *Obes Surg*. 2004;14(5):579–88.

[35] Gaudrat B, Andrieux S, Florent V, Rousseau A. Psychological characteristics of patients seeking bariatric treatment versus those seeking medical treatment for obesity: is bariatric surgery a last best hope? *Eat Weight Disord*. 2021;26(3):949–61.

[36] Mitchell JE, Selzer F, Kalarchian MA, Devlin MJ, Strain GW, Elder KA, et al. Psychopathology before surgery in the longitudinal assessment of bariatric surgery-3 (LABS-3) psychosocial study. *Surg Obes Relat Dis*. 2012;8(5):533–41.

[37] Sogg S, Mori DL. Psychosocial evaluation for bariatric surgery: the Boston interview and opportunities for intervention. *Obes Surg*. 2009;19(3):369–77.

[38] Ratcliffe D, Sogg S, Friedman KE. Letter to the editor: A comparative study of three-year weight loss and outcomes after laparoscopic gastric bypass in patients with "yellow light" psychological clearance. *Obes Surg*. 2015;25(3):539–40.

[39] Rouleau CR, Rash JA, Mothersill KJ. Ethical issues in the psychosocial assessment of bariatric surgery candidates. *J Health Psychol*. 2016;21(7):1457–71.

[40] Fabricatore AN, Crerand CE, Wadden TA, Sarwer DB, Krasucki JL. How do mental health professionals evaluate candidates for bariatric surgery? Survey results. *Obes Surg*. 2006;16(5):567–73.

[41] Marek RJ, Ben-Porath YS, Ashton K, Heinberg LJ. Minnesota multiphasic personality inventory-2 restructured form (MMPI-2-RF) scale score differences in bariatric surgery candidates diagnosed with binge eating disorder versus BMI-matched controls: MMPI-2-RF and Bed. *Int J Eat Disord*. 2014;47(3):315–9.

[42] Duarte-Guerra LS, Coêlho BM, Santo MA, Wang YP. Psychiatric disorders among obese patients seeking bariatric surgery: results of structured clinical interviews. *Obes Surg.* 2015;25(5):830–7.

[43] Dawes AJ, Maggard-Gibbons M, Maher AR, Booth MJ, Miake-Lye I, Beroes JM, et al. Mental health conditions among patients seeking and undergoing bariatric surgery: A meta-analysis. *JAMA.* 2016;315(2):150.

[44] Marek RJ, Ben-Porath YS, Heinberg LJ. Understanding the role of psychopathology in bariatric surgery outcomes: Hierarchical models and bariatric surgery outcomes. *Obes Rev.* 2016;17(2):126–41. (11) [7].

[45] de Zwaan M, Enderle J, Wagner S, Mühlhans B, Ditzen B, Gefeller O, et al. Anxiety and depression in bariatric surgery patients: a prospective, follow-up study using structured clinical interviews. *J Affect Disord.* 2011;133(1–2):61–8.

[46] Bhatti JA, Nathens AB, Thiruchelvam D, Grantcharov T, Goldstein BI, Redelmeier DA. Self-harm emergencies after bariatric surgery: A population-based cohort study. *JAMA Surg.* 2016;151(3):226–32.

[47] Yen YC, Huang CK, Tai CM. Psychiatric aspects of bariatric surgery. *Curr Opin Psychiatry.* 2014;27(5):374–9.

[48] Gondek W. Psychiatric suitability assessment for bariatric surgery. In: *Psychiatric Care in Severe Obesity.* Cham: Springer International Publishing; 2017. p. 173–86.

[49] Shelby SR, Labott S, Stout RA. Bariatric surgery: a viable treatment option for patients with severe mental illness. *Surg Obes Relat Dis.* 2015;11(6):1342–8.

[50] Mauri M, Rucci P, Calderone A, Santini F, Oppo A, Romano A, et al. Axis I and II disorders and quality of life in bariatric surgery candidates. *J Clin Psychiatry.* 2008;69(2):295–301.

[51] Jasinska AJ, Yasuda M, Burant CF, Gregor N, Khatri S, Sweet M, et al. Impulsivity and inhibitory control deficits are associated with unhealthy eating in young adults. *Appetite.* 2012;59(3):738–47.

[52] Cournot M, Marqui JC, Ansiau D, et al. Relation between body mass index and cognitive function in healthy middle-aged men and women. *Neurology.* 2006; 67:1208–1214.

[53] Gunstad J, Lhotsky A, Wendell CR, et al. Longitudinal examination of obesity and cognitive function: results from the Baltimore Longitudinal Study of Aging. *Neuroepidemiology*. 2010; 34:222–29.

[54] Alosco ML, Galioto R, Spitznagel MB, Strain G, Devlin M, Cohen R, et al. Cognitive function after bariatric surgery: evidence for improvement 3 years after surgery. *Am J Surg.* 2014;207(6):870–6.

[55] Lokken KL, Boeka AG, Yellumahanthi K, Wesley M, Clements RH. Cognitive performance of morbidly obese patients seeking bariatric surgery. *Am Surg.* 2010;76(1):55–9.

[56] Cremieus PY, Ledoux S, Clerici C, Cremieux F, Buessing M. The impact of bariatric surgery on comorbidities and medication use among obese patients. *Obes Surg* 2010;20:861-870. 28.

[57] Fried M, Dolezalova K, Buchwald JN, McGlennon TW, Sramkova P, Ribaric G. Laparoscopic greater curvature plication (LGCP) for treatment of morbid obesity in a series of 244 patients. *Obes Surg* 2012;22:1298-1307.

[58] Alosco ML, Spitznagel MB, Strain G, Devlin M, Cohen R, Paul R, et al. Improved memory function two years after bariatric surgery: Bariatric Surgery and Improved Memory. *Obesity* (Silver Spring). 2014;22(1):32–8.

[59] Pawlow LA, O'Neil PM, White MA, Byrne TK. Findings and outcomes of psychological evaluations of gastric bypass applicants. *Surg Obes Relat Dis.* 2005;1(6):523–7.

[60] Sogg S, Friedman KE. Getting off on the right foot: The many roles of the psychosocial evaluation in the bariatric surgery practice: Roles of the psychosocial evaluation. *Eur Eat Disord Rev.* 2015;23(6):451–6.

[61] Bauchowitz AU, Gonder-Frederick LA, Olbrisch ME, Azarbad L, Ryee M-Y, Woodson M, et al. Psychosocial evaluation of bariatric surgery candidates: a survey of present practices. *Psychosom Med.* 2005;67(5):825–32.

[62] Friedman KE, Applegate KL, Grant J. Who is adherent with preoperative psychological treatment recommendations among weight loss surgery candidates? *Surg Obes Relat Dis.* 2007;3(3):376–82.

[63] Beck AT, Steer RA. Relationship between the beck anxiety inventory and the Hamilton anxiety rating scale with anxious outpatients. *J Anxiety Disord.* 1991;5(3):213–23.

[64] Nevonen L, Clinton D, Norring C. Validating the EDI-2 in three Swedish female samples: eating disorders patients, psychiatric outpatients and normal controls. *Nord J Psychiatry.* 2006;60(1):44–50.

[65] Henderson M, Freeman CP. A self-rating scale for bulimia: the "BITE." *Br J Psychiatry* 1987;150:18–24.

[66] Kolotkin RL, Crosby RD, Williams GR. Health-related quality of life varies among obese subgroups. *Obes Res.* 2002;10(8):748–56.

[67] Endicott J, Nee J, Harrison W, et al. Quality of Life Enjoyment and Satisfaction Questionnaire: a new measure. *Psychopharmacol Bull* 1993;29:321–326.

[68] Foster GD, Wadden TA, Vogt RA, Brewer G. What is a reasonable weight loss? Patients' expectations and evaluations of obesity treatment outcomes. *J Consult Clin Psychol.* 1997;65(1):79–85.

[69] Stanford MS, Mathias CW, Dougherty DM, Lake SL, Anderson NE, Patton JH. Fifty years of the Barratt Impulsiveness Scale: An update and review. *Pers Individ Dif.* 2009;47(5):385–95.

[70] Rouel M, Raman J, Hay P, Smith E. Validation of the Behaviour Rating Inventory of Executive Function – Adult Version (BRIEF-A) in the obese with and without binge eating disorder. *Eat Behav.* 2016;23:58–65.

[71] Walfish S, Vance D, Fabricatore AN. Psychological evaluation of bariatric surgery applicants: procedures and reasons for delay or denial of surgery. *Obes Surg.* 2007;17(12):1578–83.

[72] Marcus MD, Kalarchian MA, Courcoulas AP. Psychiatric evaluation and follow-up of bariatric surgery patients. *Am J Psychiatry.* 2009;166(3):285–91.

[73] Ríos B. *Manejo multidisciplinario del paciente con cirugía bariátrica y metabólica* [*Multidisciplinary patient management with bariatric and metabolic surgery*]. Instituto de Investigación y Educación en Ciencias de la Salud (IIECS). 2016.

In: Enhanced Recovery after Surgery ... ISBN: 978-1-53619-976-5
Editor: Jaime Ruiz-Tovar

Chapter 2

PREOPERATIVE EVALUATION IN BARIATRIC SURGERY

María Asunción Acosta Mérida[1,2*], MD, PhD and Luis Manuel Santana Ortega[3], MD

[1]Department of Esophagogastric, Endocrinometabolic, and Obesity Surgery at the University Hospital of Gran Canaria, Dr. Negrín.
[2]Digestive Surgery at the University of Las Palmas de Gran Canaria, Canary Islands, Spain
[3]Department of Anesthesiology and Critical Care, University Hospital of Gran Canaria, Dr. Negrín.
Las Palmas de Gran Canaria, Canary Islands, Spain

ABSTRACT

An adequate preoperative evaluation is essential for the success of bariatric surgery.

Preoperative optimization aims to educate the patient, promote healthy lifestyle habits, and study and treat the comorbidities to reduce the risk of perioperative complications.

In this chapter, we will analyze the aspects of this preoperative evaluation, focusing mainly on the preoperative cardiovascular,

* Corresponding Author's Email: maacosta03@yahoo.es.

respiratory, metabolic and anesthetic evaluation of the patient candidate for bariatric surgery.

Keywords: preoperative assessment, bariatric surgery, enhanced recovery after surgery, obesity, morbidly obese patient

INTRODUCTION

Obesity is a growing concern in the whole world and one of the most important problems nowadays. It is thought to be the second preventable cause of death in United States (U.S.) [1]. Prevalence has increased quickly across the last decades. According to official statistics of the Centers for Disease Control and Prevention from 2011 to 2014, 36% of American adults and 17% of young people are [2]. This disease is associated with an increase morbidity and mortality as a result of cardiac disease, diabetes and premature death. The evidence supports the impact that obesity directly has on economic and health indicators. [3]. Obesity-related medical care costs in the U. S. in adults increased from 6.13% in 2001to 7.91% in 2015, a rise of 29% [4].

With the available information, there isn´t any specific medical treatment for obesity which provides good results, being the bariatric surgery the only known treatment with long-term outcomes for obesity and its morbidities [5, 6, 7]. The bariatric surgery reverses the the metabolic disorders in those patients, with improvements in diabetes, hypertension, sleep apnoea syndrome, arthritis and/or metabolic syndrome [8, 9] compared to dietetic and medical treatment [10]. However, obesity-related morbidities are risk factors in any surgery; so preoperative assessment is really important.

The enhanced recovery after surgery (ERAS) in bariatric surgery is focused in strategies to reduce the surgical aggression in morbidly obese patient, causing less surgical stress response associated with a better and faster patient recovery [11, 12, 13]. Many studies have showed safety and viability of this perioperative program [14, 15], but in bariatric surgery, reduction in complications and mortality has had variable results compared with other pathologies like colorectal surgery, where real benefits have been demonstrated [16]. The implantation of ERAS bariatric surgery protocols in Spain was analysed by Ruiz-Tovar et al. [17], who concluded after studied 519 patients that the main difference with standard protocols was a decrease of postoperative length of stay, neither improvements in postoperative complications nor in mortality. An ERAS program affects a long period of time, from preoperative stage to beyond surgical procedure. Some of ERAS strategies in each phase are showed below [18]:

A. Previous Phase to Income

- Patient and family information. Consent report. Information paper.
- Psychological conditioning. Assessment and suitability of patient expectations. Changes of lifestyles: Introduction of healthy lifestyle and discourage unhealthy habits
- Preoperative assessment: nutritional, cardiologic, respiratory, metabolic... Clinical, analysis study and additional tests.
- Metabolic optimization: loss weight strategies, hypocaloric diets, healthy habits. Optimization of associated morbilities.
- Functional rehabilitation programs: actions to improve of functional postoperative recovery. Chest physiotherapy.
- Specific anaesthetic issues: airway, medication ...

B. Inmediate Preoperative Phase

- Decrease fasting period: clear liquids until 2 hours before surgery. High carbohydrate drinks reduce insulin resistance. Low residue diet.
- Thromboprophylaxis

C. Intraoperative Phase

- Minimally invasive procedures: laparoscopic surgery

- Antibiotic prophylaxis, antiemetic prophylaxis, temperature control, inflatable pneumatic compression stockings…
- Monitoring, anaesthetic approach (intubation with rapid sequence, alveolar recruitment manoeuvre, “opioid-free analgesia”), multimodal analgesia, fluid balance, gastroesophageal reflux prophylaxis and so on.
- Avoid routine use of drains, catheters, nasogastric tube, …

D. Inmediate Postoperative Phase

- Early mobilization
- Early oral intake
- Multimodal analgesia
- Encouraged breathing exercises (Inspiron).

E. Postoperative Phase and Discharged

- Evaluation of discharged criteria, safety and complications
- Discharged report, outpatients recommendation and advices.
- Telephone call at 24 hours, at-home support and coordination with General Practitioner.

An appropriate preoperative assessment is basic for the bariatric surgical success [19], being a challenge due to anthropometric characteristics and high incidence of associated morbidities. This evaluation should be holistic, integral and include an assessment by multidisciplinary team. This team must be formed by surgeons, endocrinologists, dieticians, psychologists, anaesthesiologists, cardiologists, pulmonologists, gastroenterologists and nurses. Several steps must be taken during the preoperative evaluation to ensure a positive result after bariatric surgical procedure [20].

This chapter has analysed aspects of the period before the surgical hospital admission, focusing mainly on the cardiovascular, respiratory, metabolic and preoperative antesthesic evaluation to determine the fitness of the patient to undergo bariatric surgery. Other issues such as endocrine, nutritional or preoperative diets are regarded in other chapters of this book.

IMPORTANCE OF PREOPERATIVE ASSESSMENT

Despite the improvements in safety that have been achieved, bariatric surgery has complications, which range from 7% to 15% and associate a mortality range from 0.1 to 2% [21, 22, 23, 24]. It has described several risk factors to increase perioperative complications under bariatric surgery [25, 26, 27, 28]. Many of these factors are comorbidities that bariatric surgery itself aims to improve, being the last goal, the reduction of global mortality associated to obesity [29, 30, 31, 32, 33, 34, 35]. Among the few validated systems to stratified specific risks to categorize what is the risk of patients to undergo to bariatric surgery, we have:

- Obesity Surgery- Mortality Risk Score (OS-MRS): It is the most frequently used [36, 37, 38, 39]. (Table 1)

Table 1. Obesity Surgery- Mortality Risk Score

Risk Factors	Category	No. of factors	Reported Mortality
1. BMI ≥ 50 kg/m^2	A	0-1	0.2-0.3%
2. Male gender	B	2-3	1.2-1.9%
3. Hypertension	C (3-5% of patients)	4-5	2,4- 7,6%
4. Risk of pulmonary embolism (previous thromboembolism, preoperative vena cava filter, hypoventilation, pulmonary hypertension)			
5. Age ≥ 45 years			

- Stratification model of risk from Maciejewski et al. [27]: It is suggested the evaluation of 12 factors for gastric bypass: Age (40-64, ≥ 65), male gender, BMI (50-59.9, ≥ 60), SHAO, back pain, diabetes, pulmonary hypertension, ischemic heart disease, functional state and ASA IV or V according to American Society of Anaesthesiology.

The optimization of these and other "modifiable" risk factors such as arterial hypertension or dyslipidemia - recognized contributors to cardiovascular morbidity and mortality - help to balance the preoperative risks and comorbidities in regards the benefits related to bariatric surgery.

In the same way, recognition and observation of non modifiable risk factors are useful to plan the therapeutic strategy more suitable.

Appropiate preparation of the patient before surgery (election of the surgical technique, provision of information) is the basis to get a right risk-benefit balance for everyone.

Preoperative Assessment

Preoperative optimization has its goals:

1. Patient education about the own disease and implications of bariatric surgery
2. Promotion of healthy habits
3. Study and treatment of comorbidities to reduce the risk of perioperative complications.

Patient Education

An integral component of the preoperative evaluation involves a comprehensive patient education about surgical outcomes and the postoperative behavioural regimen required. A multidisciplinary assessment by a team of endocrinologists, dieticians, psychologists, and the surgeon, preoperatively to evaluate and educate the patient, helps in appropriate patient selection to ensure that the patient is physically and psychologically fit to undergo weight loss surgery (WLS) [19]. Candidate selection criteria for bariatric surgery include body mass index, presence, and effect of comorbidities to patient's overall health, and a history of prior weight loss attempts. Personalized assessment of the risk and benefits of the procedure, along with the assessment of the individual's ability to comply with postoperative care is vital to the preoperative assessment and education of the patient [19].

Many patients seeking bariatric surgery hold unrealistic expectations, without a complete understanding of the procedures and the subsequent long-term implications [40, 41, 42, 43]. Patient understanding of long-term consequences of WLS, such as postoperative lifestyle modification, psychosocial implications, need for long-term follow-up, and consistent implementation of recommended postoperative regimens, facilitates a more informed decision making.

The preoperative education is pivotal in managing expectations and dispelling any misconceptions that patients may have. It is crucial to evaluate each patient, in terms of existing comorbid conditions to establish individual patient goals and expectations. For instance, while WLS has significant benefits of sustained weight loss and improvements in metabolic comorbidities, it is important to be cognizant of the effect of existing comorbidities on perioperative morbidity [44, 45, 46, 47].

Overall, a thorough discussion of the potential postoperative morbidity and patient expectations of postsurgical weight loss, including the potential for weight regain, is strongly recommended [19].

Medical Assessment and Surgical Criteria

A complete evaluation is necessary before bariatric surgery (Table 2). This assessment should include a detailed clinical history with a review of medical and surgical backgrounds, obesity starting date and potential trigger factors, weight evolution during time, diets performed and other strategies of lost weight carried out by patient, psychological history (eating disorders, abuse, psychopathologies…), social factors which could have affected in lost weight (employment, housing, family), physical exercise or pharmacological treatment. Physical examination must include besides the general aspects, functional state assessment, anthropometric measures and other parameters associates to obesity (abdominal skirt, skin fold injuries, vasculopathy, varicose veins, hirsutism caused of polycystic ovaries and so on) [48]. Moreover, this study must be completed with the recognition of prevalent illness in morbidly obese patient such as cardiovascular and pulmonary problem, for example, obstructive sleep apnoea syndrome (OSAHS) [20].

Supplementary tests are going to review in this chapter, focus on diagnosis of cardiovascular and pulmonary pathologies. Relevance of upper digestive endoscopy and screening of Helicobacter Pylori will be studied in the next chapter.

Table 2. Complete medical history

• Obesity progress and associated factors
• Previous diets and physical exercise
• Other actions to lost weight
• Psychosocial factors
• Comorbilities
• Drugs

Preoperative Analysis Study

The following tests will be requested from obese patients, submitted to evaluation:

1. Analysis Test with High Recommendation and Strong Level of Evidence

- Complete blood count
- Coagulation
- Blood glucose profile: Study of hyperglycemia, and diabetes.
- Haemoglobin A1c: It appraises the glycemic control to medium term (3 months).
- Lipid profile: cholesterol, triglycerides, high-density lipoprotein (HDL), low-density protein (LDL)
- Renal function: electrolytes, creatinine, urea
- Liver function: gamma-glutamyl transpeptidase (GGT), alanine transaminase (ALT), alkaline phosphatase (ALP), lactic dehydrogenase (LDH), bilirubin

- Nutritional parameters: total proteins, albumin and prealbumin

* Micronutrients: There is not a consensus in which micronutrients will be requested systematically before bariatric surgery, with low level of evidence and low grade of recommendation in preoperative period. However, many obese patients have vitamin and mineral deficits which must be corrected before surgery, for example, the iron deficiency anaemia appears in around 20% [49, 50]. Table 3, presents the most frequent preoperative nutritional deficits in morbidly obese patients, candidates to surgery.

Table 3. Most frequent preoperative nutritional deficits in morbidly obese patients

Minerals	Previous deficiency	Preoperative analysis recommendation
Iron	7.7-44%	+++++ (routine) *Sideremia, ferritin, transferrin*
Calcium	25.4%	+++++ (routine) *Calcemia, ionic calcium, 25-OH-Vit D3, PTHi, 24 hour calciuria*
Zinc	0.7-28%	+++
Copper	2-67.8%	++

There is consensus in the importance of monitoring frequently micronutrients in postoperative, particularly in those patients undergo to surgery with high risk of malabsorptive criteria (strong level of evidence and grade of recommendation). The main micronutrients to follow are:

- *Vitamins*: Vitamin A, vitamin B1 (thiamine), vitamin B12, vitamin E, vitamin K, folic acid, 25-OH-Vit D3.
- *Minerals*: Iron, calcium, phosphorus, zinc, magnesium, copper and selenium.

Vitamins	Previous deficiency	Preoperative analysis recommendation
D	68-89%	+++++ (routine) *25-OH-D3*
B1 (thiamine)	30%	+++++ (routine)
B9 (Folic acid)	3.2-24%	+++++ (routine)
B12 (cobalamin)	0-13%	+++++ (routine)
A	10-15%	+++

Therefore, it is considered that a preoperative determination of micronutrients is necessary to perform an adequate perioperative optimization and for that reason we include it in this section.

2. Analysis Test with Low Recommendation and Weak Level of Evidence

- *Insulin*: The increased level during preoperative period in non diabetic patients, allows to evaluate the insulin resistance rate due to obesity and predict the development of mellitus diabetes. It could apply some index like "Homeostasis Model Assessment (HOMA-IR) to make the "insulin resistance" calculation. This permits to evaluate the improvement after bariatric surgery. This tool is used to predict the progression risk to diabetes and/or metabolic syndrome and as well, to reduce that risk after therapeutic actions such as diets, exercise or drugs.
- *Peptide C*: It is a molecule after demotion of insulin. It assesses the pancreatic endocrine reserve and a prognostic factor of mellitus diabetes referral then metabolic surgery.
- *C-Reactive protein*: It evaluates the inflammatory obese state. (It is studying its value to predict the time in what postoperative weight will be steady).
- *Hormones*: It is not recommended to do widespread hormonal analysis. In contrast, it has been individualized according to clinical circumstances of patients. If it is suspected:
    - Hypoparathyroidism: screening of thyrotropin, thyroid-Stimulating Hormone. It is recommended routine screening for primary hypothyroidism.
    - Secondary hyperparathyroidism due to calcium or vitamin D deficit, it is recommended parathyroid hormone (PTH) blood test.
    - Polycystic ovarium: screening total and free testosterone, dehydroepiandrosterone sulphate (DHEA-S), delta-4-androstenedione.
    - Cushing Syndrome: check the suppression test with 1 mg dexamethasone, cortisoluria in 24h, cortisol salivary at 11:00 pm.

Metabolic Optimization

In 1988, Gerald Reaven defined "X Syndrome" as group of pathologies that vest a high risk compared to each illness independently. Later, World Health Organization (WHO) called "Metabolic Syndrome" of the obese patient. It is characterized by insulin resistance (with hyperglycemia-hyperinsulinemia) associated with dyslipidemia and arterial hypertension. It has thought brown or intraabdominal fat could stimulate this insulin resistance.

Although different scientific societies and international consensus have stablished cutting points and parameters for the metabolic syndrome definition; according to Experts in detection, evaluation and treatment of high cholesterol, proposed by third report of the Education National Program of Cholesterol from United States (NCEP-III or ATP III), has verified the high prevalence of the syndrome, the absence of accepted criteria for diagnosis. It is defined for unless three from the following features [51]:

1. Central obesity: abdominal circumference ≥ 102 cm in men and 88 cm in women.
2. Arterial hypertension in treatment or arterial pressure ≥ 130/85mmHg.
3. Diabetes treatment or fasting glycemia ≥ 110 mg/dl.
4. Hypercholesterolemia in treatment or HDL cholesterol < 40 mg/dl men or <50/ml women.
5. Hypertriglyceridemia in treatment ≥ 150 mg/dl.

Included parameters in the definition of American Heart Association (AHA) and National Heart, Lung and Blood Institute are exposed in Table 4 [52].

If BMI is more 30 kg/m^2, it may assume there is a central obesity and it has not needed to know the circumference waist [53].

Independently of lack of consensus in diagnosis and treatment criteria, the aim will be detection and early treatment of these disorders. The importance is to stop or reverse the metabolic, inflammatory, oxidative processes and endothelial disfunction to carry on patients through the appearance of diabetes, cardiovascular events and increasing of mortality rate. Other frequent endocrine diseases are hypothyroidism, liver steatosis, vitamin deficiencies and polycystic ovarium syndrome due to androgenic growing that may not to be transformed at peripheral level in estrogens. It should have performed all possible efforts to reach the optimal glycemic perioperative to reduce the risk of postoperative complications [54].

Table 4. Metabolic syndrome according to AHA/NHLBI (unless 3 criteria)

1. Abdominal obesity with circumference. Men (> 102 cms in USA, 94 cms in Europe), women (88 cms in USA, 80 cms in Europe).
2. Tryglicerides > 150 ml/dl.
3. HDL cholesterol < 40mgr/dl in men, < 50 mgr/dl in women.
4. Arterial pressure > 130/85 mmHg
5. Fasting glucose >100 mgr/dl

Table 5. Specified patterns to amend some frequent alterations

It is recommended to treat:	
1.	**Cholesterol disorders,** according to *National Cholesterol Education Program Adult Treatment Panel III guidelines.*
2.	**Iron deficiency anaemia,** before surgery (20% in obese patients)
3.	**If hypothyroidism,** it should be treated with thyroid hormones
4.	**Keep basal glycemia ≤ 110 mg/dl,** postprandial glycemia ≤ 140 mg/dl and HbA1c 6.5- 7%. In diabetes patients with vascular complications or long time from diagnosis with difficult to reach a good glycemic control, it has accepted HbA1c 7-8%

All finding disorders (endocrinal or nutritional) with clinical relevance or prognosis value, should be corrected from the diagnosis. In Table 5 is specified patterns to amend some frequent alterations.

Cardiovascular System Assessment

1. Perioperative Cardiac Risk Evaluation

Obesity is a known risk factor for cardiovascular diseases such as coronary arteries illness, arrythmias, left ventricular hypertrophy and heart failure [55]. Metabolic demands are increased by fat accumulation, creating a growth of blood volume, cardiac output and systolic volume. Moreover, it exits a high preload which associates initially a distension of left ventricular and then eccentric hypertrophy ventricular. Therefore, the sum of these disorders along with factors that produce the metabolic syndrome, all together cause arterial hypertension, heart failure, pulmonary hypertension, arteriosclerosis and coronary disease. This fact produces a high preoperative risk in candidate patient to weight lost surgery.

- Morbidly obese patients have more cardiac risk than general population.
- It should look for: ischemic heart disease, pulmonary and systemic hypertension, signs of left or right ventricular failure.
- The patients that most benefit from undergoing bariatric surgery are those with severe diseases, therefore, with high surgical risk For that reason, routine assessment before surgery of high-risk patients allows to:
    - **Correct modifiable risk factors** before surgery
    - **Inform patient about the surgical procedure** which adapts to their surgical risk.
    - **Contraindicate surgery** if risks are higher than expected benefits.
- High-risk cardiovascular patients will be checked by cardiologists to complete a functional study, according to patient features.

Preoperative heart evaluation is a challenge in every candidate patient for non-cardiac surgery, being necessary to categorize a presurgical heart risk. It is known that obese population have a major adverse cardiovascular event [56]. Mortality due to cardiovascular causes in severe obese patients reach 90% in old studies [57], but the detection of cardiovascular risk (CVR) in this population is difficult and requires long term follow-up. The cardiovascular mortality risk to 5 or 10 years could be evaluated by some equations:

- *BMI equation of Framingham:* it allows to evaluate a specific risk related to obesity. Variables include age, gender, smoking history, diabetes, systolic and diastolic pressure, antihypertensive drugs used, total cholesterol and blood HDL analysis. The result of each patient was used to prevent the risk to have cardiovascular event past 10 years, pursuant to specific equations to each gender [58].
- *PROCAM Model (Münster Heart Study)* includes lipid parameters which do not appear in Framingham equation [59].
- *Coronary risk evaluation of European System Model (SCORE project):* it evaluates the cardiovascular risk in population between 40-65 years [60].

There are modifiable risk factors like adult obstructive sleep apnoea, insulin resistance and diabetes, smoking, weight lost before surgery and hypoalbuminemia. Other factors are not modifiable such as age, men gender, BMI, cardiovascular disease and functional disorder [61].

Bariatric surgery in patients with previous cardiovascular disease is associated with increase surgical risk. Recently, Pirlet et al. [56] suggest a significant increase of global and cardiac mortality in group studied with previous coronary arterial disease (CAD) and as well, high rate of major adverse cardiovascular and cerebrovascular event (MACCE), mainly for myocardial infarction without ST elevation. In the multivariant model, CAD, age >55 years, dyslipidemia, diabetes treated with insulin, cerebrovascular event history, atrial fibrillation, pacemaker and chronic renal failure were independent predictors of MACCE. The authors themselves indicate that, curiously, 4 of these parameters (CAD history, diabetes with insulin, cerebrovascular event and chronic renal failure) are included in the 6 risk factors of the reviewed cardiac risk index that recommends to know which patients should require further tests before surgery [62, 63, 64].

Some MACCE could be cause of postoperative mortality. This is important in bariatric surgery due to cardiovascular risk factors associated to obesity. Therefore, benefits of weight lost surgery in major risk population, as severe morbid obesity and CAD, will need more studies because of current data are inconclusive. In addition, the American Heart Association (AHA) assessment classifies intraabdominal surgery as an intermediate risk procedure, so effectively optimizing comorbidities is essential to prevent poor surgical results in bariatric surgery patients. [65, 66, 67].

2. Relevant Risk Factors

The cardiovascular risk factors more frequent in obese patients may be:

A. Ischemic Heart Disease

The increase of cardiac ischemic events in obese patient is related chronic hypercholesterolemia and hypertriglyceridemia, high rate of diabetes, hypercoagulability syndrome and so on. It has caused an alteration of small vessels which predispose to coronary obstructions that will be presented clinically as angina pectoris, myocardial infarction or sudden death. For frequency, ischemic heart disease (IHD) is a second cause of early death in morbidly obese patient.

IHD treatment is difficult because once vascular damage established is rarely reversible. Many patients undergo surgery with endovascular stents or previous cardiac surgery.

B. Dyslipidemia

Sixty-four percent of adults with severe obesity seeking bariatric surgery have dyslipidemia, which includes any or all the following: a high level of low-density lipoprotein, high triglycerides, and a low level of high-density lipoprotein [68]. Therefore, hypertriglyceridemia, hypercholesterolemia (especially at the expense of HDL fraction) are usual. These lipidemic disorders have a multifactorial origin. It has been determined several causes of its development, such as hypercaloric diet (specially by the increse of saturated fats) or the capacity of intraabdominal brown fat to produce endogenous cholesterol and long chain triglycerides. It is associated with endoluminal vascular deposits (fatty deposits) of atheromas and with arterial hypertension and IHD.

Dyslipidemias are complicated to treat as a result of a partial response with the common drugs prescribed as well as the difficulties that these patients have to perform exercises and the level of sedentarism.

C. Arterial Hypertension

In the same way that previous pathologies, there are more incidence of arterial hypertension in obese patients compared with general population. Sixty-eight percent of adults with severe obesity seeking bariatric surgery have hypertension. Systematic reviews indicate that bariatric surgery is associated with a 1-year hypertension remission rate ranging from 43% to 83% [69]. Among the possible physiolopathological mechanisms are found the renin- angiotensin system alteration and the association with diabetes, which produce together vascular damage and increase of peripheral resistances. All factors coexist in a difficult vicious circle to break independently, which should be treated of integral way within metabolic syndrome linked to obesity.

D. Venous Stasis with Hypercoagulability

Early high blood level of fibrinogen has been found in morbid obesity, with values more than double compared to normal. Another finding is the slowing venous circulation at infradiaphragmatic zone, especially in lower extremities. The venous stasis, hyperfibrinogenaemia and alterations of other coagulation factors are some elements associated to major thrombosis venous incidence, thrombophlebitis and in some cases, thromboembolic events in morbidly obese patients. It should be highlighted that pulmonary thromboembolism is the first death cause in this kind of patients.

3. Cardiologic Assessment

Additionally to all previous comments, it is crucial to make a right cardiac evaluation of patients candidates to undergo weight loss surgery with the purpose to investigate cardiac pathologies and cardiovascular risks through exhaustive clinical history. Past medical history of aterial hypertension, dyslipidemia, diabetes, heart failure, arrythmias, coronary diseases, cerebrovascular events, renal failure, thrombotic incidents, among other disease must be assessed. [70]. Higher-risk patients should weigh the risk-to-benefit ratio of preoperative interventions and focus on improved long-term outcomes rather than simply perioperative outcomes [71].

Initial assessment is performed by anaesthesiologist in preanesthetic evaluation. This assessment includes usually a 12 derivations electrocardiogram (ECG) and clinical history of pasts and functional state. In this ECG should be defined the cardiac rhythm, identifies clinically silent cardiovascular disease such as prior Q-wave myocardial infarction, and provides a baseline for postoperative comparison. Among patients with CAD undergoing major surgery, preoperative ST-segment depressions greater than 0.5mm are associated with increased risk of postoperative death or myocardial infarction (event rate of 11.2% in patients with ST-segment depressions vs 2.6%in those without such depressions; P = .001) [72,73].

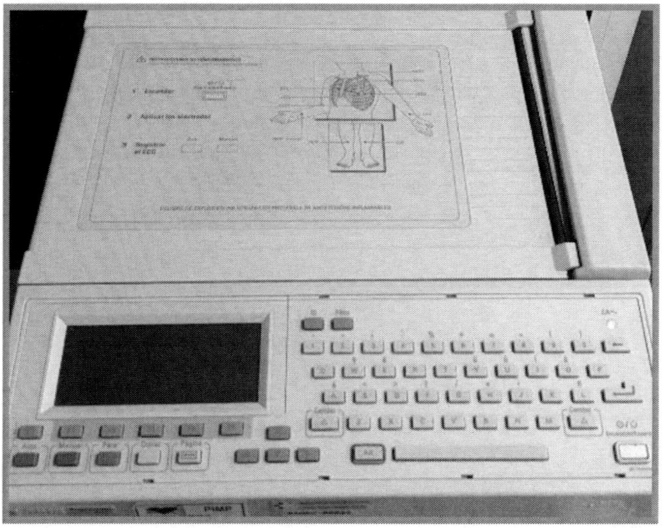

It should be consulted to cardiologists when patients have a high suspect index of cardiological risk, defined by presenting 3 or more cardiovascular risk factors (high recommendation, strong level of evidence) from the revised cardiac risk index (RCRI) which is relatively simple to use. One point is assigned for each of the following 6 components: ischemic heart disease, cerebrovascular disease, heart failure, insulin-dependent diabetes, chronic kidney disease (serum creatinine level 2.0mg/dL), and high-risk surgery (intraperitoneal, intrathoracic, or vascular), Table 6.

Table 6. High-risk cardiac conditions considered contraindications to Noncardiac Surgery

• Acute coronary syndrome • Acute decompensated heart failure • Tachyarrthythmias or bradyarrthythmias associated with hypotension or requiring urgent medical attention (e.g., Ventricular tachycardia or high-grade atrioventricular block) • Symptomatic severe aortic stenosis (mean gradient > 40 mmHg or peak velocity >4 m/s

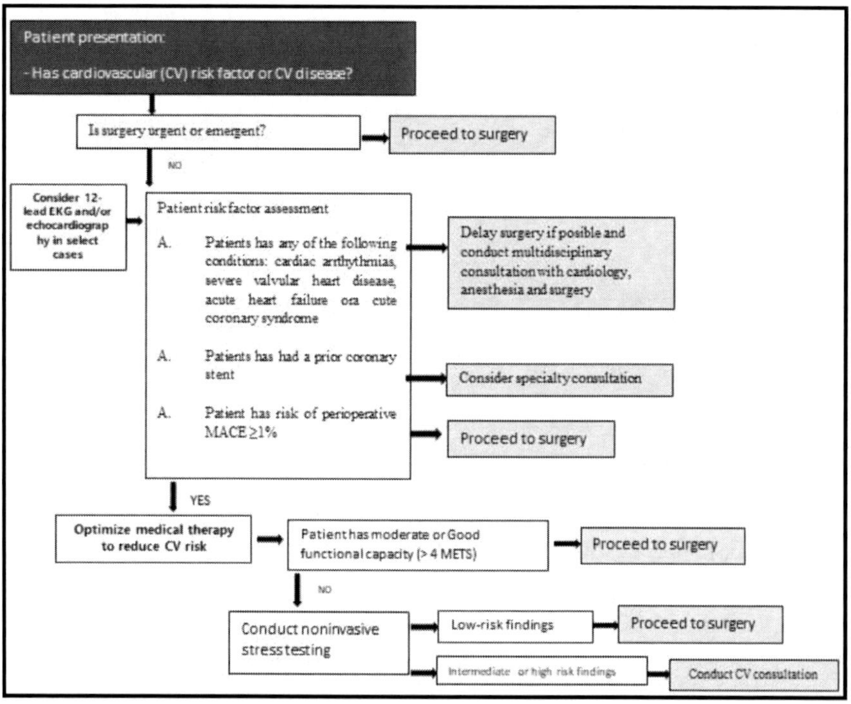

Figure 1. Model with algorithm used to to stratify the perioperative cardiovascular risk.

Cardiologist checks the patient functional state and will perform complementary tests to evaluate the cardiac reserve. Classical methods are ergometric (treadmill exercise, scintigraphy) could be not possible in morbidly obese patients due to limitations by weight and accurate interpretation of images [74, 75]. In the ultrasonography diagnosis, the election is the transthoracic echocardiography (TTE). The main will be to evaluate ventricular function, structural pathology and rule out valvular diseases. Overall, except in special circumstances, routine preoperative evaluation of ventricular function is not recommended [70].

If there are doubts with TTE findings, there are other options to get an accurate diagnosis. One odd is the pharmacological stress echography with or without ultrasound contrast. Dobutamine is a popularly used drug to produce a control cardiac stress due to inotropes and chronotropic features [76, 77]. Another option is transoesophageal echocardiography to improve the poor window (for growth of distance between transductor and heart in TTE) that obese patient are used to having. However, it is an invasive technique because of the introduction of the echography tube through the oesophagus. Sedative drugs should be used to tolerate the procedure [78].

4. Preoperative Strategies

Regarding the measures to be taken in these patients related to bariatric surgery, it is remarkable to consider the next:

- Routine coronary revascularization is not recommended before noncardiac surgery to reduce perioperative MACE. In contrast, European guidelines suggest that prophylactic coronary revascularization may be considered before high-risk surgery if there is substantial stress-induced ischemia. Although preoperative coronary revascularization may be performed for a compelling indication independent of surgery, such as for those with acute coronary syndrome, performing surgery within 12 months after coronary stent placement is associated with increased perioperative risks [70].
- Despite recommendations to delay noncardiac surgery after percutaneous coronary intervention (PCI), 3.5% of patients or more undergo noncardiac surgery within 6 months of stent placement. Individuals requiring surgery within 1 year after PCI are at increased risk of perioperative events compared with those without coronary stents (8.9%vs 1.5%, respectively; adjusted OR, 2.6 [95% CI, 1.4-4.9]; $P < .001$). Ischemic risks are

inversely related to the length of time between stent placement and noncardiac surgery and are directly related to prothrombotic surgical trauma and early discontinuation of dual antiplatelet therapy. In some cases, clinically significant perioperative stent thrombosis and myocardial infarction can occur. Patients undergoing coronary stent placement should have surgery delayed until the risks associated with delaying surgery outweigh the thrombotic risks of stopping dual antiplatelet therapy. Elective noncardiac surgery should be delayed for at least 2 weeks after balloon angioplasty, 30 days after baremetal stent implantation, and 12 months after drug-eluting stent placement, although evidence suggests that surgery 3 to 6 months after drugeluting stent PCI or longer may be safe [70]. Elective noncardiac surgery afterdrug-eluting stent PCI may be considered after 6 months or longer if the risk of further delay is greater than the expected risks of myocardial infarction and stent thrombosis. Shorter delays to surgery after PCI require further study.

- After coronary stent placement, continuation of single antiplatelet therapy with aspirin is recommended in the AHA/ACC guidelines [79], whereas European guidelines favour individualized decisions based on bleeding and thrombotic risks [62].
- The perioperative management of b-blockers remains a controversial topic, with a multitude of studies published as the POISE Trial to reassess their safety versus risk profile. Overall, the results suggest a personalized approach to perioperative b-blocker use, with consideration given to the patient's cardiovascular risk factors, the type of surgery, anticipated perioperative hemodynamic changes, and the existence of off-label indications for b-blocker use [80]. Patients already taking β-blockers should continue treatment during the perioperative period in the absence of bradycardia or hypotension (it has had criteria according to recommendations, Figure 2). Initiation of β-blockers before surgery may be warranted in select patients with CAD or with multiple risk factors and at high risk for perioperative myocardial infarction. Although high dose β-blocker therapy should not be initiated on the day of surgery, it

may be reasonable to initiate β-blocker therapy more than one week prior to surgery to determine tolerability and safety [70].

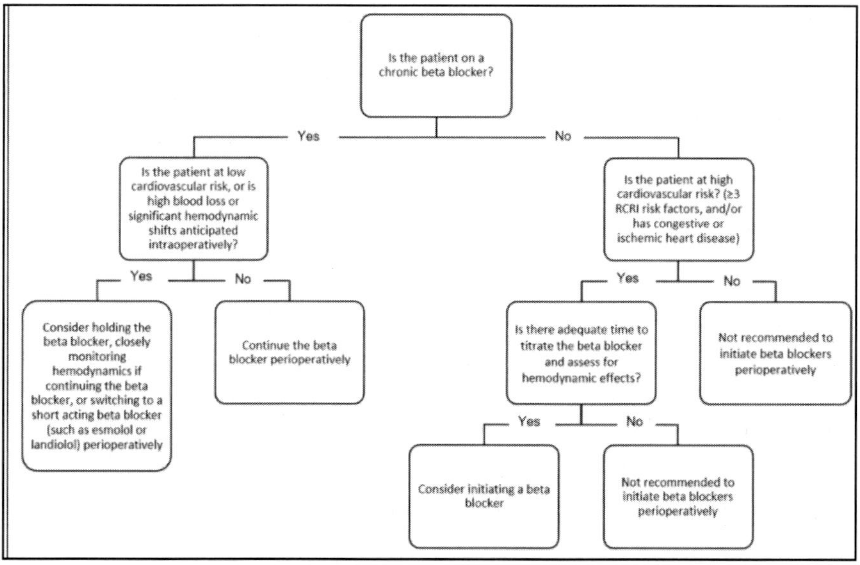

Figure 2. Criteria for β-blockers treatment during the perioperative period in the absence of bradycardia or hypotension.

- Although randomized trials do not support prescribing *statins prior to surgery*, the AHA/ACC guidelines suggest that preoperative initiation of statin therapy is reasonable prior to vascular surgery, and the authors' opinion is that statin therapy may be beneficial with few adverse effects in patients with indications for lipid-lowering therapy, such as those with diabetes or atherosclerotic cardiovascular disease who are scheduled for higher-risk surgery.
- Routine administration of perioperative *antiplatelet* therapy prior to noncardiac surgery is not recommended because it is not associated with benefit and results in an increased risk of bleeding. Low-dose aspirin may be appropriate for a subset of patients when ischemic risks outweigh the bleeding risks, such as for patients with coronary artery stents [70].
- For patients taking *warfarin or a direct oral anticoagulant* for stroke prevention in atrial fibrillation, perioperative interruption of

oral anticoagulation is safe, and bridging with heparin should not be routinely performed. Patients with mechanical mitral valves and those at increased risk for thrombotic events with mechanical aortic valves should receive bridging anticoagulation with heparin prior to noncardiac surgery.

Respiratory Evaluation

Mechanic restriction due to fatty deposit in oropharyngeal cavity, neck and thoracic wall is itself, a risk factor to develop respiratory disease. Obese patients present a decrease tidal volume and functional residual capacity compared to general population, and as result, major risk to hypoxemia. Tachypnoea may be a sign which shows problems to increase the tidal volume in situations where it is needed to increase the supply of oxygen. Moreover, it is added the high metabolic activity in fat with growing of carbon dioxide production.

Routine pulmonary function testing could help to assess the pulmonary reserve and identify those potential patients to develop postoperative pulmonary complications such as atelectasis, laryngospasm and reintubation [81, 82]. Besides, it exists a high asthma incidence produces for the increase respiratory work and alterations in airway size with poor response to bronchodilators.

1. More Frequent Respiratory Pathologies Associated to Obesity

A. Obesity Hypoventilation Syndrome (OHS)

OHS is defined by the triad of obesity, daytime hypoventilation, and sleep-disordered breathing without an alternative neuromuscular, mechanical, or metabolic cause of hypoventilation. It is a disease entity distinct from simple obesity and obstructive sleep apnoea (OSAHS). OHS is often undiagnosed but its prevalence is estimated to be 10 –20% in obese patients with obstructive sleep apnoea and 0.15– 0.3% in the general adult population.

This syndrome is characterized by the combination of obesity (body mass index (BMI) >30 kg/m2), daytime awake hypercapnia (partial pressure of arterial carbon dioxide (PaCO2) > 45 mmHg at sea level) and hypoxemia (partial pressure of arterial oxygen (PaO2) >70 mmHg at sea level), in the presence of sleep-disordered breathing without other known causes of hypoventilation [83].

- The obesity hypoventilation syndrome (OHS) and obstructive apnea-hypopnea sleep syndrome (OSAHS) are associated to morbid obesity (>80%), although underdiagnosed.
- Routine preoperative spirometry should not be applied.
- OSAHS evaluation questionnaires (Epworth sleepiness scale, Berlin questionnaire or STOP-BANG questionnaire) allow discriminate OSAHS high-risk patients, who should make a polysomnography.
- OSAHS diagnosis involves starting continuous positive airway pressure (CPAP) during 2 or 3 months before bariatric surgery and then, after surgery, several months from immediate postoperative period until resolution of this comorbility.
- Preoperative respiratory physiotherapy may contribute to reduce complications after surgery, and for that it is strongly recommended. Incentive spirometry is included in this strategy

These patients are more liable to respiratory infections and pneumonia due to deposit of secretions in airways that may get superinfected. They should be treated preoperatively with respiratory physiotherapist.

B. Obstructive Apnea-Hypopnea Sleep Syndrome (OSAHS)

OSAHS is characterized by recurrent episodes of partial or complete upper airway collapse during sleep that is highlighted by a reduction in, or complete cessation of, airflow despite documented on going inspiratory efforts. Due to the lack of adequate alveolar ventilation that results from the upper airway narrowing, oxygen saturation may drop, and partial pressure of CO2 may occasionally increase. The events are mostly terminated by arousals. Clinical consequences are excessive daytime sleepiness related to the sleep disruption [84]. OSAHS is affected to general citizens, being its estimated prevalence between 3.1 to 7.5% in men and 1.2 to 4.5% in premenopausal women. While postmenopausal women have a similar prevalence compared to men [85]. Some studies suggest a high percentage of people with this pathology, being underestimated and without diagnosis between 80-95% at present [86]. So, it is very important to detect these cases and study them.

OSAHS is associated to loss of quality of life, hypertension and development of cardiovascular and cerebrovascular diseases [87, 88, 89]. It must be dismissed in all preoperative assessment for bariatric surgery. Until 40% morbidly obese patients present some grade of alterations said before. It should be suspected in patients more than 40, with cervical-thoracic obesity, smokers and snorers. When OSAHS is diagnosed, it should be treated with starting continuous positive airway pressure (CPAP) to avoid apnoeas and allow a continuous rest and mender sleeping.

2. Preoperative Pulmonary Function Testing

A. Chest X-ray

It is basic to make a tracing and comparison in view of postoperative complications [90].

B. Spirometry

Routine spirometry for all candidate patients to undergo to weight loss surgery is questionable. It is suggested a selective benefit only if there is a high risk for pulmonary complications [91]. Spirometry measures respiratory flows and volumes. It could be simple or forced. The maximal flow-volume curve is helpful in quality assurance, in detecting mild airflow obstruction, and in detecting central airway obstruction. For best results, both inspiratory and expiratory loops are obtained.

- *Simple spirometry*: Spirometry requires a voluntary maneuverer in which a patient inhales maximally from tidal breathing at rest to total lung capacity (TLC) and then rapidly exhales to the fullest extent until no further volume is exhaled at residual volume (RV), followed by a maximum inspiration back to TLC (Figure 3).

Spirometry allows static lung volume measurements which it be defined such as volumes and capacities [92]:

- Tidal volume (TV): It is the amount of air that can be inhaled or exhaled during one respiratory cycle. This depicts the functions of the respiratory centres, respiratory muscles and the mechanics of the lung and chest wall. The normal adult value is 10% of vital capacity (VC), approximately 300-500ml (6-8 ml/kg); but can increase up to 50% of VC on exercise.
- Inspiratory Reserve Volume (IRV): It is the amount of air that can be forcibly inhaled after a normal tidal volume. IRV is usually kept in reserve but is used during deep breathing. The normal adult value is 1900-3300ml.
- Expiratory Reserve Volume (ERV): It is the volume of air that can be exhaled forcibly after exhalation of normal tidal volume. The normal adult value is 700-1200ml. ERV is reduced with obesity, ascites or after upper abdominal surgery.

- *Residual Volume (RV)*: It is the volume of air remaining in the lungs after maximal exhalation. Normal adult value is averaged at 1200ml (20-25 ml/kg). It is indirectly measured from summation of FRC and ERV and cannot be measured by spirometry.
- *Total Lung Capacity (TLC)*: It is the maximum volume of air the lungs can accommodate or sum of all volume compartments or volume of air in lungs after maximum inspiration. The normal value is about 6,000mL. TLC is calculated by summation of the four primary lung volumes (TV, IRV, ERV, RV).
- *Vital Capacity (VC)*: It is the total amount of air exhaled after maximal inhalation. The value is about 4800mL and it varies according to age and body size. It is calculated by summing tidal volume, inspiratory reserve volume, and expiratory reserve volume. VC = TV+IRV+ERV. VC indicates ability to breathe deeply and cough, reflecting inspiratory and expiratory muscle strength. VC should be 3 times greater than TV for effective cough.

- *Forced spirometry*: After maximal inhalation it is applied to the patient to exhale all air more quickly possible. Once reaches an adequate forced vital capacity, the flow is going to depend on elastic pressure and airway resistance (not from patient effort), Figure 4. It is used to evaluate several respiratory pathologies through next following flows and volumes [93].
  - Forced vital capacity (FVC): it is the amount of air that can be forcibly exhaled from lungs after taking the deepest breath possible.
  - Forced expiratory Volume in 1 second (FEV1): It is the amount of air exhaled in one second. It is used to measure the mechanical properties of the lungs. The absolute value of the FEV1 obtained by the patient is then compared to his or her peers according to age, gender, height, and ethnicity.
  - FEV1/FVC ratio: it indicates a percentage of exhaled total volume in the first second.
  - Expiratory flow at 25–75% of FVC (FEF25–75%): It was introduced as maximum mid-expiratory flow (MMEF). This measurement was intended to reflect the most effort-independent portion of the curve and the portion most sensitive to airflow in peripheral airways.

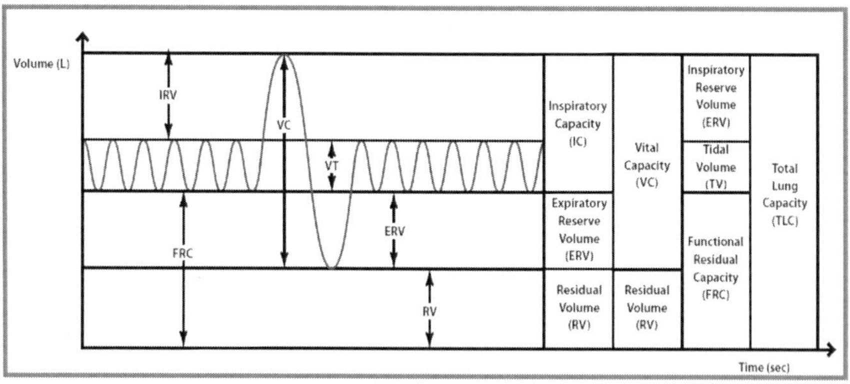

Figure 3. Simple spirometry.

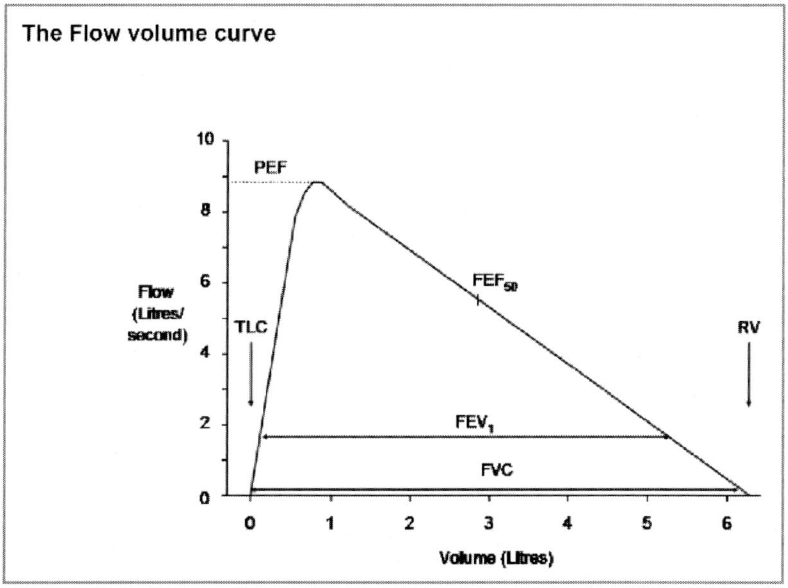

Figure 4. The flow volume curve.

C. Polysomnography (PSG)

Reference diagnostic proof of OSAHS. It exists other simplified methods such as home PSG and respiratory polygraphy which have been accepted and validated. Apnea-Hypoapnea index (AHI) is used to diagnose by PSG through several cutting points. With an AHI ≥5, OSAHS is mild and it should be recommended hygienic-dietary measures; if AHI is ≥ 15, the OSAHS is moderate and it requires sleeping unit control [94, 95]. The low diagnostic of OSAHS is associated with the PSG is an expensive test and within the reach of few centres [96].

D. OSAHS Preoperative Assessment Tools

As the PSG is difficult to make, it has developed instruments to screen quickly and easily potential patients, detecting them through evaluation questionnaires:

- Epworth sleepiness scale [97].
- Berlin questionnaire [98].
- American Society Anaesthesiologists list (ASA Checklist) [99].

- Preoperative sleep apnoea prediction score (P-SAP score) [100].
- STOP-BANG questionnaire [101]. Table 7. Each variable sum 1 point. If a patient sums ≥3 points it is considered high odd to suffer OSAHS (Intermediate risk 3-4, high risk 5-8). A 0-2 mark has an upper negative predictive value associated to OSAHS low risk. This questionnaire has easy application with 8 simple questions of YES/NOT answer. For that is not required of experience. Those patients with ≥ 5 points may be indicated to apply a OSAHS confirmed diagnosis analysis without need to a previous consultation to sleeping specialist physician, allowing an early treatment.

In the Nagappa et al. [102] meta-analysis is confirmed that high performance of the STOP-Bang questionnaire in the sleep clinic and surgical population for screening of OSAHS. The higher the STOP-Bang score, the greater is the probability of moderate-to-severe OSAHS. In an effort to unify the subject populations, all studies were divided into major groups: sleep clinic, surgical and general populations. The other reason for the heterogeneity may be variation in the prevalence of OSAHS in the different populations.

In summary, detection of OSAHS high risk patients according to screening by questionnaires should be assessed more using a night PSG [19]. After confirmed diagnosis, patients could benefit of preoperative non-invasive ventilation for example, CPAP or bi-level positive airway pressure (BiPAP) [103]. Preoperative respiratory physiotherapy could contribute to reduce complications after bariatric surgery, so it is strongly recommended.

Incentive spirometry, which involves having the patient take a sustained maximal inspiration that must be slow, deep inspiration from the Functional Residual Capacity up to the total lung capacity, followed by ≥ 5 seconds breath hold. This with other directed respiratory exercises, are important tools to prevent atelectasis in early postoperative. It should be started in the preoperative period and reintroduce again after surgery in the postoperative recovery unit.

Table 7. STOP-BANG Questionnaire

Please answer the following questions by checking "yes" or "no" for each one	**Yes**	**No**
Snoring (Do you snore loudly?)		
Tiredness (Do you often feel tired, fatigued, or sleepy during the daytime?)		
Observed Apnea (Has anyone observed that you stop breathing, or choke or gasp during your sleep?)		
High Blood Pressure (Do you have or are you being treated for high blood pressure?)		
BMI (Is your body mass index more than 35 Kg per m^2?)		
Age (Are you older than 50 years?)		
Neck Circumference (Is your neck circumference greater than 40 cm?)		
Gender (Are you male?)		
Score1 point for each response Scoring interpretation: 0-2 low risk, 3-4 intermediate risk, 5-8 high risk		

Preoperative Anaesthetic Considerations

Preoperative anaesthetic assessment of patients scheduled for bariatric surgery is a challenge due to be patients with important obesity, associated comorbidities and less than 60 years in most of the cases [104]. They are going to present difficulties in intraoperative management and appear postoperative complications [105].

So, anaesthetic consultation is basis to find and treat associated pathologies, without forgetting that many of these patients have been treated during long-term period with weight lost diets or they have taken slimming drugs and herbal products to decrease the appetite. All this could have anaesthetic implications. Some "anorectics" such as phentermine and fenflurazine, now more obsolete, generate severe cardiologic and pulmonary problems. Other, like Sibutramine (Reductil®) inhibits the noradrenaline, serotonin and dopamine reuptake, it could cause hypertension and cardiac arrythmias (forbidden in Europe); and the Orlistat (Xenical®) blocks fat digestion and absorption due to inhibition of gastrointestinal tract lipases. It could induce liposoluble vitamin deficients and coagulopathy by low level of vitamin K.

- Anaesthetic consultation has as a goal to prevent perioperative complications.
- Electrocardiogram and thoracic X-ray preoperative study with analysis is performed.
- Functional capacity, cardiovascular risk and OSAHS according to predictor tests already commented are evaluated. After results, it could be required additional assessment by cardiologist or pulmonologist before surgery.
- There will be ptimization of the usual medication of the candidates for bariatric surgery and preoperative premedication will be planes, including the adjusted thromboembolic prophylaxis.
- The major risk of difficult airway, both ventilation and orotracheal intubation, forces to make a planification of its management. If awake intubation with fibreoptic bronchoscope is anticipated, it should explain to the patient previously to get a maximum collaboration in anaesthetic induction, already in theatre.

Main goals to consider in the preoperative period of an obese patient are:

1. Preoperative Anaesthetic Study

An assessment of more frequent comorbidities and the application of conventional preoperative analysis: biochemistry with liver and thyroid function tests, blood count, coagulation, and electrocardiogram, is carried out. According to the functional state, a consultation to the cardiologist or pulmonoligst may be carried out.

Spirometry test is not systematically requested, except in cases where a pulmonary pathology other than the mild-moderate restrictive pattern of morbid obesity is suspected due to decreased compliance, since it usually does not modify the anaesthetic attitude. In contract, it is recommended polysomnography based on the findings of the OSAHS risk assessment questionnaires (such as the "STOP_BANG" questionnaire), a snorer or clinically suspected patient due to the high prevalence of OSAHS (50-70%), to be able to prescribe CPAP or BiPAP preoperatively and improve postoperative results. If the use of CPAP is considered necessary when it is diagnosed in the pre-anaesthesia consultation, the surgery will be delayed 2 to 3 months and, maintained for several months later, from the immediate postoperative period until the resolution of this comorbidity.

2. Adjustment of Medications Prior to Hospital Admission

- Set the necessary insulin dose in diabetic patients
- Withdraw metformin 24-48 h before surgery due to the risk of producing lactic acidosis.
- Withdraw antihypertensive drugs such as ACE inhibitors and angiotensin II receptor antagonists (ARAS) 24 h before surgery, cause of they produce intraoperative hypotension that is difficult to treat.
- Take inhaled bronchodilators the morning of surgery if the patient takes them regularly.
- Use CPAP or BiPAP pre and postoperatively.
- It is advisable to stop smoking 8 weeks before surgery.
- For the management of antiaggregants, statins and anticoagulants, review section 3.5 in the cardiological evaluation of this chapter.

3. Airway Evaluation

It is known that the airway management of morbidly obese patients is more complex. In the general population, intubation difficulty is 1% and it doubles in obese people, while ventilation difficulty triples from 5% to 18%. The degree of difficulty of intubation and/or ventilation must be assessed since BMI, in itself, is not a predictor of poor intubation but it does favour its difficulty [20].

Difficulty in securing the airway is the main cause of anaesthesia-related morbidity [106].

Numerous simple and easy to perform tests have been described in the literature. Neither are exact and, by itself, they do not ensure whether a patient will be difficult to intubate. However, if they are added together, you get great reliability. The tests that we systematically carry out are:

A. *Predictors of Difficult ventilation*
   - Presence of beard
   - BMI> 30 Kg/m2
   - Age> 57 years
   - Lack of teeth
   - Snorer or OSAHS

B. *Predictors of Difficult intubation*
   - Mallampati Test ≥ 3. The Mallampati score is the most important parameter. It evaluates the visibility of the base of the uvula, facial pillars and soft palate; and classifies patients into four classes. In class 1, these structures are easily visible, and class 4 identifies an anatomical condition with less visible structures. Mallampati classes 1 and 2 are correlated with relatively easy intubation, and classes 3 and 4 are associated with a higher probability of difficult intubation.
   - Upper lip bite test: 2-3
   - Interdental distance (DID) < 2.5 cm
   - Neck Circumference (CC) > 40 cm
   - Thyromental distance (TMD) < 6.5 cm
   - Sternomental distance. (DEM) < 12.5 cm
   - Kim's ratio: CC/TMD > 5. This ratio is currently considered quite reliable as a predictor of intubation difficulty if it is > 5.

It is highlighted that studies show that only a large neck circumference (greater than 40 cm) and a Mallampati score greater than or equal to 3 are predictors of potentially difficult intubation, while BMI, or weight, does not always predict a difficult intubation [107]. The only predictor that anaesthetists may modify before surgery is the presence of a beard, so the risks are explained in the preanesthesia consultation and all patients are asked to shave it. With all these conditions, we must apply well-structured protocols during the induction and intubation of the morbidly obese that are discussed later.

It is important to have an action plan for airway management. Patients should be explained that there is the possibility of awake fibreoptic bronchoscope intubation, use of pre-induction high-flow nasal cannulas, and/or rapid-sequence induction [104].

4. Premedication

The necessary medication should be planned and prescribed from the anaesthetic consultation, including:

1. *Sedation*: Lorazepam 1mg. the previous night.
2. *Ant reflux prophylaxis*: Although it has always been thought that the morbidly obese patient had a high residual volume, there are studies that cast doubt on this statement and ensure that the amounts necessary to produce an aspiration syndrome must be greater than those usually found in these patients. However, due to the high prevalence of gastroesophageal reflux and hiatal hernia, it is advisable to do prophylaxis with:
   - Ranitidine 150 mg orally (PO) the night before surgery.
   - Sodium Citrate 30 ml orally (PO) 1 hour before surgery.
3. *Prophylaxis Deep vein thrombosis*:
   - Enoxaparin 60 mg/24h sc if the patient has a BMI <50 and 60 mg/12h if BMI> 50. Another option is to use Fondaparinux 2.5 mg day 6 hours after surgery.
   - Placement of the elastic stockings on ward, on which the intermittent pneumatic venous compression device will be placed in the operating room.
4. *Antibiotic prophylaxis*: Increasing the body mass of a severely obese patient, possibly leading to an increase in the volume of distribution of certain categories of antibiotics, which will require dose adjustment to higher values.

5. Other Issues

A. Difficulty of Venous Access in Obese Patients

Prior to anaesthesia, the extremities should be closely examined for good veins or considered a central line insertion. Intravenous access is vital for induction of anaesthesia, administration of medications and fluid therapy. At the same time, the pharmacist should recommend the appropriate dose of drugs based on body weight [108].

B. Venous Thromboembolism (VTE)

It is a major cause of postoperative morbidity in patients undergoing WLS. While the optimal approach to VTE prophylaxis in these patients is unclear, most receive some way of prophylaxis, including lower extremity compression stockings, drug prophylaxis or both. The standard antithrombotic regimen reduces VTE risk [109], with more evidence that suggests superiority of low molecular weight heparin treatment over unfractionated heparin [110, 111]. There is no evidence on the usefulness of routine venous Doppler, and it is not currently recommended [112, 113, 114].

Key Points

Key points of preoperative evaluation in bariatric surgery
• A proper preoperative evaluation is critical to the success of bariatric surgery. It allows to guarantee the selection of eligible candidates and achieve good outcomes after surgery. • The study will be adapted to each patient, according to their comorbidities, expectations, medical and psychological aspects involved in perioperative management, including the possibility of regaining weight. • The management of obesity requires a holistic approach and the intervention of an interprofessional team (doctors, psychologists, dietitians, nurses, ...). • Specialized medical, psychological, nutritional and anaesthesiology evaluation are mandatory in the preoperative study of the patient who undergoes bariatric surgery (Level II). • An exhaustive medical history will be taken, with analysis and complementary tests, including abdominal ultrasound and upper gastrointestinal endoscopy. Additional tests (spirometry, polysomnography, echocardiography, ...) must be individualized. (Level III). • Deficits and comorbidities will be detected, identifying those who require specific treatment and close management in the perioperative period.

- Although there must be a preoperative weight loss plan and optimization of lifestyle habits; the inability to obtain adequate weight loss should not disqualify the patient as a candidate for bariatric surgery (Level II).
- Morbidly obese patients have a higher cardiological risk than the rest of the population. Those with several high cardiovascular risk factors will be referred to the cardiologist to complete a directed functional study.
- Obesity hypoventilation syndrome (OHS) and obstructive sleep apnoea-hypopnea syndrome (OSAHS) are highly associated with morbid obesity.
- OSAHS risk assessment questionnaires, such as the STOP-BANG, allow to discriminate which ones would be indicated to request polysomnography. If OSAHS is confirmed, treatment with continuous positive air pressure (CPAP) should be maintained at least 1 month before the intervention and restarted from the immediate postoperative period.
- Preoperative respiratory physiotherapy can help reduce complications after bariatric surgery and it is therefore strongly recommended. Incentive spirometry is part of this strategy.
- The preoperative assessment in the anaesthesia consultation is of great relevance for the detection and optimization of comorbidities in the patient candidate for bariatric surgery.

References

[1] Hill, JO. "Obesity and the environment, where do we go from here?" *Science*, 299, (2003), 853–855.

[2] Ogden, CL. "Prevalence of obesity among adults and youth: United States, 2011– 2014". *NCHS Data Brief*, 219, (2015), 1–8.

[3] Shafiee, G. "Socioeconomic inequality in cardio-metabolic risk factors in a nationally representative sample of Iranian adolescents using an Oaxaca-Blinder decomposition method: the CASPIAN-III study." *J Diabetes Metab Disord*, 18, no. 1, (Jun 2019), 145-153.

[4] Biener, A. "The impact of obesity on medical care costs and labor market outcomes in the US." *Clin Chem*, 64, (2018), 108–117.

[5] Gloy, VL. "Bariatric surgery versus non- surgical treatment for obesity: a systematic review and meta-analysis of randomised controlled trials." *BMJ*, 347, (2013), f5934.

[6] Sjostrom, L. "Swedish Obese Subjects Study Scientific G. Lifestyle, diabetes, and cardiovascular risk factors 10 years after bariatric surgery." *N Engl J Med*, 351, (2004), 2683–2693.

[7] Ricci, C. "Long-term effects of bariatric surgery on type II diabetes, hypertension and hyperlipidemia: a meta-analysis and meta-regression study with 5-year follow-up." *Obes Surg*, 25, (2015), 397–405.

[8] Gil-Rendo, A. "J. Laparoscopic Sleeve Gastrectomy for High-Risk Patients in a Monocentric Series: Long-Term Outcomes and Predictors of Success." *Obes Surg*, 29, no. 11, (Nov 2019), 3629-3637.

[9] Sjostrom, L. "Bariatric surgery and reduction in morbidity and mortality: experiences from the SOS study." *Int J Obe*, 32, Suppl 7, (2008), 93–7.

[10] De Paris, FGC. "Assessment of Changes in Body composition During the First Postoperative Year After Bariatric Surgery." *Obes Surg.*, 29, no. 9, (Sep 2019), 3054-3061.

[11] Wilmore, DW. "Management of patients in fast track surgery." *BJM.*, 322, (2001), 473–476.

[12] Teeuwen, PH. "Enhanced recovery after surgery (ERAS) versus conventional postoperative care in colorectal surgery." *J Gastrointest Surg.*, 14, (2010), 88–95.

[13] Spanjersberg, WR. "Fast track surgery versus conventional recovery strategies for colorectal surgery." *Cochrane Database Syst Rev*, 2, (2011), CD007635.

[14] Jacobsen, HJ. "High-volume bariatric surgery in a single center: safety, quality, cost-efficacy and teaching aspects in 2000 consecutive patients." *Obes Surg.*, 22, (2012), 158–166.

[15] Lemanu, DP. "Optimizing perioperative care in bariatric surgery patients." *Obes Surg*, 22, (2012), 979–990.

[16] Greco, M. "Enhanced recovery program in colorectal surgery: a meta-analysis of randomized controlled trials." *World J Surg*, 38, no. 6, (2014), 1531–41.

[17] Ruiz-Tovar, J. "Implementation of the Spanish ERAS program in bariatric surgery." *Minim Invasive Allied Technol*, 27, no. 6, (Mar 2018), 1-8.

[18] Preet Mohinder Singh. "Efficiency and Safety Effects of Applying ERAS Protocols to Bariatric Surgery: a Systematic Review with Meta-Analysis and Trial Sequential Analysis of Evidence." *Obes Surg*, 27, (2017), 489–501.

[19] Schlottmann, F. "Preoperative Evaluation in Bariatric Surgery." *J Laparoendosc Adv Surg Tech A*, 28, no. 8, (Aug 2018), 925-929.

[20] Benalcazar, DA. "Obesity surgery pre-op assessment and preparation". *Treasure Island (FL): StatPearls Publishing*, (Jan 2021). PMID: 31536273.

[21] Picot, J. "The clinical effectiveness and cost-effectiveness of bariatric (weight loss) surgery for obesity: a systematic review and economic evaluation." *Health Technol Assess*, 13, no. 41, (2009), 1–4.

[22] Sanni. "Postoperative complications in bariatric surgery using age and BMI stratification: a study using ACS-NSQIP data." *Surg. Endosc*, 28, no. 12, (2014), 3302-3309.

[23] Dumon, KR. "Bariatric surgery outcomes." *Surg. Clin. North Am.*, 91, no. 6, (2011), 1313-1318.

[24] Cardoso, L. "Short- and long-term mortality after bariatric surgery: A systematic review and meta-analysis." *Diabetes Obes Metab*, 19, no. 9, (2017), 1223–1232. doi:10.1111/dom.12922.

[25] Nickel, F. "Predictors of Risk and Success of Obesity Surgery." *Obes Facts*, 12, No. 4, (2019), 427-439.

[26] Sharma, AM. "A proposed clinical staging system for obesity." *Int J Obes*, 33, no. 3, (Mar 2009), 289–95.

[27] Maciejewski, ML. "Risk stratification of serious adverse events after gastric bypass in the Bariatric Outcomes Longitudinal Database." *Surg Obes Relat Dis*, 8, no. 6, (Nov-Dic 2012), 671–7.

[28] Chiappetta, S. "The importance of the Edmonton obesity staging system in predicting postoperative outcome and 30-day mortality

after metabolic surgery." *Surg Obes Relat Dis*, 12, no. 10, (Dec 2016), 1847–55.

[29] Sjostrom, L. "Effects of bariatric surgery on mortality in Swedish obese subjects." *N Engl J Med*, 357, no. 8, (2007), 741–52.

[30] Boyer, M. "*Acute and chronic impact of bariatric surgery on plasma LDL cholesterol and PCSK9 levels in patients with severe obesity.*," 102, (2017), 4023–4030.

[31] Kwok, CS. "Bariatric surgery and its impact on cardiovascular disease and mortality: a systematic review and meta-analysis." *Int J Cardiol*, 173, (2014), 20–28.

[32] Fisher, DP. "Association between bariatric surgery and macrovascular disease outcomes in patients with type 2 diabetes and severe obesity." *JAMA*, 320, (2018), 1570–1582.

[33] Benotti, PN. "Gastric bypass surgery produces a durable reduction in cardiovascular disease risk factors and reduces the long-term risks of congestive heart failure." *J Am Heart Assoc*, 23, no. 6, (May 2017). DOI: 10.1161/jaha.116.005126,

[34] Zhou, X. "Effects of Bariatric Surgery on Mortality, Cardiovascular Events, and Cancer Outcomes in Obese Patients: Systematic Review and Meta-analysis." *Obes Surg*, 26, no. 11, (2016), 2590–2601.

[35] Kindel, TL. "Bariatric surgery as a treatment for heart failure: review of the literature and potential mechanisms." *Surg Obes Relat Dis*, 14, no. 1, (2018), 117–122.

[36] DeMaria, EJ. "Obesity surgery mortality risk score: proposal for a clinically useful score to predict mortality risk in patients undergoing gastric bypass." *Surg Obes Relat Dis*, 3, (2007), 34–40.

[37] DeMaria, EJ. "Validation of the obesity surgery mortality risk score in a multicenter study proves it stratifies mortality risk in patients undergoing gastric bypass for morbid obesity." *Ann Surg*, 246, (2007), 578–82.

[38] Gupta, PK. "Development and validation of a bariatric surgery morbidity risk calculator using the prospective, multicenter NSQIP dataset." *J Am Coll Surg*, 212, (2011), 301–9.

[39] Nguyen, NT. "Proposal for a bariatric mortality risk classification system for patients undergoing bariatric surgery." *Surg Obes Relat Dis*, 9, no. 2, (2013), 239–46.

[40] Sherf-Dagan, S. "The effect of pre-surgery information online lecture on nutrition knowledge and anxiety among bariatric surgery candidates." *Obes Surg*, 28, no. 7, (Jul 2018), 1876-1885.

[41] Bauchowitz, A. "Evaluation of expectations and knowledge in bariatric surgery patients." *Surg Obes Relat Dis*, 3, (2007), 554–558.

[42] Giusti, V. "Impact of preoperative teaching on surgical option of patients qualifying for bariatric surgery." *Obes Surg*, 14, (2004), 1241–1246.

[43] Wee, CC. "Expectations for weight loss and willingness to accept risk among patients seeking weight loss surgery." *JAMA Surg*, 148, (2013), 264–271.

[44] Sjöstrom, L. "Lifestyle, diabetes, and cardiovascular risk factors 10 years after bariatric surgery." *N Engl J Med*, 351, (2004), 2683–2693.

[45] Buchwald, H. "Bariatric surgery: A systematic review and meta-analysis." *JAMA*, 292, (2004), 1724–1737.

[46] Colquitt, JL. "Surgery for weight loss in adults." *Cochrane Database Syst Rev*, 2014, CD003641.

[47] Greenburg, DL. "Effects of surgical weight loss on measures of obstructive sleep apnea: A meta-analysis." *Am J Med*, 122, (2009), 535–542.

[48] Aills, L. "ASMBS allied health nutritional guidelines for the surgical weight loss patient." *Surg Obes Relat Dis*, 4, (2008), S73–S108.

[49] Mohapatra, S. "Malnutrition in obesity before and after bariatric surgery." *Dis Mon*, 66, no.2, (Feb 2020), 100866.

[50] Martín García, E. "Vía clínica de cirugía bariátrica 2017 (AEC, SECO, GERM)". ISBN: 978-84-697-7104-4.

[51] Third report of the National Cholesterol Education Program (NCEP) expert panel on detection, evaluation, and treatment of high blood cholesterol in adults (Adult Treatment Panel III). Final report. *Circulation*, 106, (2002), 3143-3421.

[52] Grundy, SM. "Diagnosis and management of the metabolic syndrome: an American Heart Association/National Heart, Lung, and Blood Institute Scientific Statement." *Circulation*, 112, (2005), 2735-2752.

[53] Alberti, KGMM. "Metabolic syndrome –a new world-wide definition. A consensus statement from the international diabetes federation." *Diabet Med*, 23, (2006), 469-480.

[54] Mechanick, JI. "Clinical practice guidelines for the perioperative nutritional, metabolic, and nonsurgical support of the bariatric surgery patient—2013 update: Cosponsored by American Association of ClinicalEndocrinologists, the Obesity Society, and American Society for Metabolic & Bariatric Surgery." *Endocr Pract*, 19, (2013), 337–372.

[55] Zalesin, KC. "Impact of obesity on cardiovascular disease." *Med Clin North Am*, 95, (2011), 919–937.

[56] Pirlet, C. "Comparison of Short and Long Term Cardiovascular Outcomes After Bariatric Surgery in Patients With vs Without Coronary Artery Disease." *Am J Cardiol*, 125, (2020), 40−47.

[57] Mechanick, JI. "American Association of Clinical Endocrinologists, The Obesity Society, and American Society for Metabolic & Bariatric Surgery Medical Guidelines for Clinical Practice for the perioperative nutritional, metabolic, and nonsurgical support of the bariatric surgery patient." *Surg Obes Relat Dis*, 4, no. Suppl 5, (2008), S109-84.

[58] D'Agostino, RB Sr. "General cardiovascular risk profile for use in primary care: the Framingham Heart Study." *Circulation*, 117, no. 6, (2008), 743-53.

[59] Assmann, G. "Simple scoring scheme for calculating the risk of acute coronary events based on the 10-year follow-up of the prospective cardiovascular Munster (PROCAM) study." *Circulation*, 105, (2002), 310-5.

[60] Conroy, RM. "Estimation of ten- year risk of fatal cardiovascular disease in Europe: the SCORE project." *Eur Heart J*, 24, (2003), 987-1003.

[61] Quilliot, D. "Evaluation of risk factors for complications after bariatric surgery." *J Visc Surg.*, 155, no. 3, (2018), 201–210.

[62] Kristensen, SD. "2014 ESC/ESA Guidelines on non-cardiac surgery: cardiovascular assessment and management: The Joint Task Force on non-cardiac surgery: cardiovascular assessment and management of the European Society of Cardiology (ESC) and

the European Society of Anaesthesiology (ESA)." *Eur Heart J*, 35, (2014), 2383-2431.

[63] Lee, TH, Marcantonio, ER. "Derivation and prospective validation of a simple index for prediction of cardiac risk of major noncardiac surgery." *Circulation*, 100, (1999), 1043–1049.

[64] Poirier, P. "American Heart Association Obesity Committee of Council on Nutrition PA, Metabolism CoCP, Critical Care CoCS, Anesthesia CoC. Cardiovascular evaluation and management of severely obese patients undergoing surgery: a science advisory from the American Heart Association." *Circulation*, 120, (2009), 86–95.

[65] Fleisher, LA. "2009 ACCF/AHA focused update on perioperative beta blockade incorporated into the ACC/AHA 2007 guidelines on perioperative cardiovascular evaluation and care for noncardiac surgery: A report of the American college of cardiology foundation/American heart association task force on practice guidelines. *Circulation*, 120, (2009), e169-e276.

[66] O'Rourke, RW. "Perioperative morbidity associated with bariatric surgery." *Arch Surg*, 141, (2006), 262–268.

[67] Vest, AR. "Bariatric surgery and cardiovascular outcomes: A systematic review." *Heart*, 98, (2012), 1763–1777.

[68] Courcoulas, AP. "Seven-Year Weight Trajectories and Health Outcomes in the Longitudinal Assessment of Bariatric Surgery (LABS) Study." *JAMA Surg*, 153, no. 5, (2018), 427-434.

[69] Arterburn, DE. "Benefits and Risks of Bariatric Surgery in Adults: A Review." *JAMA.*, 324, no. 9, (Sep 2020), 879-887.

[70] Nathaniel, R. "Perioperative Cardiovascular Risk Assessment and Management for Noncardiac Surgery." *JAMA.*, 324, no. 3, (2020), 279-290.

[71] Vahé S Tateosian. "Preoperative Cardiac Evaluation for Noncardiac Surgery." *Anesthesiol Clin*, 36, no. 4, (2018), 509-521.

[72] Jeger, RV. "Long-term prognostic value of the preoperative 12-lead electrocardiogram before major noncardiac surgery in coronary artery disease." *Am Heart J*, 151, no. 2, (2006), 508-513.

[73] Landesberg, G. "Perioperative ischemia and cardiac complications in major vascular surgery: importance of the preoperative twelve-lead electrocardiogram." *J Vasc Surg*, 26, no. 4, (1997), 570-578.

[74] Hammond, KL. "Practical issues in the surgical care of the obese patient." *Ochsner J*, 13, (2013), 224–227.
[75] Uppot, RN. "Effect of obesity on image quality: Fifteen year longitudinal study for evaluation of dictated radiology reports." *Radiology*, 240, (2006), 435–439.
[76] Shah, BN. "Stress echocardiography in patients with morbid obesity." *Echo Res Pract*, 3, (2016), 13-18.
[77] Supariwala, A. "Feasibility and prognostic value of stress echocardiography in obese, morbidly obese, and super obese patients referred for bariatric surgery." *Echocardiography*, 31, (2014), 879–885.
[78] Kanchi Muralidhar. "Practice guidelines for perioperative transesophageal echocardiography: recommendations of the Indian association of cardiovascular thoracic anesthesiologists." *Ann Card Anaesth*, 16, no. 4, (Oct-Dec 2013), 268-78.
[79] Fleisher, LA. "American College of Cardiology; American Heart Association. 2014 ACC/AHA guideline on perioperative cardiovascular evaluation and management of patients undergoing noncardiac surgery: a report of the American College of Cardiology/American Heart Association Task Force on practice guidelines." *J Am Coll Cardiol*, 64, no. 22, (2014), 77-137.
[80] Wang, X. "Perioperative β-blocker use: what is new in 2020?" *Curr Opin Anaesthesiol*, 33, no. 3, (2020), 417-422.
[81] Hamoui, N. "The value of pulmonary function testing before bariatric surgery." *Obes Surg*, 16, (2006), 1570–1573.
[82] Van Huisstede, A. "Pulmonary function testing and complications of laparoscopic bariatric surgery." *Obes Surg*, 23, (2013), 1596–1603.
[83] Edmond H L Chau. "Obesity hypoventilation syndrome: a review of epidemiology, pathophysiology, and perioperative considerations." *Anesthesiology*, 117, no. 1, (2012), 188-205.
[84] Kapur, VK. "Clinical practice guideline for diagnostic testing for adult obstructive sleep apnea: an American Academy of Sleep Medicine Clinical Practice Guideline." *JAMA*, 13, (2017), 479-504.
[85] Nogueira, F. "Guías prácticas de diagnóstico y tratamiento del síndrome de apneas e hipopneas obstructivas del sueño." *Medicina (B Aires)*, 73 (2013), 349-62.

[86] Durán-Cantolla, J. "El síndrome de apneas-hipopneas durante el sueño (SAHS) en España. Disponibilidad de recursos para su diagnóstico y tratamiento en los hospitales del estado español." *Arch Bronconeumol*, 40, (2004), 259-67.
[87] Baldwin, CM. "The association of sleep disordered breathing and sleep symptoms with quality of life in the Sleep Heart Health Study." *Sleep*, 24, (2001), 96-105.
[88] Durán, J. "Obstructive sleep apnea-hypopnea and related clinical features in a population-based sample of subjects aged 30 to 70 yr." *Am J Respir Crit Care Med*, 163, (2001), 685-9.
[89] Nieto, FK. "Association of sleep-disordered breathing, sleep apnoea, and hypertension in a large community-based study." *JAMA*, 283, (2000), 1829-36.
[90] Preoperative Tests (Update): "Routine Preoperative Tests for Elective Surgery. NICE Guideline, No. 45. National Guideline Centre (UK)." *National Institute for Health and Care Excellence (UK)*, Apr 2016.
[91] Clavellina-Gaytan, D. "Evaluation of spirometric testing as a routine preoperative assessment in patients undergoing bariatric surgery." *Obes Surg*, 25, (2015), 530–536.
[92] Hall, J. "Guyton and Hall Textbook of Medical Physiology." Fourteenth Edition. Philadelphia. Elsevier., 2020. International ISBN: 978-0-323-67280-1.
[93] Heckman, EJ. "Pulmonary function tests for diagnosing lung disease." *JAMA*, 313, no. 22, (2015), 2278-9.
[94] Bibbins-Domingo, K. "Screening for obstructive sleep apnea in adults: US Preventive Services Task Force Recommendation Statement." *JAMA*, 317, (2017), 407.
[95] Lloberes, P. "Diagnóstico y tratamiento del síndrome de apneas-hipopneas del sueño." *Arch Bronconeumol*, 47, (2011), 143-156.
[96] González-Mangado, N. "Síndrome de apnea-hipopnea del sueño." *Arch Bronconeumol*, (2015), 1-21
[97] Johns, MW. "A new method for measuring daytime sleepiness: the Epworth sleepiness scale." *Sleep*, 14, (1991), 540-55.
[98] Ahmadi, N. "The Berlin questionnaire for sleep apnoea in a sleep clinic population: Relationship to polysomnographic measurement of respiratory disturbance." *Sleep Breath*, 12, (2008), 39-45.

[99] Chung, F. "Validation of the Berlin questionnaire and American Society of Anesthesiologists checklist as screening tools for obstructive sleep apnea in surgical patients." *Anesthesiology*, 108, (2008), 822-30.

[100] Ramachandran, SK. "Derivation and validation of a simple perioperative sleep apnea prediction score." *Anesth Analg*, 110, (2010), 1007-15.

[101] Chung, F. "STOP questionnaire: a tool to screen patients for obstructive sleep apnea." *Anesthesiology*, 108, (2008), 812-21.

[102] Nagappa, M. "Validation of the STOP-Bang Questionnaire as a screening tool for obstructive sleep apnea among different populations: a systematic review and meta-analysis." *PLoS One*, 10, (2015), e0143697.

[103] Berry, RB. "Rules for scoring respiratory events in sleep: Update of the 2007 AASM Manual for the Scoring of Sleep and Associated Events. Deliberations of the Sleep Apnea Definitions Task Force of the American Academy of Sleep Medicine." *J Clin Sleep Med*, 8, (2012), 597-619.

[104] Audrey De Jong. "How can I manage anaesthesia in obese patients?" *Anaesth Crit Care Pain Med*, 39, no. 2, (Apr 2020), 229-238.

[105] Soleimanpour, H. "Anesthetic Considerations in Patients Undergoing Bariatric Surgery: A Review Article." *Anesth Pain Med*, 7, no. 4, (Aug 2017), e57568.

[106] Juvin, P. "Difficult tracheal intubation is more common in obese than in lean patients." *Anesth Analg*, 97, no. 2, (Aug 2003), 595-600.

[107] Moon, TS. "The influence of morbid obesity on difficult intubation and difficult mask ventilation." *J Anesth*, 33, no. 1, (Feb 2019), 96-102.

[108] Cascella, M. "Towards a better understanding of anesthesia emergence mechanisms: Research and clinical implications." *World J Methodol*, 12, no. 8, (Oct 2018), 9-16.

[109] Becattini, C. "Venous thromboembolism after laparoscopic bariatric surgery for morbid obesity: Clinical burden and prevention." *Surg Obes Relat Dis*, 8, (2012), 108-115

[110] Birkmeyer, NJO. "Comparative effectiveness of unfractionated and low-molecular-weight heparin for prevention of venous thromboembolism following bariatric surgery." *Arch Surg*, 147, (2012), 994-998.

[111] Ikesaka, R. "Efficacy and safety of weight-adjusted heparin prophylaxis for the prevention of acute venous thromboembolism among obese patients undergoing bariatric surgery: A systematic review and meta-analysis." *Thromb Res*, 133, (2014), 682-687.

[112] American Society for Metabolic and Bariatric Surgery Clinical Issues Committee. "ASMBS updated position statement on prophylactic measures to reduce the risk of venous thromboembolismin bariatric surgery patients." *Surg Obes Relat Dis*, 9, (2013), 493-497.

[113] Bartlett, MA. "Prevention of venous thromboembolism in patients undergoing bariatric surgery." *Vasc Health Risk Manage*, 11, (2015), 461-477.

[114] Prystowsky, JB. "Prospective analysis of the incidence of deep venous thrombosis in bariatric surgery patients." *Surgery*, 138, (2005), 759-763.

In: Enhanced Recovery after Surgery ... ISBN: 978-1-53619-976-5
Editor: Jaime Ruiz-Tovar

Chapter 3

Relevance of Upper Digestive Endoscopy and Screening of Helicobacter Pylori in Bariatric Surgery

Soledad García Gómez-Heras**, *MD, PhD* and *Ana Vilches-López
Human Histology, Basic Health Department,
Health Science Falculty, Rey Juan Carlos University, Madrid, Spain

Abstract

Helicobacter pylori (H. pylori) is the most prevalent chronic bacterial infection and is associated with diverse gastric disorders: peptic ulcer disease, chronic gastritis, gastric adenocarcinoma, and gastric mucosa associated lymphoid tissue (MALT) lymphoma.

Testing for it is not routinely performed, only reserved for those cases in which the clinician suspects a disorder or in whose pathogenesis can be involved. The choice of test used to diagnose H. pylori depends on whether a patient requires an upper endoscopy for evaluation of symptoms or surveillance.

This infection is very common in morbidly obese patients, with a prevalence of 23% to 70% in bariatric patients. Its eradication before the surgery is mandatory, as the infection has been associated with postoperative complications, and the eradication of H. pylori has been related to a reduction of all these entities. It can be diagnosed with different techniques. However, the upper digestive endoscopy is the only diagnostic test that can inform us about the edoscopic and its histologic implication in these patients.

Keywords: upper digestive endoscopy, helicobacter pylori, bariatric surgery

INTRODUCTION

Helicobacter pylori (H. pylori) is the most prevalent chronic bacterial infection and is associated with diverse gastric disorders, such as peptic ulcer disease, chronic gastritis, gastric adenocarcinoma, and gastric mucosa associated lymphoid tissue (MALT) lymphoma [1-4].

Testing for H. pylori are not routinely performed and are reserved for those cases in which the clinician suspects a disorder, in whose pathogenesis H. pylori can be involved, and plans to offer treatment to improve the results. Indications for H. pylori testing includes [5-8]:

- uninvestigated dyspepsia in patients <60 years even without alarm features
- patients planned to receive chronic treatment with Non-steroideal aintiinflammatory drugs (NSAID): H. pylori infection is a risk factor for the development of ulcers and for ulcer bleeding in patients on low-dose aspirin treatment. H. pylori also increases the risk of NSAID-related peptic complications.
- Unexplained iron deficiency: H. pylori can cause iron deficiency and iron deficiency anemia by interfering with absorption of oral iron.

In addition, endoscopic diagnosis of mucosa associated lymphoid tissue (MALT) lymphoma, active peptic ulcer disease or past history of peptic ulcer, and gastric cancer are also indications for testing, as H. pylori can be involved in the pathogenesis and development of these pathologies.

DIAGNOSTIC TESTS FOR H. PYLORI

The choice of test used to diagnose H. pylori depends on whether a patient requires an upper endoscopy for evaluation of symptoms or surveillance. Among patients undergoing upper endoscopy, the choice of test to diagnose H. pylori is a biopsy urease test. If a gastric mucosal biopsy is not obtained at the time of endoscopy or upper endoscopy is not performed, a urea breath test or stool antigen assay can be used to diagnose H. pylori. Serologic testing for H. pylori should be avoided altogether. If performed in areas of low prevalence of H. pylori, positive results should be confirmed with a test for active infection prior to initiating eradication therapy [9, 10].

- *Biopsy urease testing*: Gastric biopsy specimens are placed in a medium that contains urea and a pH reagent. Urease cleaves urea to liberate ammonia, producing an alkaline pH and a resultant color change. Commercially available urease testing kits differ in the use of medium (agar versus membrane pad) and testing reagents and the time to obtain a final result (1 to 24 hours). The sensitivity and specificity of biopsy urease testing is approximately 90- 95% [3]. With the rapid urease testing kits, results are obtained in one hour. One hour sensitivity and specificity of rapid urease tests are comparable to those seen with agar gel tests at 24 hours and superior to agar gel tests at one hour [11]. It is recommended that samples obtained from both the gastric antrum and the fundus to increase the sensitivity of the test. Increasing the number of gastric biopsy specimens from one to four also increases the sensitivity of the test [12, 13].
- *Histology*: Gastric biopsies can diagnose of H. pylori infection and associated lesions (e.g., atrophic gastritis, intestinal metaplasia, dysplasia, and MALT lymphoma). Biopsies for histology should be taken from both the antrum and body of the stomach, especially when looking for evidence of multifocal atrophic gastritis and/or intestinal metaplasia. The accuracy of histologic diagnosis of H. pylori infection can be improved by using special stains such as Giemsa or specific immune stains

[14]. The sensitivity and specificity of histology for the H. pylori infection are 95% and 98%, respectively.

- *Bacterial culture and sensitivity testing*: Biopsies for culture should be obtained before the forceps are contaminated with formalin. The tissue should be placed into a container with a few drops of saline. This preparation will allow for culture and antibiotic sensitivity testing. While bacterial culture has high specificity, it has low sensitivity, as H. pylori is difficult to culture. Microcapillary culturing methods and improved transport media may improve sensitivity [15].
- *Urea breath testing (UBT)*: UBT is based upon the hydrolysis of urea by H. pylori to produce CO_2 and ammonia. Oral intake of urea with a labeled carbon isotope (non-radioactive 13C or radioactive 14C) is administrated. H. pylori liberates labeled CO_2 that can be detected in breath samples. The tests can be performed in 15 to 20 minutes and have similar cost and accuracy. The dose of radiation in the 14C test is approximately 1 microCi, which is equivalent to one day of background radiation exposure. Even though this dose of radiation is small, the non-radioactive 13C test is preferred in young children and pregnant women. The sensitivity and specificity of UBT are approximately 88-95% and 95-100%, respectively [16, 17].
- *Stool antigen assay*: The detection of bacterial antigen indicates an ongoing H. pylori infection. Stool antigen testing can therefore be used to establish the initial diagnosis of H. pylori and to confirm eradication [3]. Of the available tests, stool antigen testing is the most cost-effective in areas of low to intermediate prevalence of H. pylori. The sensitivity and specificity of the laboratory-based monoclonal enzyme immunoassay are comparable to the UBT [18, 19].
- *Serology*: Laboratory-based ELISA test to detect immunoglobulin G (IgG) antibodies is inexpensive and noninvasive. However, serologic tests require validation at the local level, which is impractical in routine practice. In addition, concerns over its accuracy have limited its use. Guidelines recommend that serologic testing should not be used in low prevalence populations as the low accuracy of serology would result in

inappropriate treatment in significant numbers of patients [2, 3]. Serology does not reliably distinguish between active and past infection. A quantitative ELISA test is generally used in research settings. It allows for determination of IgG titers of paired sera from the acute and convalescent (three to six months or longer) phase and can confirm eradication of the infection. However, this is not performed in clinical practice.

Gastric Pathology Associated to H. pylori Infection

H. pylori has been related to gastric pathology, such as peptic ulcer, chronic gastritis, gastric atrophy, intestinal metaplasia and gastric adenocarcinoma. Among them, chronic gastritis, gastric atrophy and intestinal metaplasia can be considered as premalignant lesions, amenable for H. pylori eradication treatment and eventual endoscopic follow-up, to determine a progression to malignant neoplasms.

In 1994, the International Agency for Research on Cancer considered the H. pylori as carcinogen agent for the type I gastric cancer (GC). It is important to emphasize that more than 90% of patients with GC suffer an active or past infection by H. pylori [20]. According to the model of the pathogenesis of the stomach carcinogenesis proposed by Correa [21], the sequential changes in the gastric mucosa are: first a chronic gastritis (CG), evolving to a gastric atrophia (GA) and to a gastric intestinal metaplasia (GIM) which could eventually lead to a GC. These clinical situations are often associated with an H. pylori infection [22].

All these pathologies are diagnosed by UGE, with biopsy and histopathological study, whose classification is based on the Sydney System (SS) [23], a score system protocol that stages the GA and the GIM, as precancerous lesions. The SS includes endoscopic and histological aspects.

1. Chronic Gastritis due to H. pylori

Gastritis denotes inflammation associated with gastric mucosal injury. Gastritis is usually caused by infectious agents, being H. pylori the most frequently microorganim involved [24]. Most patients with H. pylori infection will show features of both acute and chronic gastritis (chronic active gastritis).

H. pylori resides primarily in the unstirred layer of gastric mucus, adjacent to epithelial cells at the mucosal surface and in gastric pits [25]. Gastric glands are usually not involved. H. pylori does not attach to small intestinal or other gastric epithelial cell types. The organisms are uncommonly found in the lamina propria. The usual natural history of H. pylori gastritis is of an antral predominant early stage of infection with only minimal corpus involvement. This stage is associated with exaggerated gastrin release and reduced somatostatin release, often precipitating an increase in acid secretion, enough to cause duodenal ulcers in some patients [26]. With continued inflammation, gastrin producing (G) cells and acid producing parietal cells are gradually lost, precipitating a decreased in acid secretion and the development of atrophy with intestinal metaplasia [27].

It remains unclear if chronic gastritis causes abdominal pain in the absence of peptic ulcer disease. However, it has been associated with functional dyspepsia. Patients with chronic H. pylori gastritis can present with complications of peptic ulcer disease or gastroduodenal complications of chronic infection including gastric atrophy, intestinal metaplasia, gastric cancer, and mucosa-associated lymphoid tissue (MALT) lymphoma.

Chronic H. pylori infection has been associated with other extragastrointestinal diseases including:

- Iron deficiency anemia [28]. The most plausible mechanism is decreased iron absorption due to H. pylori-associated gastric atrophy and hypochlorhydria
- Vitamin B12 deficiency [28] – H. pylori infection can lead to chronic (metaplastic) atrophic gastritis resulting in hypochlorhydria and vitamin B12 malabsorption. Also, the bacteria may elicit production of antibodies that cross-react with

the gastric parietal $H^+ K^+$ ATPase. Eradication of chronic H. pylori infection has been associated with increases in vitamin B12 levels.

The endoscopic appearance of chronic gastritis is normal in as many as 50% of patients [29]. Other patients may have nonspecific endoscopic features including mucosal erythema, friable gastric mucosa, and diffuse antral nodularity.

As previously mentioned, histopathology plays a major role in diagnosing H. pylori infection, establishing the presence, severity, and extent of gastritis, and detecting associated complications of H. pylori infection (e.g., intestinal metaplasia, MALT lymphoma, and gastric carcinoma). H. pylori is almost always accompanied by gastritis and the diagnosis of H. pylori should be suspect in its absence. The organisms can be detected in both the antrum and the body of the stomach in the around 80% of chronically infected patients [30]. Localization of H. pylori to the body alone is usually due to concurrent proton pump inhibitors (PPI) use or marked gastric atrophy and intestinal metaplasia.

Given the variable distribution of H. pylori in the stomach, diagnostic accuracy can be increased when biopsies are taken from multiple sites in the stomach. The updated SS [31] recommends that biopsy specimens be taken from five different sites for optimal assessment of both gastritis and H. pylori status: lesser and greater curvature of the antrum, lesser and greater curvature of the corpus, and the incisura angularis.

The chronic inflammatory elements in H. pylori gastritis primarily consist of lymphocytes and plasma cells, scattered macrophages, and often eosinophils [32]. Lymphoid follicles are frequently present and represent an immune response to the bacteria; their presence provides a useful marker for H. pylori infection. Similarly, a prominence of plasma cells is a valuable clue to H. pylori infection.

The intensity of the inflammation varies among patients and sometimes from specimen to specimen in the same patient. Although casual observation reveals no obvious relation between the numbers of organisms and the severity of the chronic inflammation, a correlation with bacterial density and active gastritis has been described [33]. Inflammation associated with chronic H. pylori gastritis improves dramatically after eradication of the organisms with appropriate antibiotics. Studies have shown that atrophy associated to chronic gastritis usually it is not resolve in one year but that significant improvement has been recognized after 10 years [34]. Organism eradication may also help to prevent the development of further gastric atrophy and intestinal metaplasia [35].

2. Gastric Atrophia (GA) and Gastric Intestinal Mertaplasia (GIM) due to Helicobacter Pylori

The term metaplastic chronic atrophic gastritis, also referred to as gastric atrophy (GA), is used to describe a form of chronic gastritis that, in addition to inflammation, is associated with mucosal thinning, loss of specialized cells in gastric glands, and changes in epithelial cell types (i.e., metaplasia). It results in the replacement of the normal oxyntic mucosa in the gastric corpus by atrophic and metaplastic mucosa, leading to a corpus predominant atrophic gastritis, reduced or absent acid and pepsin production, and loss of intrinsic factor, which may progress to a severe form of vitamin B12-deficiency anemia known as pernicious anemia.

There is evidence that H. pylori might serve as a trigger of GA and that H. pylori infection at a younger age triggers the development of autoimmune gastritis, which progresses clinically over time from iron deficiency anemia (perhaps due to iron malabsorption because of hypochlorhydria/achlorhydria) to cobalamin deficiency with macrocytosis [36].

The association between GA and H. pylori infection in many patients has led to speculation that H. pylori may, in some cases, induce GA via antigenic cross-reactivity.

Patients with GA may be asymptomatic, but many of them have dyspepsia with postprandial distress [37]. Patients with GA may be symptomatic from vitamin B12 malabsorption and pernicious anemia [37]. The presence of symptoms attributable to anemia depends on the rate that deficiency has developed, the severity of the deficiency, the hemoglobin level, and the person's overall health. Patients with B12 deficiency usually have vague or nonspecific symptoms (e.g., fatigue, irritability, cognitive decline), which are likely to be due to anemia. B12 deficiency can cause glossitis (including pain, swelling, tenderness, and loss of papillae of the tongue). B12 deficiency can also cause neurologic, cognitive, or psychiatric changes. The most common neurologic manifestation is symmetric paresthesias or numbness and gait problems.

Patients with GA are at increased risk for the development of gastric neuroendocrine tumors and adenocarcinomas. Thus, this entity can be considered as a premalignant disorder [38]. Neuroendocrine tumors arise from transformation of enterochromaffin-like (ECL) cells (which are responsible for histamine secretion) within the oxyntic mucosa due to chronic stimulation by high circulating levels of gastrin. The hypochlorhydria or achlorhydria associated with GA induces hyperplasia of the antral/pyloric G cells (the cell type responsible for producing gastrin) and hypergastrinemia. Gastrin exerts a trophic effect on endocrine cells within the metaplastic and atrophic body mucosa, which increase in number and may give rise to hyperplastic nodules both within and around the glands [39]. The relationship between gastrin-induced ECL cell hyperplasia and neuroendocrine tumor formation is supported by the observation that antrectomy, with resultant loss of G cell mass and normalization of plasma gastrin concentrations, can lead to reversal of endocrine hyperplasia and reduced carcinoid tumor size [40].

Gastric adenocarcinoma develops in patients with GA via intervening steps of intestinal metaplasia and dysplasia [41, 42]. A retrospective study of 150 patients diagnosed with GA on endoscopic gastric biopsy, found a high prevalence (5.3%) and incidence (14.2 cases per 1000 person-years) of gastric adenocarcinoma, far exceeding that of the general population (0.073 cases per 1000 person-years) [43]. Patients with GA are at a 10- to 15-fold increased risk for gastric cancer, particularly the intestinal type [42]. It is hypothesized that increased macrophage-derived inflammatory drivers present in GA may be responsible for the progression from metaplasia to carcinoma in this population.

Histopathologic studies indicate that chronic H. pylori infection progresses over decades through stages of chronic superficial gastritis, GA, GIM, dysplasia, and cancer [42]. The mechanisms whereby some patients with H. pylori infection develop intestinal metaplasia and carcinoma, while others do not, are multifactorial and likely involve an interplay of bacterial virulence factors and host susceptibility factors.

The diagnosis of GA is based on the histologic evaluation of gastric biopsies which demonstrate atrophy of the gastric mucosa with the loss of glandular cells and their replacement by metaplastic epithelium.

The endoscopic appearance of GA is normal during the early disease stages. Only in cases with extensive atrophy are the rugal folds flattened and the submucosal vessels visible. Mucosa may appear pseudopolypoid as polypoid areas represent islands of preserved oxyntic mucosa adjacent to areas of atrophy. Chromoendoscopy may be superior to white-light endoscopy [44].

Biopsy is the most reliable method to diagnose GA and diagnose H. pylori. Assessment of its severity and determining the subtype of GA requires gastric biopsy mapping with an adequate number of biopsies from specific sites.

Two main types of metaplasia are seen in chronic atrophic gastritis: pseudopyloric metaplasia and gastric intestinal metaplasia (GIM). Metaplasia, especially of the intestinal type, is virtually a universal feature of chronic atrophic gastritis and is often the most dependable defining morphologic feature. GIM is a precursor lesion to dysplasia and gastric cancer. Other types of metaplasia may be seen in GA, including pancreatic (acinar), ciliated cell, and squamous. These are rare and of uncertain clinical significance.

Endoscopic surveillance in patients with GA is controversial and has not been uniformly recommended [44]. Recommendations for endoscopic surveillance in patients with GA are based on the severity of atrophy, extent of intestinal metaplasia, and risk factors for gastric cancer (e.g., family history of gastric cancer). The American Society for Gastrointestinal Endoscopy (ASGE) 2015 guidelines do not recommend surveillance in all patients with GIM, but state that patients with GIM who are at increased risk of gastric cancer due to ethnic background or family history may benefit from screening [46].

There is no specific treatment for GA. H. pylori, if identified, should be eliminated as early as possible. Eradication of H. pylori may lead to partial regression of atrophic gastritis. Whether eradication of H. pylori can affect the natural history of GIM and its associated cancer risk is uncertain. H. pylori eradication before the development of extensive GIM may be effective in reducing gastric cancer incidence, but there may be a point of no return during the sequence of H. pylori-induced carcinogenesis, coinciding with the presence of extensive GA [47].

RELEVANCE OF UPPER DIGESTIVE ENDOSCOPY (UGE) IN PATIENTS PRIOR TO BARIATRIC SURGERY

Bariatric surgery has become the most powerful tool as a long-term solution to both obesity and its associated pathologies. Currently, Roux-en-Y gastric bypass (RYGB) and sleeve gastrectomy (SG) are the two most popular bariatric procedures performed [48, 49]. There is no ideal or worldwide standardized bariatric operative procedure. The decision of which technique is most appropriate for a patient depends often on the surgeon´s preferences and experience. However, several factors strongly influence the decision of the procedure performed, including gastrointestinal disorders or even asymptomatic endoscopic findings [50].

Many upper digestive pathologies are directly associated with morbid obesity, such as hiatal hernia, gastroesophageal reflux disease (GERD) and their complications, including erosive esophagitis, Barrett's esophagus, and esophageal adenocarcinoma [51]. These pathologies are more common among obese population, because the esophageal sphincter is affected, due to the excessive visceral fat that increases intra-abdominal pressure. Consequently, the gastric pressure is increased, the gastric emptying is altered and there is a trend towards reflux of gastric content to the esophagus [51].

The performance of a routine UGE is still controversial. Despite UGE is associated with a low complications rate [52], some groups defend that it is unnecessary to expose patients to a routine UGE, given the low prevalence of asymptomatic findings that may change the surgeons´ decision of the bariatric technique to be performed [53, 54].

The European Association for Endoscopic Surgery (EAES) recommends to perform UGE or contrast-enhanced esophago-gastro-duodenal series to all patients in the preoperative assessment prior to bariatric surgery [52]. The Society of American Gastrointestinal and Endoscopic Surgeons (SAGES) and the American Society of

Gastrointestinal Endoscopy (ASGE) recommend UGE to be individualized in cases when a gastric pathology is suspected or H. pylori infection is present, deciding the selected bariatric procedure after the UGE investigation [55]. The guidelines of the American Society for Metabolic & Bariatric Surgery (ASMBS) only recommend it in selected cases with the symptomatic gastric disease. Independently of the planned bariatric technique, they recommend a mandatory UGE for those patients with preoperative symptoms of GERD or gastritis [52].

All these societies pay special attention to the presence of GERD and mostly recommend to carry out a UGE when clinical symptoms are present. In a recent study conducted by our group, 18% of the patients planned to undergo bariatric surgery showed clinical symptoms of GERD. In all of them, a certain degree of esophagitis has been confirmed and additionally, 2.7% of the patients presented features of esophagitis despite they were clinically asymptomatic. The preoperative diagnosis of asymptomatic esophagitis is a challenging issue, as the patients may be indicated to undergo a SG, which can aggravate the esophagitis and will induce symptoms, which can be difficult to be controlled with conservative treatment [55]. A meta-analysis reported that the increase of postoperative GERD after SG can reach up to 19% of the patients and the appearance of de novo reflux rate was 23% [56]. In our experience, we observed a worsening of GERD symptoms after SG, even in those cases with hiatal hernia after repair of the hiatus, requiring in many cases a further conversion to RYGB for uncontrolled symptomatology [50].

However, UGE is not considered the best diagnostic method for GERD, and the gold standard test for its confirmation is the pH-metry [57]. pH-metry is often reserved for patients with clinical manifestations for GERD, but without endoscopic features of esophagitis. Schwameis et al. reported that all the patients with esophagitis grade C and D presented abnormal values at pH-metry, whereas 79% and 75% of patients with grade A and B esophagitis, respectively, presented abnormal pH scores. Consequently, they recommend pH testing prior to antireflux surgery in patients with grade A or B esophagitis [58]. It can be assumed that up to 25% of esophagitis cannot be secondary to acid reflux, but probably be due to bile reflux caused by duodeno-gastro-esophageal reflux because of pyloric incompetence. Even in these cases, it is also recommended to perform a RYGB rather than a SG, in order to distance the bile from the esophagus.

In our published series, the endoscopic findings of esophagitis changed the surgical decisión in only 0.89% of the cases, based on endoscopic findings of esophagitis [50]. Actually, SG is the most frequent procedure performed worldwide and its proportion is progressively increasing. Thus, our estimated percentage could be significantly increased when applied to populations undergoing preferently SG. Saarinen et al. described in their study that a great majority (92%) of the clinically significant findings in UGE are relevant if the chosen operation is SG (hiatal hernia, esophagitis, Barrett's esophagus) [59].

UGE also evaluates other conditions that may change the planned surgical procedure, such as peptic ulcers or polyps. The routine performance of UGE may lead to minimizing complications in the postoperative period, especially related to ulcer´s perforations or the development of malignancies on ulcers or polyps [51]. In our series, the decision of surgical technique was changed in 3.8% of the cases, based on these items. The presence of polyps or ulcers is especially relevant when a technique is applied, involving gastric or duodenal exclusion, such as RYGB [50].

Duodenal and especially gastric ulcers have been associated with the coexistence of neoplasms in up to 14% of the cases and with a close follow-up new-onset neoplasms arising on the ulcer has been observed in up to 4.9% of the cases [60]. Several studies have demonstrated that with the eradication of H. pylori, this risk significantly decreases. On the other hand, ulcers are also at risk of bleeding, and having endoscopic access to control it is recommendable. Consequently, given the risk of complications related to the ulcer, it seems to be mandatory, first to diagnose them preoperatively and second to have endoscopic access to them, in order to control an eventual evolution to neoplasms or the appearance of complications (perforations or bleedings) [61]. In addition, it has been described that gastric and duodenal ulcers are also associated with postoperative complications. Therefore, it is recommendable to know their presence before deciding the most appropriate technique [62].

More controversial is the issue referring to gastric or duodenal polyps. In our series, the prevalence of these entities is 5.7%, similar to that reported by other series of non-bariatric patients [50, 63]. Among our patients presenting gastric polyps, 78% were hyperplastic polyps and 22% adenomatous ones. 75% of the duodenal polyps showed hyperplasia and 25% adenoma. Adenomatous polyps are at risk of evolving to a malignant entity, however, the malignant transformation of hyperplastic ones is rare [64]. Thus, it can be assumed that all patients with adenomatous polyps or those ones not completely excised at preoperative UGE, are not suitable candidates for RYGB, because of leaving a gastric remnant without the possibility of endoscopic control.

Altogether, the endoscopic findings have changed the decision of the bariatric technique to be performed in 3.17% of our patients. Iman Ghaderi 2019 [65] reported a 3.34% of changes in the selection of the technique and given this small rate, they do not recommend routine preoperative UGE. In contrast, a German group reported a change in the operative strategy in only 1.6%, but they found essential the performance of preoperative UGE, as it allows the identification of a wide range of abnormal endoscopic findings, which may have a significant impact on decision-making [66]. Other authors have reported greater percentages of changes in decision. Parikh et al. observed 7.6% of preoperative endoscopic findings that influenced, altered, or delayed the surgical treatment of obesity [67]. Schneider et al. described that preoperative endoscopy led to a change of the bariatric approach in 16% of the patients, specifically 16.5% in the RYGB group and 15.9% in the SG group [68].

Relevance of H. pylori Screening in Patients Prior to Bariatric Surgery

H. pylori infection is very common in Morbidly obese patients, with reported higher prevalence than in lean population. In the last years, epidemiological studies revealed that the prevalence of H. pylori in bariatric patients ranges from 23% to 70% [69]. The eradication of H. pylori before the bariatric approach is mandatory, as the infection has been associated with postoperative complications, and the eradication of H. pylori has been related to a reduction of all these entities [69]. As previously mentioned, H. pylori has been involved with gastric pathology, such as peptic ulcer, chronic gastritis, GA, GIM and gastric adenocarcinoma. Thus, it is not advisable to carry out bariatric techniques with gastric exclusion in patients without prior eradication of H. pylori, as a part of the stomach would remain with difficult access for postoperative endoscopic control [70], despite recent challenges have shown the possibility of access and intervention on the blind-ended gastric remnant [71]. Moreover, gastric disorders are often at risk of bleeding, and having endoscopic access to control is advisable. Consequently, given the risk of complications related to the gastric disorders, it seems mandatory to diagnose them preoperatively, treat them if possible and to guarantee endoscopic access to them, in order to control an eventual evolution to neoplasms or the appearance of complications (perforation or bleeding) [61]. As previously discussed, H. pylori infection can be diagnosed with other techniques, different than biopsy. However, the endoscopic and, even more relevant, the histologic implication of the H. pylori infection remains unknown when UGE is not performed.

The analysis of H. pylori infection in our series showed that 36.1% of the patients presented preoperative H. pylori infection. After antibiotic therapy (before the bariatric surgery), H. pylori was eradicated in 94.7% of the cases. The global prevalence of chronic gastritis was 47%, GA 3.6% and GIM 7.7%. All the patients with diagnosis of H. pylori infection presented chronic gastritis. Similarly, 4.5% of the patients with H. pylori infection presented GA, but H. pylori accounts only for 44.7% of the total number of GA. Finally, 8.5% of the patients with H. pylori infection presented GIM, but H. pylori was involved in only 40% of the cases. In those cases, with H. pylori infection, we observed that the greater the grade of H. pylori infection, the higher the rate of GA and GIM. Though the global eradication rate of H. pylori was 94.7%, in those cases with GA, the eradication rate decreased to 47.1%, and in those patients with GIM, the eradication rate decreased to 37.8%. A relevant finding of the present study is that H. pylori is not the only factor involved in the development of gastric pathology. This reveals that other factors are present and should be investigated, and that gastric pathology cannot be discarded just with H. pylori eradication. Furthermore, it has been observed that the percentage of cases with severeH. Pylori infection tends to be higher in patients with GA and GIM, than in the patients without these lesions. Probably, in these cases, both the bacterial load and the genotype of H. pylori can influence the changes found in the histopathologic analysis and the patients' outcome. Futhermore, it is remarkable, that the H. pylori eradication rate is significantly lower, when GA or GIM are present. We hypothesized that this can be associated with the infection grade or if the inflammatory response of the organism prevents an adequate effect of the antibiotic treatment.

References

[1] NIH Consensus Conference. Helicobacter pylori in peptic ulcer disease. NIH Consensus Development Panel on Helicobacter pylori in Peptic Ulcer Disease. *JAMA* 1994; 272:65-69.

[2] Malfertheiner P, Megraud F, O'Morain CA, et al. Management of Helicobacter pylori infection--the Maastricht IV/ Florence Consensus Report. *Gut* 2012; 61:646-664.

[3] Chey WD, Wong BC, Practice Parameters Committee of the American College of Gastroenterology. American College of Gastroenterology guideline on the management of Helicobacter pylori infection. *Am J Gastroenterol* 2007; 102:1808-1825.

[4] Laine L. Helicobacter pylori, gastric ulcer, and agents noxious to the gastric mucosa. *Gastroenterol Clin North Am* 1993; 22:117-125.

[5] DuBois S, Kearney DJ. Iron-deficiency anemia and Helicobacter pylori infection: a review of the evidence. *Am J Gastroenterol* 2005; 100:453-459.

[6] Rostami N, Keshtkar-Jahromi M, Rahnavardi M, et al. Effect of eradication of Helicobacter pylori on platelet recovery in patients with chronic idiopathic thrombocytopenic purpura: a controlled trial. *Am J Hematol* 2008; 83:376-381.

[7] Parsonnet J, Harris RA, Hack HM, Owens DK. Modelling cost-effectiveness of Helicobacter pylori screening to prevent gastric cancer: a mandate for clinical trials. *Lancet* 1996; 348:150-154.

[8] Levi F, Lucchini F, Negri E, et al. Trends in cancer mortality in the European Union and accession countries, 1980-2000. *Ann Oncol* 2004; 15:1425.

[9] Gisbert JP, Abraira V. Accuracy of Helicobacter pylori diagnostic tests in patients with bleeding peptic ulcer: a systematic review and meta-analysis. *Am J Gastroenterol* 2006; 101:848-863.

[10] Gisbert JP, Esteban C, Jimenez I, Moreno-Otero R. 13C-urea breath test during hospitalization for the diagnosis of Helicobacter pylori infection in peptic ulcer bleeding. *Helicobacter* 2007; 12:231-237.

[11] Laine L, Lewin D, Naritoku W, et al. Prospective comparison of commercially available rapid urease tests for the diagnosis of Helicobacter pylori. *Gastrointest Endosc* 1996; 44:523-526.

[12] Weston AP, Campbell DR, Hassanein RS, et al. Prospective, multivariate evaluation of CLOtest performance. *Am J Gastroenterol* 1997; 92:1310-1315.

[13] Siddique I, Al-Mekhaizeem K, Alateeqi N, et al. Diagnosis of Helicobacter pylori: improving the sensitivity of CLOtest by increasing the number of gastric antral biopsies. *J Clin Gastroenterol* 2008; 42:356-360.

[14] Wright CL, Kelly JK. The use of routine special stains for upper gastrointestinal biopsies. *Am J Surg Pathol* 2006; 30:357-361.

[15] Mégraud F, Lehours P. Helicobacter pylori detection and antimicrobial susceptibility testing. *Clin Microbiol Rev* 2007; 20:280-322.

[16] Leide-Svegborn S, Stenström K, Olofsson M, et al. Biokinetics and radiation doses for carbon-14 urea in adults and children undergoing the Helicobacter pylori breath test. *Eur J Nucl Med* 1999; 26:573-580.

[17] Howden CW, Hunt RH. Guidelines for the management of Helicobacter pylori infection. Ad Hoc Committee on Practice Parameters of the American College of Gastroenterology. *Am J Gastroenterol* 1998; 93:2330-2338.

[18] Kelly SM, Pitcher MC, Farmery SM, Gibson GR. Isolation of Helicobacter pylori from feces of patients with dyspepsia in the United Kingdom. *Gastroenterology* 1994; 107:1671-1674.

[19] Braden B, Teuber G, Dietrich CF, et al. Comparison of new faecal antigen test with (13)C-urea breath test for detecting Helicobacter pylori infection and monitoring eradication treatment: prospective clinical evaluation. *BMJ* 2000; 320:148.

[20] Kim N. Chemoprevention of gastric cancer by Helicobacter pylori eradication and its underlying mechanism. *J Gastroenterol Hepatol.* 2019;34: 1287–1295.
[21] Correa P, Haenszel W, Cuello C, et al. A model for gastric cancer epidemiology. *Lancet* 1975; 2:58-60.
[22] Huang RJ, Choi AY, Truong CD, et al. Diagnosis and Management of Gastric Intestinal Metaplasia: Current Status and Future Directions. *Gut Liver* 2019;13: 596-603.
[23] Sipponen P, Price AB. The Sydney System for classification of gastritis 20 years ago, *J Gastroenterol Hepatol.* 2011; 26:31-34.
[24] Yardley JH, Hendrix TR. Gastritis, duodenitis, and associated ulcerative lesions. In: *Textbook of Gastroenterology,* Yamada T, Alpers DH, Owyang C, et al. Lippincott, Philadelphia 1995. p.1456.
[25] Hazell SL, Lee A, Brady L, Hennessy W. Campylobacter pyloridis and gastritis: association with intercellular spaces and adaptation to an environment of mucus as important factors in colonization of the gastric epithelium. *J Infect Dis* 1986; 153:658-663.
[26] Graham DY, Opekun A, Lew GM, et al. Helicobacter pylori-associated exaggerated gastrin release in duodenal ulcer patients. The effect of bombesin infusion and urea ingestion. *Gastroenterology* 1991; 100:1571-1575.
[27] Väänänen H, Vauhkonen M, Helske T, et al. Non-endoscopic diagnosis of atrophic gastritis with a blood test. Correlation between gastric histology and serum levels of gastrin-17 and pepsinogen I: a multicentre study. *Eur J Gastroenterol Hepatol* 2003; 15:885-891.
[28] Tsay FW, Hsu PI. H. pylori infection and extra-gastroduodenal diseases. *J Biomed Sci* 2018; 25:65.
[29] Elitsur Y, Raghuverra A, Sadat T, Vaid P. Is gastric nodularity a sign for gastric inflammation associated with Helicobacter pylori infection in children? *J Clin Gastroenterol* 2000; 30:286-288.
[30] Paull G, Yardley JH. Pathology of C pylori-associated gastric and esophageal lesions. In: *Campylobacter Pylori in Gastritis and Peptic Ulcer Disease,* Blaser MJ, Igaku-Shoin, New York 1989. p.73.
[31] Dixon MF, Genta RM, Yardley JH, Correa P. Classification and grading of gastritis. The updated Sydney System. International

Workshop on the Histopathology of Gastritis, Houston 1994. *Am J Surg Pathol* 1996; 20:1161-1181.

[32] Karttunen T, Niemelä S, Lehtola J, et al. Campylobacter-like organisms and gastritis: histopathology, bile reflux, and gastric fluid composition. *Scand J Gastroenterol* 1987; 22:478-486.

[33] Riddell R, Jain D. Stomach and proximal duodenum: inflammatory and miscellaneous disorders. In: *Lewin, Weinstein and Riddell's Gastrointestinal Pathology and its Clinical Implications,* 2nd ed, Bernstein C, Guha S. Lippincott Williams & Wilkins, Philadelphia 2014. p.590.

[34] van der Hulst RW, van der Ende A, Dekker FW, et al. Effect of Helicobacter pylori eradication on gastritis in relation to cagA: a prospective 1-year follow-up study. *Gastroenterology* 1997; 113:25-30.

[35] Sung JJ, Lin SR, Ching JY, et al. Atrophy and intestinal metaplasia one year after cure of H. pylori infection: a prospective, randomized study. *Gastroenterology* 2000; 119:7-14.

[36] Hershko C, Ronson A, Souroujon M, et al. Variable hematologic presentation of autoimmune gastritis: age-related progression from iron deficiency to cobalamin depletion. *Blood* 2006; 107:1673-1679.

[37] Carabotti M, Lahner E, Esposito G, et al. Upper gastrointestinal symptoms in autoimmune gastritis: A cross-sectional study. *Medicine (Baltimore)* 2017; 96:e5784.

[38] Lahner E, Esposito G, Pilozzi E, et al. Occurrence of gastric cancer and carcinoids in atrophic gastritis during prospective long-term follow up. *Scand J Gastroenterol* 2015; 50:856-865.

[39] Sundaresan S, Kang AJ, Merchant JL. Pathophysiology of Gastric NETs: Role of Gastrin and Menin. *Curr Gastroenterol Rep* 2017; 19:32.

[40] Hirschowitz BI, Griffith J, Pellegrin D, et al. Rapid regression of enterochromaffinlike cell gastric carcinoids in pernicious anemia after antrectomy. *Gastroenterology* 1992; 102:14091418.

[41] Fenoglio-Preiser CM. Autoimmune gastritis. In: *Gastrointestinal Pathology,* 3rd ed, Lippincott, Williams & Wilkins, Philadelphia 2008. p.188.

[42] Fox JG, Wang TC. Inflammation, atrophy, and gastric cancer. *J Clin Invest* 2007; 117:60-69.

[43] Mahmud N, Stashek K, Katona BW, et al. The incidence of neoplasia in patients with autoimmune metaplastic atrophic gastritis: a renewed call for surveillance. *Ann Gastroenterol* 2019; 32:67-72.

[44] Pimentel-Nunes P, Libânio D, Marcos-Pinto R, et al. Management of epithelial precancerous conditions and lesions in the stomach (MAPS II): European Society of Gastrointestinal Endoscopy (ESGE), European Helicobacter and Microbiota Study Group (EHMSG), European Society of Pathology (ESP), and Sociedade Portuguesa de Endoscopia Digestiva (SPED) guideline update 2019. *Endoscopy* 2019; 51:365-388.

[45] ASGE Standards of Practice Committee, Evans JA, Chandrasekhara V, et al. The role of endoscopy in the management of premalignant and malignant conditions of the stomach. *Gastrointest Endosc* 2015; 82:1-8.

[46] Dinis-Ribeiro M, Areia M, de Vries AC, et al. Management of precancerous conditions and lesions in the stomach (MAPS): guideline from the European Society of Gastrointestinal Endoscopy (ESGE), European Helicobacter Study Group (EHSG), European Society of Pathology (ESP), and the Sociedade Portuguesa de Endoscopia Digestiva (SPED). *Endoscopy* 2012; 44:74-94.

[47] Zhao H, Jiao L. Comparative analysis for the effect of Roux-en-Y gastric bypass vs sleeve gastrectomy in patients with morbid obesity: Evidence from 11 randomized clinical trials (meta-analysis).*Int J Surg.* 2019; 72:216-223.

[48] Canil AM, Iossa A, Termine P, Caporilli D, Petrozza V, Silecchia G. Histopathology Findings in Patients Undergoing Laparoscopic Sleeve Gastrectomy. *Obes Surg.* 2018; 28:1760-1765.

[49] García-Gómez-Heras S, Garcia A, Zubiaga L, et al. Prevalence of Endoscopic Findings Before Bariatric Surgery and Their Influence on the Selection of the Surgical Technique. *Obes Surg* 2020;30:4375-4380.

[50] Abou Hussein B, Khammas A, Shokr M, Majid M, Sandal M, Awadhi SA, Mazrouei AA, Badri F. Role of routine upper

endoscopy before bariatric surgery in the Middle East population: a review of 1278 patients. *Endoscopy International Open* 2018; 06: E1171–E1176.

[51] Sauerland S, Angrisani L, Belachew M, Chevallier JM, Favretti F, Finer N, et al. Obesity surgery: Evidence-based guidelines of the European Association for Endoscopic Surgery (EAES). *Surg Endosc* 2005; 19:200–221.

[52] Dhariwal A, Plevris JN, Lo NT, Finlayson ND, Heading RC, Hayes PC. Age, anemia, and obesity associated oxygen desaturation during upper gastrointestinal endoscopy. *Gastrointest Endosc.* 1992; 38:684–688.

[53] Bennett S, Gostimir M, Shorr R, Mallick R, Mamazza J, Neville A. The role of routine preoperative upper endoscopy in bariatric surgery: a systematic review and meta-analysis. 2016. *Surg Obes Relat Dis;* 12:1116–1125.

[54] SAGES guideline for clinical application of laparoscopic bariatric surgery. *Surg Obes Relat Dis* 2009, 5:387–405.

[55] Evans JA, Muthusamy VR, Acosta RD, Bruining DH, Chandrasekhara V, Chathadi KV, et al. The role of endoscopy in the bariatric surgery patient. *Gastrointest Endosc.* 2015; 29:1007–1017.

[56] Yeung KTD, Penney N, Ashrafian L, Darzi A, Ashrafian H. Does Sleeve Gastrectomy Expose the Distal Esophagus to Severe Reflux?: A Systematic Review and Meta-analysis. *Ann Surg* 2020; 271:257-265.

[57] Pérez de la Serna y Bueno J, Ruiz de León San Juan A. pH-metry/impedance-24 hours pH-metry. *Rev Esp Enferm Dig.* 2015;107:243.

[58] Schwameis K, Lin B, Roman J, Olengue K, Siegal S, DeMeester SR. Is pH Testing Necessary Before Antireflux Surgery in Patients with Endoscopic Erosive Esophagitis? *J Gastrointest Surg* 2018; 22:8-12.

[59] Saarinen T, Kettunen U, Pietiläinen KH, Juuti A. Is preoperative gastroscopy necessary before sleeve gastrectomy and Roux-en-Y gastric bypass? *Surg Obes Relat Dis* 2018; 14:757-763.

[60] Rosai J. Stomach. In: Rosai J. Ackerman´s Surgical Pathology. *St Louis, Mosby,* 1996::616-666.

[61] Kashiwagi H. Ulcers and gastritis. Endoscopy. 2003;35:9-14.
[62] Fernandes SR, Meireles LC, Carrilho-Ribeiro L, Velosa J. The Role of Routine Upper Gastrointestinal Endoscopy before Bariatric Surgery. *Obes Surg* 2016. 26:2105–2110.
[63] Genta RM, Schuler CM, Robiou CI, Lash RH. No association between gastric fundic gland polyps and gastrointestinal neoplasia in a study of over 100,000 patients. *Clin Gastroenterol Hepatol,* 2009; 7:849-854.
[64] Carmack SW, Genta RM, Schuler CM, Saboorian MH. The current spectrum of gastric polyps: A 1-year national study of over 120,000 patients. *Am J Gastroenterol.* 2009; 104: 1524-1532.
[65] Ghaderi I, Gondal AB, Samamé J, Serrot F, Galvani CA. Preoperative Endoscopic and Radiologic Evaluation of Bariatric Patients: What Do They Add? *J Gastrointest Surg.* 2020;24:764-771.
[66] Moulla Y, Lyros O, Mehdorn M, et al. Preoperative Upper-GI Endoscopy Prior to Bariatric Surgery: Essential or Optional? *Obes Surg.* 2020; 30:2076-2084.
[67] Parikh M, Liu J, Vieira D, Tzimas D, Horwitz D, Antony A, et al. Preoperative endoscopy prior to bariatric surgery: systematic review and meta-analysis of the literature. *Obes Surg.* 2016; 26:2961–2966.
[68] Schneider R, Lazaridis I, Kraljevic M, et al. The impact of preoperative investigations on the management of bariatric patients; results of a cohort of more than 1200 cases. *Surg Obes Relat Dis* 2018; 14:693-699.
[69] Yardimci E, Bozkurt S, Baskoy L, et al. Rare Entities of Histopathological Findings in 755 Sleeve Gastrectomy Cases: a Synopsis of Preoperative Endoscopy Findings and Histological Evaluation of the Specimen, *Obes. Surg* 2018;28: 1289–1295.
[70] Öner RI, Özdaş S. Histopathological Findings in Morbid Obese Patients Undergoing Laparoscopic Sleeve Gastrectomy: Does H. pylori Infection Effective on Pathological Changes? *Obes Surg* 2018;28: 3136–3141.
[71] Mala T. The Gastric Remnant in Roux-en-Y Gastric Bypass: Challenges and Possibilities. *J Clin Gastroenterol* 2016; 50:527-531.

In: Enhanced Recovery after Surgery … ISBN: 978-1-53619-976-5
Editor: Jaime Ruiz-Tovar

Chapter 4

Preoperative Nutritional Optimization

Pablo Priego*[*], *MD, PhD
Department of General Surgery,
Division of Esophagogastric and Bariatric Surgery,
Ramón y Cajal University Hospital, Madrid, Spain

Abstract

Optimizing postoperative patient outcomes and nutritional status begins preoperatively. A preoperative nutritional assessment with a specialist dietitian is essential when preparing for bariatric surgery, not only for identify preoperative nutritional deficiencies, but also to help the patient recognize the need for positive lifestyle changes and develop a plan to incorporate nutritional and lifestyle changes before surgery. Enrollment in a preoperative weight loss program including a low-calorie diet has been suggested with a grade B recommendation. Planned and structured physical activity program before surgery shoud be implanted in order to improve physical aptitudes and reduce postoperative complications. The paper of inmunonutrition is controversial.

* Corresponding Author's Email: papriego@hotmail.com.

Keywords: bariatric surgery; preoperative; optimization; nutrition care; nutritional deficiencies; weight loss; physical activity; inmunonutrition

INTRODUCTION

Candidates for bariatric and metabolic surgery very often present with various comorbidities (diabetes mellitus type 2, hypertension, pneumopathies, cardiopathies, arthropathies, anxious depressive syndrome, ...) that can decompensate during the perioperative period, increasing the risk of postoperative morbimortality [1].

Because all of this, the management of the obese patient by a multidisciplinary team is mandatory. This may include a number of health professionals including endocrinologists, specialist nurses, specialist dieticians, and psychologists as well as the surgeons and anaesthetists.

Optimizing postoperative patient outcomes and nutritional status begins preoperatively. The American Society for Metabolic and Bariatric Surgery (ASMBS) Nutrition Committee has recently uptdated the Allied Health Nutritional Guidelines for the Surgical Weight Loss Patient. These guidelines recommend that obese patients waiting for bariatric surgery should undergo a preoperative clinical nutrition evaluation by a specialist dietician in order to identify preoperative nutritional deficiencies, as well as to evaluate patients' ability to incorporate nutritional changes before and after bariatric surgery [2].

The aim of this chapter is to summarize the current scientific literature.

PREOPERATIVE NUTRITIONAL EVALUATION

A preoperative nutritional assessment with a specialist dietitian is essential when preparing for bariatric surgery. This contact should be adapted to each individual patient. The preoperative nutritional assessment is designed not only for identify preoperative nutritional deficiencies, but also to help the patient recognize the need for positive lifestyle changes and develop a plan to incorporate nutritional and lifestyle changes before surgery [3].

Most nutritional evaluations involve a clinical interview that include a review of anthropometrical data, weight history (family history of obesity), previous weight-loss regimens, medical history, available laboratory values, psychological history (including history of eating disorders), social history, substance abuse history (alcohol, drugs), nutrition-focused physical findings (such as poor dentition), dietary intake (number and types of meals per day, liquid intake), eating patterns (grazing, binge eating, picking, nibbling) physical activity, surgery expectations and psychosocial factors that affect weight loss [4].

It is advised to determine the patient's eating habits. These may be influenced by several factors. *Environmental* factors include occupation, socioeconomic status, and family traditions. *Psychological* factors include low self-confidence, depression, anxiety, stress, and solitariness. *Social* factors include society placing more value on physical appearance and not on inner qualities, and stress related to size/body shape due to past discrimination. *Biological and biochemical* factors are related to the gastrointestinal hormone imbalances that affect hunger and appetite.

It is important for patients to understand that, regardless of the reasons behind them, current eating patterns will likely result in poor weight loss, weight regain, and malnutrition after surgery. Preoperative nutritional counseling should focus on addressing these behaviors, working with the patient to avoid or manage them, and having the patient demonstrates compliance with the recommended changes.

Obesity is frequent in people who live in low socioeconomic areas. In these regions, access to nutrient-rich foods is often limited. Planning grocery lists and affordable recipes with a low-income patient would be an appropriate intervention. Indeed, this healthy disorder is also seen in people who work overnight shifts or who have alternating shifts and late shift workers have higher rates of weight gain after starting their jobs. These workers feel inappropriate to eat in the middle of the night, resulting in eating large portions before work and after work, as well as grazing on empty-calorie foods during the night. A conductual and nutritional work will set the patient up for long-term success after bariatric surgery [3].

Table 1. Supplementation for the prevention and treatment of nutritional deficiencies

Vitamins and minerals	Routine supplementation for deficiency prevention	Treatment for deficiency
Multivitamin-mineral	Two adult multivitamin-mineral supplements/d (only 1 supplement/d is required after LAGB containing iron, folic acid, zinc, cooper, selenium and thiamin (200% of the RDA)	-
Calcium citrate	600 mg Ca supplement/d (1200 mg/d after BPD) or more[1]	-
Vitamin D	3000 IU/d [as ergocalciferol (vitamin D_2), or cholecalciferol (vitamin D_3); titration should be done to reach normal concentrations of 30 ng/ml	50000 IU vitamin D_2 or D_3 1 time/wk for 8 wk, followed by maintenance therapy of 1500-2000 IU/d to achieve normal concentrations
Iron[2]	45-60 mg elemental Fe/d from multivitamin and supplements (after LAGB, iron supplementation is necessary if iron intake from food is insufficient)	150-200 mg elemental Fe supplements/d
Vitamin B12	250-300 µg/d or 1000 µg/wk sublingual, 1000 µg/mo i.m., or 3000 µg every 6 mo i.m. after RYGB and BPD. After LSG and LAGB, the use of vitamin B12 supplements should be considered as needed to maintain vitamin B12 concentrations and should be included in the multivitamin supplement	1000-2000 µg/d sublingual Intramuscular or subcutaneous vitamin B12 is necessary when oral therapy does not repair deficiency
Thiamin	DRI for thiamin should be included in the routine multivitamin supplement	500 mg thiamin/d i.v. for 3-5 d, then 250 mg/d for 3-5 d or until the symptoms disappear and then further treatment by oral administration of 100 mg/d as needed
Folic acid	400 µ/d should be included in the routine multivitamin; pregnant women or those planning to conceive should take 800-1000 µg folic acid/d included in a multivitamin supplement or separately	1000 µg folic acid/d

Vitamins and minerals	**Routine supplementation for deficiency prevention**	**Treatment for deficiency**
Fat soluble vitamins (A, K and E)[3]	6000 IU vitamin A should be included in the routine multivitamin; for pregnant women or those planning to conceive, the β-carotene form of vitamin A is preferred over retinol After BPD 10000 IU vitamin A/d, 300 µg vitamin K/d and 400 IU vitamin E/d (included in a multivitamin or separately)	Vitamin A deficiency without corneal changes: 10000-25000 IU/d orally to achieve clinical improvement When changes in the cornea appear: 50000-100000 IU i.m. for 3 d followed by 50000 IU/d for 2 wk i.m. is recommended Vitamin K deficiency: 10 mg i.m. or submuscular, followed by 1-2 mg/wk parenterally or orally Vitamin E deficiency: 800-1200 IU/d to reach normal serum concentrations
Zinc	The routine daily multivitamin should contain 15 mg/d ≥1 mg Cu per 8-15 mg Zn to prevent cooper deficiency is recommended	60 mg Zn 2 times/d
Cooper	The routine daily multivitamin should contain 2 mg Cu	Severe deficiency requires 2-4 mg Cu/d i.v. for 6 d
Vitamin C	The routine daily multivitamin should follow the DRI recommendation for vitamin C	100 mg vitamin C 3 times/d or 500 mg/d for 1 mo

LAGB: Laparoscopic adjustable gastric band; BPD: Laparoscopic biliopancreatic diversion; LSG: Laparoscopic sleeve gastrectomy; RYGB: Laparoscopic Roux-en Y-Gastric Bypass

[1]Daily intake of calcium from food and supplements should reach 1200-1500 mg/d (1800-2400 mg after BPD). Singles doses should not exceed 600 mg and should be separated by ≥2 h intervals form iron supplements or a multivitamin that contains iron.

[2]Women of childbearing age or at increased risk of anemia should consume 50-100 mg elemental Fe/d.

[3]Patients should begin taking fat-soluble vitamin supplements 2-4 wk after surgery.

(From Dagan SS, Goldenshluger A, Globus I, Schweiger C, Kessler Y, Sandbank GK, Ben-Porat T, Sinai T. Nutritional Recommendations for Adult Bariatric Surgery Patients: Clinical Practice. *Adv Nutr* 2017; 8(2):382-394).

Sometimes, patients have a past or present history of eating disorders that likely require additional psychological counseling in addition to nutritional counseling. Hence, coordination between the dietitian and the mental health care provider is essential. Outcomes following bariatric surgery after these eating disorders are controversial. Questions inquiring about eating disorders should be included in the nutrition evaluation. If the specialist dietitian identifies the patient has tendencies towards these behaviors, they should undergo psychological treatment before proceeding with surgery.

Dietitians use various tools to help assess a patient's food and beverage intake, including the 24-hour recall and food frequency questionnaires. When counseling patients preoperatively, it is important to put the emphasis on how dietary and lifestyle changes positively affect long-term weight maintenance. Patients often argue they can not eat all kind of foods postoperatively. Developing a menu before surgery that includes a variety of soft proteins (e.g., low-fat dairy, beans, nut butters, fish), whole grains, fruits, vegetables, and healthy fats will empower patients to try new foods and recipes after surgery that are appropriate for the texture that they are able to tolerate. Patients should also be advice to eliminate intake of sugar-sweetened beverages in the preoperative period and including mostly water and sugar-free beverages. Patients often have the misconception that skipping breakfast will lead to eating fewer calories in the day, when in fact, skipping breakfast can lead to cravings of high-calorie foods later in the day. Therefore, patients should be encouraged to include breakfast daily in order to better maintain weight loss after surgery [3].

Nutritional complications after bariatric surgery due to micro or macronutrient deficiencies are relatively frequent. Indeed, related adverse clinical outcomes including osteomalacia and osteoporosis, anemia and neurologic disorders have been reported. Although these deficiencies have been attributed to a reduce in oral intake (e.g., due to persistent vomiting, food aversion, modified eating behavior and nonadherence to dietary recommendations) and/or malabsorption following these procedures, several studies have demonstrated similar deficiencies in obese patients who are in waiting list for bariatric surgery. As such, routine investigation of the nutritional status, including micro and macronutrient levels, prior to bariatric surgery has been suggested to recognize existing deficiencies and, as soon as possible, correct them prior to surgery. This is particularly important as preoperative malnutrition has been associated with worse surgical outcome [5].

Although is truly know that nutritional deficiencies are rare in developed countries due to the high socioenocomic level and abundant food supply; this food normally tends to comprise fast foods and a lower intake of fresh fruits and vegetables. For this reason, these kinds of diets tend to contain fewer 'quality' calories compared with a mediterranean balanced diet. As such, although obese patients frequently consume high food energy, these calories may not contain all of their micronutrient needs, leading to deficiencies.

Obese patients are at increased risk for nutritional abnormalities in the preoperative setting; they have been found to be deficient in thiamine, folate, zinc, iron, ferritin, selenium, beta-carotene, magnesium, and vitamins A, B-12, C and D [6]. Therefore, daily multivitamin supplementation is recommended during the preoperative diet. The management of specific nutritional deficiencies is described in Table 1.

PREOPERATIVE WEIGHT MANAGEMENT

Enrollment in a preoperative weight loss (WL) program including a low-calorie diet has been recommended by some bariatric surgery centers, especially in USA and is still requested by some insurance companies. The suggested benefits of WL before surgery were: 1) to facilitate surgery itself by reducing the volume of intra-abdominal fat and liver size; and 2) to achieve better long-term WL results. However, success in preoperative WL should not be a condition for accepting patients to surgery [7].

There are few randomized studies and systematic reviews published in the literature design to evaluate the preoperative WL and all of them led to contradictory results. Although it is true that the volume of the liver can be reduced, the positive clinical relevance of this effect was weak at the most [8]. The long-term effect on WL was either weak or absent. Moreover, the ASMBS has downgraded preoperative WL to a grade B recommendation "due to inconsistent results" in the last version of its guidelines [2].

However, before planning these preoperative WL programms, we have to consider the pre-existing nutritional deficiencies of the patient, in order not to worse them. Anderin et al. [9], showed that patients with preoperative WL > 9.5% had reduced rate of postoperative complications compared to patients with WL < 0.5%. Moreover, the proportion of complications reduction was the highest in patients with a body mass index (BMI) >45.8. Van Nieuwenhove et al. [10], showed that

14-day very low-calorie diet regimen before surgery could notably reduce the surgeon's subjective perception of the difficulty of the procedure and the number of 30-day postoperative complications. We firmly believe that the routine use of a preoperative WL regimen should be recommended in our patients planned for bariatric surgery, especially for superobese patients (BMI ≥50), where it seems that the benefits can be significant.

Anyway, and although a number of studies have evaluated the effects of a preoperative WL program on postoperative WL and operative difficulty and morbidity, few have evaluated the effects of this WL on nutritional parameters such as changes in micronutrient levels, body composition and bone density prior to surgery. Nielsen et al. [11] has conducted a study in which published their results with all patients received 1000 kcal/day for 7 or 11 weeks before surgery; 77% of the patients not only reached the WL goal of 8% by 7 weeks but also an improvement in metabolic parameters (decreased fasting glucose, insulin, low-density lipoprotein, triglycerides and blood pressure).

To date, there is no consensus with regard to the recommended duration of preoperative diet and its macronutrient composition [12]. When several preoperative diets were compared, a "low-carbohydrate diet" was found to be more effective than a low-fat diet" with regard to short-term WL, improvement in insulin sensitivity, and reduction in lipid concentrations. Moreover, this "low-carbohydrate diet" has also showed a positive effect in patients with metabolic syndrome or nonalcoholic fatty liver disease. "The very-low-calorie diet," (450–800 kcal/d) was related to a 10% preoperative WL, a 9% reduction in BMI, and a 15–20% reduction in liver volume. However, the use of a very-low-calorie diet as a sole method for multiple weeks before surgery may induce a catabolic state, which could potentially harm recovery after surgery [13].

According to the ASMBS, the maximum length of a preoperative diet is 3 months, because a longer period may decrease motivation. Recommendations for the duration of the diet range from 2 to 6 weeks not only for reducing liver volume but also to reduce visceral adipose tissue before surgery. Despite the proven short-term benefits of preoperative WL, the evidence on long-term outcomes is still controversial [14].

Is There a Role for Preoperative Carbohydrate Load?

Carbohydrate load minimizes postoperative insulin resistance, postoperative hyperglycaemia, losses of protein; fat-free mass depletion and muscle function, and reduce anxiety and postoperative nausea and vomiting. Nowadays, carbohydrate load has been integrated in the Enhanced Recovery After Surgery (ERAS) program, and should be indicated from 12 to 2 hours before bariatric surgery [1, 15, 16].

What about Physical Activity?

It is an established fact that both overweight and obesity are associated with a decrease in cardiovascular fitness, muscle strength, physical function and ability to perform activities of daily living. There is a clear relationship between the physical training of patients with obesity and the attainment of clinical benefits. Thus, not only will improvements be obtained in the area of health, but also in the reduction of the economic costs of medical care, work absenteeism and hospitalization rates [17].

Diet, physical exercise and lifestyle modification are the fundamental basis for the prevention and management of obesity [18]. However, the implementation of a physical exercise program in this type of patient is a major challenge for medical and sports professionals. For example, obese patients present limitations in their mobility, decreased quality of muscle contraction, fatigue and reduced exercise capacity [19].

The American College of Sports Medicine and the American Heart Association [20] recommend a minimum of 30 minutes of moderate-intensity aerobic physical activity (PA) 5 days per week or a minimum of 20 minutes of vigorous aerobic activity 3 days per week for healthy adults. In addition, they recommend resistance training with 8-12 repetitions at least 2 days per week [21].

Several studies have investigated the sedentary behavior of patients on the waiting list for bariatric surgery [22]. The results show that the time spent sedentary by these individuals' ranges from 9.5 to 11 hours per day, with television or computer work being the most frequently performed activities.

Preoperative measurement of PA is the crucial step in understanding whether PA levels at this time could contribute to variability or predict weight outcomes after surgery. Bond et al. [23], demonstrated an increased of PA and preparation to PA in gastric bypass (GB) patients during the preoperative stage. To this end, they distributed a PA questionnaire at an initial preoperative visit and then again 1-2 weeks before surgery. With an average of 3 months between visits, patients demonstrated increases in moderate and vigorous activities between visits. Most patients were in the action and preparation phase, with very few in the contemplation or precontemplation phases. Although a formal activity intervention was not initiated, these data suggest that a preoperative intervention targeting PA has the potential to increase participation in PA.

It is an evident fact that patients with lower physical aptitudes have a higher postoperative risk than when compared to individuals with good physical preparation. Thus, in a study on patients undergoing BG, Hennis et al. [24] observed that patients with a low preoperative anaerobic threshold measured by a stress test had a longer hospital stay and a higher number of postoperative complications. Ultimately, improvement of physical fitness by preoperative PA intervention could help to achieve better postoperative outcomes.

Brandenburg et al. [25] demonstrated that the application of a preoperative physical exercise program for 6 weeks with the aim of improving postoperative outcomes was well received by patients. Thus, the study found that 1 year after the intervention, patients reported that the program had helped them to make postoperative lifestyle changes. However, there were no correlations between patient satisfaction and perceived usefulness of the program and postoperative WL.

Another study that attempts to determine the efficacy of applying intervention programs preoperatively to increase PA in the context of bariatric surgery is the Bari-Active study [26]. In this randomized study, a group of patients in which a 6-week behavioral PA plan was implemented was compared with a group of control patients, and changes before and after surgery were evaluated in relation to the number of minutes of moderate to vigorous PA, quality of life and physical function as well as the number of daily steps. PA consisted of individual weekly sessions aimed at increasing the intensity of exercise by walking more than 30 minutes each day, and increasing the number of steps by 5000 each day. An increase of 21 minutes per day in moderate to vigorous PA was found after 6 weeks for the surgery group, while the control group showed no change in the number of minutes spent in PA. Similarly, the step count increased by more than 2,000 in the surgery group compared with 200 in the control group. Despite all this increase in activity, only 30% and 14.3% of participants in the surgery and control groups met the recommendations for at least 150 minutes per week of moderate to vigorous activity at the end of the study. In addition, physical and mental health improved more for the surgery group than for the control group. However, the study did not examine the effect of the intervention on postoperative outcomes.

In the study by Brandemburg et al. [25], the implementation of a lifestyle behavior program (including exercise) before surgery found that only 45% of respondents exercised at least 3 days/week and only 20% exercised at least 5 days/week 1 year after bariatric surgery. Finally, in the study by Lier et al. [27], a revealing finding was that 31% of subjects who were offered counseling sessions chose not to participate, indicating the difficulty of providing an intervention to this cohort of patients.

Is There a Role for Inmunonutrition?

The term "Immunonutrition" (IMN) describes the enteral administration of certain substrates (arginine, omega-3 fatty acids, nucleotides, glutamine and antioxidants) with a putative immunomodulating function. Animal models and human studies have suggested that the individual components have beneficial (or potentially beneficial) effects on immune function. Most of the reported evidence of IMN in surgical patients has been focused on malignant pathologies, reporting decreases in postoperative complications [28-30].

Ruir-Tovar et al. [31], developed a prospective randomized clinical trial with bariatric patients undergoing laparoscopic sleeve gastrectomy (LSG). Patients were randomly assigned into 3 groups: those patients receiving a preoperative regular diet of 900 kcal/day (group 1), those receiving a preoperative balanced energy high-protein formula (group 2) and those receiving preoperative Immunonutrition (group 3). Sixty patients were included in the study, 20 in each group. Preoperative excess WL was 7.7% in group 1, 12.3% in group 2 and 15.3% in group 3 ($p = 0.014$). Median postoperative pain was 3.5 in group 1, 3 in group 2 and 2 in group 3 ($p = 0.048$). C-reactive protein determined 24 h after surgery was significantly lower in group 3 than in the other groups. AST and ALT values were significantly lower in group 3 than in the other groups, without significant differences between groups 1 and 2. In conclusion, preoperative diet with Immunonutrition formulas during 2 weeks achieves a greater preoperative WL, lower postoperative pain and lower values of CRP and liver enzymes than high-protein formulas or regular diet, all of them with similar caloric intake.

Other prospective randomized clinical trial of the same group [32] with the use of a nutritional supplement enriched with Omega-3 fatty acids (O3FA), in patients with GB showed similar results with a greater preoperative WL, reduced postoperative pain and decreased postoperative levels of C reactive protein.

However, not other studies have published in the literature, so the grade of recommendation for preoperative inmunonutrition is weak.

CONCLUSION

Nutritional complications after bariatric surgery due to micro or macronutrient deficiencies are relatively frequent. The ASMBS recommends that obese patients waiting for bariatric surgery should undergo a preoperative clinical nutrition evaluation by a specialist dietician in order to identify preoperative nutritional deficiencies, as well as to evaluate patients' ability to incorporate nutritional changes before and after bariatric surgery. Therefore, daily multivitamin supplementation is recommended during the preoperative diet.

Although, the ASMBS has downgraded preoperative weight loss to a grade B recommendation "due to inconsistent results" in the last version of its guidelines, enrollment in a preoperative weight loss program including a low-calorie diet should be recommended especially for superobese patients (BMI ≥50), where it seems that the benefits can be significant.

Planned and structured physical activity program before surgery shoud be implanted in order to improve physical aptitudes and reduce postoperative complications.

Carbohydrate load has been integrated in the Enhanced Recovery after Surgery (ERAS) program, and should be indicated from 12 to 2 hours before bariatric surgery, however, more studies need to be performed before recommending the role of inmunonutrition in the preoperative nutritional optimization of these obese patients.

References

[1] Martín García-Almenta E, Ruiz-Tovar J, Sánchez Santos R. *Vía clínica de cirugía bariátrica* 2017. Im3diA comunicación S. L.

[2] Parrott J, Frank L, Dilks R, Craggs-Dino L, Isom KA, Greiman L. ASMBS Integrated Health Nutritional Guidelines For The Surgical Weight Loss Patient — 2016 Update: Micronutrients. *Surg Obes Relat Dis.* 2017; 13(5):727-741.

[3] Matharoo GS, Renick E, Afthinos JN, Straker T, Gibbs KE. Preoperative evaluation of bariatric surgery patients. *Essentials and controversies in Bariatric Surgery* 2014, Chih-Kun Huang, IntechOpen, doi: 10.5772/58605.

[4] Dagan SS, Goldenshluger A, Globus I, Schweiger C, Kessler Y, Sandbank GK, Ben-Porat T, Sinai T. Nutritional Recommendations for Adult Bariatric Surgery Patients: Clinical Practice. *Adv Nutr* 2017; 8(2):382-394.

[5] Roust LR, DiBaise JK. Nutrition deficiencies prior to bariatric surgery. *Curr Opin Clin Nutr Metab Care* 2017; 20(2) : 138-144.

[6] Via MA, Mechanick JI. *Nutritional and Micronutrient Care of Bariatric SurgeryPatients: Current Evidence Update.*

[7] Thibault R, Huber O, Azagury DE, Pichard C. Twelve key nutritional issues in bariatric surgery. *Clin Nutr* 2016; 35(1):12-17.

[8] Owers CE, Abbas Y, Ackroyd R, Barron N, Khan M. Perioperative Optimization of Patients Undergoing Bariatric Surgery. *J Obes* 2012; 2012:781546. doi: 10.1155/2012/781546.

[9] Anderin C, Gustafsson UO, Heijbel N, Thorell A. Weight Loss Before Bariatric Surgery and Postoperative Complications: Data From the Scandinavian Obesity Registry (SOReg). *Ann Surg* 2015; 261(5):909-13.

[10] Van Nieuwenhove Y, Dambrauskas Z, Campillo-Soto A, van Dielen F, Wiezer R, Janssen I, et al. Preoperative Very Low-Calorie Diet and Operative Outcome after Laparoscopic Gastric Bypass. A Randomized Multicenter Study. *Arch Surg* 2011; 146(11):1300-1305.

[11] Nielsen LV, Nielsen MS, Schmidt JB, et al. Efficacy of a liquid low-energy formula diet in achieving preoperative target weight loss before bariatric surgery. *J Nutr Sci* 2016; 5:e22.

[12] *Ministry of Health. Bariatric surgery criteria of the Ministry of Health [Internet]* [cited 2016 Sep 4]. Available from: http://www.health.gov.il/hozer/mr33_2013.pdf.

[13] Van Wissen J, Bakker N, Doodeman HJ, Jansma EP, Bonjer HJ, Houdijk AP. Preoperative methods to reduce liver volume in bariatric surgery: a systematic review. *Obes Surg* 2016; 26:251–256.

[14] Colles SL, Dixon JB, Marks P, Strauss BJ, O'Brien PE. Preoperative weight loss with a very-low-energy diet: quantitation of changes in liver and abdominal fat by serial imaging. *Am J Clin Nutr* 2006; 84: 304–311.

[15] Henriksen MG, Hessov I, Dela F, Hansen HV, Haraldsted V, Rodt SA. Effects of preoperative oral carbohydrates and peptides on postoperative endocrine response, mobilization, nutrition and muscle function in abdominal surgery. *Acta Anaesthesiol Scand* 2003; 47(2):191-199.

[16] Braga M, Ljungqvist O, Soeters P, Fearon K, Weimann A, Bozzetti F. ESPEN Guidelines on Parenteral Nutrition: surgery. *Clin Nutr* 2009; 28(4):378-386.

[17] Lagerros YT, Rossner S. Obesity management: what brings success? *Therap Adv Gastroenterol* 2013; 6:77-88.

[18] Galani C, Schneider H. Prevention and treatment of obesity with lifestyle interventions: review and meta-analysis. *Int J Public Health.* 2007; 52:348-359.

[19] Tallis J, James RS, Seebacher F. The effects of obesity on skeletal muscle contractile function. *J Exp Biol* 2018; 221:jeb 163840.

[20] American College of Sports Medicine. *ACSM's Guidelines for Exercise Testing and Prescription. 7th ed.* Philadelphia, PA: Lippincott Williams & Wilkins; 2006.

[21] US Department of Health and Human Services. *2008 Physical activity guidelines for Americans.* 2008. http://health.gov/paguidelines/guidelines/acessed 09/25/2017.

[22] Bond DS, Thomas JG, Unick JL, Raynor HA, Vithiananthan S, et al. Self-reported and objectively measured sedentary behavior in bariatric surgery candidates. *Surg Obes Relat Dis* 2013; 9: 123-128.

[23] Bond DS, Evans RK, DeMaria EJ. Physical activity stage of readiness predicts moderate-vigorous physical activity participation among morbidly obese gastric bypass surgery candidates. *Surg Obes Relat Dis* 2006; 2: 128-132.

[24] Hennis PJ, Meale PM, Hurst R. Cardiopulmonary exercise testing predicts postoperative outcome in patients undergoing gastric bypass surgery. *Br J Anaesth* 2012; 109: 566-571.

[25] Brandenburg D, Kotlowski R. Practice makes perfect? Patient response to a prebariatric surgery behavior modification program. *Obes Surg* 2005; 15: 125-132.

[26] Bond DS, Thomas JG, King WC, Vithiananthan S, Trautvetter J, et al. Exercise improves quality of life in bariatric surgery candidates:results from the Bari-Active trial. *Obesity (Silver Spring)* 2015; 23: 536-542.

[27] Lier H, Biringer E, Stubhaug B, Tangen T. The impact of preoperative counseling on postoperative treatment adherence in bariatric surgery patients: A randomized controlled trial. *Patient Educ Couns* 2012; 87: 336-342.

[28] Cerantola Y, Hubner M, Grass F, et al. Immunonutrition in gastrointestinal surgery. *Br J Surg* 2011; 98:37–48.

[29] Zhang Y, Gu Y, Guo T, et al. Perioperative immunonutrition for gastrointestinal cancer: a systematic review of randomized controlled trials. *Surg Oncol* 2012; 21:e87–95.

[30] Braga M, Wischmeyer PE, Drover J, et al. Clinical evidence for pharmaconutrition in major elective surgery. JPEN *J Parenter Enteral Nutr* 2013; 37:66–72.

[31] Ruiz-Tovar J, Zubiaga L, Diez M, Murcia A, Boix E, Muñoz JL, Llavero C; OBELCHE group. Preoperative Regular Diet of 900 kcal/day vs Balanced Energy High-Protein Formula vs Immunonutrition Formula: Effect on Preoperative Weight Loss and Postoperative Pain, Complications and Analytical Acute Phase Reactants after Laparoscopic Sleeve Gastrectomy. *Obes Surg* 2016; 26(6):1221-1227.

[32] Ruiz-Tovar J, Blanca M, Garcia A, Gonzalez J, Gutierrez S, Paniagua A, Prieto MJ, Ramallo L, Llanos L, Duran M. Preoperative administration of Omega-3 fatty acids on postoperative pain and acute-phase reactants in patients undergoing Roux-en-Y gastric bypass: A randomized clinical trial. *Clin Nutr* 2019; 38(4):1588-1593.

In: Enhanced Recovery after Surgery ... ISBN: 978-1-53619-976-5
Editor: Jaime Ruiz-Tovar

Chapter 5

Physical Prehabilitation

Artur Marc Hernández[1], PhD,
Eva Hernández-García[2], PhD
and Jaime Ruiz-Tovar[3], MD, PhD
[1]Faculty of Humanities and Social Sciences,
University Isabel I, Burgos, Spain
[2]University College London, London, United Kingdom
[3]Department of Surgery, University Rey Juan Carlos,
Móstoles, Madrid, Spain

Abstract

At present, bariatric surgery is considered a safe and effective technique, however, there is a certain percentage of patients who suffer from perioperative complications. There are different factors, such as comorbidities associated with obesity, preoperative weight or physical fitness that are associated with perioperative complications. In order to reduce these complications and improve the results of surgery, in recent years several protocols have been used in patients awaiting bariatric surgery.

These protocols are mainly focused on the performance of a nutritional intervention with the aim of generating weight loss before bariatric surgery. However, different studies, that show the benefits that a structured exercise program can generate in bariatric surgery candidates, are emerging nowadays. On the one hand, exercise can contribute to reduce the comorbidities associated with obesity and total weight of individuals. On the other hand, through exercise, the physical fitness of patients can be improved. In turn, it is necessary to know the different factors related to physical fitness that are associated with perioperative complications in order to reduce them.

Therefore, in this chapter we will review the profile of patients awaiting bariatric surgery, showing the association between different variables of this profile and perioperative complications. In turn, different tools will be shown to assess the physical fitness in bariatric candidates and main guidelines will be provided to be able to apply a safe and effective exercise program in this population.

Keywords: bariatric surgery, exercise, perioperative complications, physical activity, physical fitness

1. INTRODUCTION

1.1. Lifestyle and Morbid Obesity

Bariatric surgery is performed on individuals with a bosy mass index (BMI) greater than 40 kg□m^{2} or 35 kg□m^{-2} associated with some comorbidity. Although genetic factors have some influence, the origin of these high BMI levels has a multifactorial component, mainly due to changes in the population's lifestyle. In recent decades, different technological advances have occurred, such as the mechanization of industries, the introduction of technological developments in jobs or new methods of transportation, which have completely transformed society. These changes began in the 1960s, when physical activity in different jobs began to require lower caloric expenditure. For instance, in the United States, between 1960 and 2008, the number of jobs in which moderate physical activity was performed decreased from 48% to 20% [1]. This involved greatly an increase in sedentary jobs, reducing by 140 kilocalories (kcal) daily energy consumption at work [1]. In turn, the emergence of new technologies has also influenced on the physical activity levels. Currently, the use of mechanized transport has greatly increased [2], while the energy expenditure derived from domestic tasks has decreased from 4,663 kcal per week to 2806 kcal per week between

1965 and 2010 [3]. On the other hand, from 1970, it became easier to acquire food and initiated the commercialization of food products rich in carbohydrates and fats, with high caloric intake, resulting in an increase in the total number of calories that individuals ingested daily [4]. In some countries such as Sweden, the daily caloric intake increased from 2,820 to 3,250 kcal between 1960 and 2010 [5], while in other countries such as the United States, it increased by 425 kcal per day between 1970 and 2009 [6]. Worldwide, a large increase in calories consumed daily has also been found, increasing from 2358 kcal per day to 2903 kcal perday between 1964 and 1999, estimating an excess caloric intake daily of 3000 kcal per day by 2030 [7].

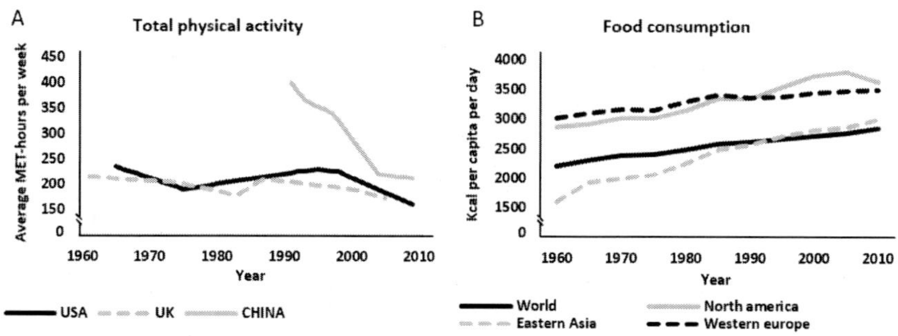

Figure 1. (A) Total physical activity in USA (1965-2009), UK (1961-2005) and China (1991-2009) [13] (B) Global and regional per capita food consumption between 1961-2010 [14].

Therefore, present-day society interacts with an environment that predisposes a positive energy balance, which can lead to weight gain, since these occur when the energy ingested is greater than the energy consumed over a prolonged period of time [8]. Unfortunately, exposure to these new changes has exacerbate obesity rates among population. Globally, it has been determined that the number of obese women increased from 69 to 390 million between 1975 and 2016, while this increase was from 31 to 281 million in men [9]. So currently, the prevalence of overweight has reached 38.5% in men and 39.4% in women, while obesity has reached 10.1% and 14.8% in men and women respectively [10]. This trend is expected to continue over time. It has been estimated that by 57.8% of the population will present overweight or obse by 2030 [11]. Indeed, it is expected that obesity rate reaches up to 9% of the population in some countries such as the United States [12].

1.2. Obesity and Physical Activity

To facilitate the understanding of some aspects of this chapter, different terms of great relevance in the subject being addressed must be defined. First, the terms of physical activity and exercise must be differentiated, since these tend to be confused in today's society, being used on many occasions as synonyms, while there is a great difference between them [15]:

- *Physical activity:* any bodily movement produced by contraction of skeletal muscles that results in a substantial increase in energy expenditure at rest. It is positively associated with physical condition.
- *Exercise:* repetitive, structured, planned bodily movements performed to improve or maintain one or more components of physical fitness. It is very positively associated with physical condition.

Equally, it is also necessary to differentiate between the terms "physical inactivity" and "sedentary behavior" [16]:

- *Sedentary behaviour:* a specific behavior or activity, which is characterized by a very low energy expenditure, being less than 1.5 METs (<20% VO2 max). Such behavior occurs while sitting, reclining, or lying down. This definition excludes the dream state.
- *Physical inactivity:* it occurs when individuals do not reach the minimum recommendations for physical activity. In adults: 150 minutes of moderate-vigorous activity or 75 minutes of vigorous activity.

Once these terms are defined, the association between physical activity and obesity will be analyzed. Although, as previously described, the origin of obesity has a multifactorial component, obesity levels are largely associated with levels of physical activity, and it has been shown that approximately 40% of obese individuals are considered physically inactive [17, 18]. This great impact of physical activity not only affects BMI levels, but also the percentage of fat mass. For example, it has been determined that in women with a similar BMI, active women had 18.9% fat mass, while this percentage decreases to 28.8% in sedentary women. Similarly, other studies have shown that men who consider themselves physically active, only 1.3% have obesity and 1.4% have more than 28.8% of fat mass, while in sedentary men this figure increases to 5.4% and 8.8%, respectively [19].

1.3. Physical Activity in Bariatric Patients

The data previously described show the great importance that physical activity can have on the BMI and the body composition of the individuals. In turn, physical inactivity is associated with weight regain after surgery. Therefore, it is essential to identify patients who are physically inactive. On the one hand, this will allow intervening in this population and modify their behavior in this regard, trying to get them to adhere to more active habits. Moreover, recognizing if there are sedentary subjects or if patients have modified their behavior regarding their lifestyle, it can be a criterion for the decision on intervening surgically in the patient.

At present, the assessment of physical activity levels is still a criterion that has not been consolidated in the ERAS protocols in bariatric patients. However, this can be an important factor, since it has been reported that physical activity levels are associated with medium and long-term weight regain after bariatric surgery. For example, a study analyzing the causes of weight regain in bariatric patients found that 80.8% of patients who gained weight were sitting for more than 3 hours a day [20]. In this same study, it was determined that 26.9% of patients who had weight regain were physically inactive, while this figure decreased to 15% in patients without weight regain [20]. Equally, other studies have shown that by 49% of the patients who did not perform physical activity prior to surgery had weight regain after surgery [21].

These data highlight the importance of maintaining an active lifestyle prior to surgery in order to maintain the weight lost after surgery.

In addition to the benefits in terms of weight control, physical activity prior to surgery will provide important benefits, such as an earlier recovery and a reduction in operative complications, factors that will be develop carefully in this chapter.

2. Surgical Complications

In the last decades, surgical techniques have improved to a great extent, and have greatly reduced the morbidity and mortality of surgery, however, there is still a certain percentage of perioperative complications. In a meta-analysis carried out on this topic, wich included approximately 16,000 patients, the mortality rate and surgical complications of different bariatric techniques were analyzed. It was observed that adjustable gastric banding had a perioperative mortality of 0.07%, a postoperative mortality of 0.021, with 13% of postoperative complications. These figures were 0.29, 0.34 and 17% for sleeve gastrectomy, and 0.38, 0.72 and 21% for gastric bypass, respectively [22]. As can be noted, the mortality rate is currently quite low, nevertheless, there is still a high rate of postoperative complications (between 13 and 21%), especially in sleeve gastrectomy and gastric bypass. In turn, it should be noted that both surgical techniques are the most frequently performed, with 304,550 sleeve gastrectomies per year and 191,326 gastric bypasses per year, meaning 53.6% and 30% of surgeries performed annually [23]. Therefore, between sleeve gastrectomy and gastric bypass, 83.6% of the annual bariatric surgeries are performed, what indicates that a high number of patients may suffer operative complications.

2.1. Variables Associated with Surgical Complications

Then, these surgical complications can affect many patients, so it is necessary to identify which factors are causing these complications. Although there are several components that can influence surgical complications such as age, surgeon's experience or gender [24–26], this chapter will focus on aspects that can be modified through physical activity and exercise, such as comorbidities associated with obesity, total weight or physical condition. Next, we will highlight to what extent these factors can influence surgical complications.

2.1.1. Comorbidities Related to Obesity

Obesity-related comorbidities have shown to be highly related with perioperative complications in bariatric patients. On the one hand, these comorbidities are directly related to postoperative mortality, and variables such as hypertension, diabetes or hyperlipidemia have been reported to be associated with 30-days mortality [25, 27, 28]. In fact, some studies have concluded that diabetes increases the probability of postoperative mortality by 2.88 times [29]. Furthermore, obesity-related comorbidities influence postoperative complications. In this regard, it has been reported that patients with diabetes are 1.6 times more likely to suffer postoperative complications compared to patients without diabetes [29], while patients with hypertension or hypercholesterolemia have shown a relative risk of postoperative complication of 1.58 and 1.82, respectively [30].

This results in the incidence of surgical complications being higher in patients with these comorbidities. For example, it has been shown that, in patients undergoing gastric bypass, of the patients with postoperative complications, 37% have diabetes and 63% have hypertension [31]. Similar data was obtained for the sleeve gastrectomy, in which it was observed that 31.6% and 62.3% of the patients with postoperative complications suffered from diabetes and hypertension, respectively [31]. Other studies have shown that 31% and 55% of patients with diabetes and hypertension present postoperative complications, while these figures drop to 22% and 48% (respectively) in patients without complications [24].

In turn, other comorbidities such as obstructive sleep apnea have also shown to be associated with postoperative complications. Some studies have reported that 57.6% of patients presenting from this pathology suffered moderate complications after surgery, while this percentage decreases to 42.4% in patients without complications [32]. Furthermore, the risk of operative complications increases with the presence of different comorbidities in the same patient. For example, in short-term complications, it has been reported that the complication ratio is 10.2% in patients with only one risk factor. However, the percentage of complication ratio is 14.9% with the presence of two risk factors, while reaches 20.6% in patients with three or more risk factors [33]. Likewise, the mortality rate increases with the number of comorbidities, being 0.04% for patients with only one comorbidity, and increasing to 1.6% in patients with five comorbidities [34]. Therefore, obesity-related comorbidities are related with mortality and postoperative complications, and thus it is necessary to an early intervention of them to ensure the safety of patients.

2.1.2. Physical Fitness

Physical fitness is another factor becoming of great relevance regarding the surgical complications. Physical fitness have been defined by how "a state characterized by (a) an ability to perform daily activities with vigor, and (b) demonstration of traits and capacities that are associated with low risk of premature development of the hypokinetic diseases (i.e., those associated with physical inactivity)" [35]. In general, physical fitness is defined by different components. On one hand, the skill-related components refer to athletic capacities, as agility, power or coordination [36]. However, the relevant components for the development of this chapter are those found within the group of health-related components, which is composed of cardiorespiratory and muscular endurance, muscle strength, body composition and flexibility [36]. The components of physical fitness more relevant in bariatric patients, and their importance in the prevention of obesity-related comorbidities are presented below.

2.1.2.1. Weight and Body Mass Index

Preoperative weight is another variable that can greatly influence surgical complications. Preoperative BMI increases the risk of mortality at 30 days, with an odds ratio of 1.65 for patients with BMI ranged between 40-49 kg·m^{-2}, 2.48 for BMI ranged between 50-59 kg·m^{-2} or 5.31 for patients with BMI ranged between 60-69 kg·m^{-2} [27]. In fact, a study reported that the average weight in patients who died was 185 kg, while patients who did not suffer mortality presented an average of 151 kg [24]. In turn, other studies have determined that a BMI greater than 50 is an indicator of postoperative complications [37], and it has been concluded that, for every point increase in BMI, the risk of suffering a postoperative complication increases by 2% [31]. In the same way as the mortality ratio, the ratio of surgical complications increases with the weight of the patient, with an average of 161.5 kg for patients presenting postoperative complications compared to 150.6 kg for patients without complications [24].

The data shows the need to generate a weight reduction before surgery, highlighting the weight control necessary in the months before surgery. In fact, it has been concluded that 27.9% of patients who presented a weight gain between 0-5% before surgery suffered postoperative complications, while these values decreased to 23.5% for patients with 0-5% weight loss and up to 14.2% in patients with 6-10% weight loss [38]. Similarly, other studies have shown other benefits of preoperative weight loss, and it has been determined that in patients who achieved ≥8% excess weight loss, a shorter operative duration and hospital length of stay have been reported [39]. However, it has not been shown that losses greater than 10% of the total weight generate additional benefits. On the contrary, some studies have shown an increased risk of mortality and complications compared to patients who have lost between 5-10% of total weight [38]. In addition, is important to note that weight losses can be accompanied by loss of fat-free mass, especially if these losses occur in a short period of time, which could lead to sarcopenic obesity [40]. This loss of fat-free mass, which would be mainly due to a loss of muscle mass, could lead to a reduction in the functional capacity and the basal metabolic rate of patients, as well as an increase in insulin resistance, predisposing individuals to a possible increase in fat mass and the development of diabetes [41–43]. Therfore, an adequate weight loss must be achieved before surgery, using strategies to maintain fat free mass levels, which can be achieved through the exercise [44, 45].

Finally, it should be considered that there are different variables in patients awaiting surgery which hinder the surgical process, such as visceral fat or non-alcoholic fatty liver disease. This causes various disadvantages. First, there may be greater liver fragility generated by fatty tissue deposits, which increases the risk of bleeding and injury caused by surgical manipulation [46, 47]. Second, a higher liver volume, concretely a higher volume of the left liver lobe, hindered an adequate visualization of the top portion of the stomach and the retroesophageal area, also making it difficult the approach to the gastroesophageal junction [46, 48]. This will lead to several drawbacks. On the one hand, a greater amount of visceral fat is associated with a longer surgical time [49]. On the other hand, liver disease presents an odds ratio of 2.26 with respect to 30-day mortality, while steatohepatitis has been shown as a predictor of the conversion from laparoscopy to open surgery [49, 50].

2.1.2.2. Cardiorespiratory Fitness

Cardiorespiratory fitness is defined as a component of the body related to the ability to supply oxygen continuously through the circulatory and respiratory systems [51], that is the capacity of these systems to provide "fuel" during physical activities. This capacity can be determined by different cardiorespiratory tests, from which different variables will be obtained. On the one hand, there is the maximum oxygen uptake (VO_{2max}), which is defined as the maximum amount of O_2 that an individual is able to use of per unit of time [52]. In turn, the anaerobic threshold must be defined, which occurs when the oxygen that the body provides to the muscle is not enough to satisfy energy demands, which causes anaerobic glycolysis to intervene significantly to supply energy to the body [53]. These variables have been defined due to their relevance in perioperative complications.

In recent decades, emerging research has concluded that cardiorespiratory fitness can be a factor of great importance in patients awaiting abdominal surgery. This is mainly due to the fact that aerobic capacity determines the cardiorespiratory reserve of individuals, which is associated with operative complications from any cause and can influence the impact of surgical stress on the patient [54]. For example, it has been reported that, after major surgery, oxygen consumption at rest increases by 50%, increasing from 110 $ml \cdot min^{-1} \cdot m^{-2}$ to 170 $ml \cdot min^{-1} \cdot m^{-2}$, maintaining these requirements over various days [55]. Therefore, there is an O_2 deficit after surgery, caused by this increased demand [56]. In case the body cannot provide adequate oxygen to meet these demands caused by surgery, these postoperative complications may appear [56]. This is clearly showed in the study performed by

Shoemaker et al. (1992), in which patients with 9.2 $L \cdot m^{-2}$ oxigen deficit had no postoperative complications, while patients with 21.6 $L \cdot m^{-2}$ oxigen deficit suffered from operative complications and subjects with 33.2 $L \cdot m^{-2}$ oxigen deficit suffered from mortality [57].

Therefore, it is necessary that the patients who are going to undergo major surgery have an optimal cardiorespiratory reserve, in order to be able to meet the body's oxygen demands after surgery without exceeding the body's physiological parameters [58].

Currently, there are few studies that analyse these aspects in bariatric patients, however, the studies found in the scientific literature provide interesting results. In a study it was concluded that patients who had a hospital length of stay greater than 3 days had lower anaerobic threshold and VO_{2peak} than patients who had a hospital length of stay ≤ 3 days (anaerobic threshold: 10.4 $ml \cdot kg^{-1} \cdot min^{-1}$ vs 11.3 $ml \cdot kg^{-1} \cdot min^{-1}$, VO_{2peak}: 16.1 $ml \cdot kg^{-1} \cdot min^{-1}$ vs 15.0 $ml \cdot kg^{-1} \cdot min^{-1}$) [59]. In this same study, it was also determined that patients with lower postoperative complications had a higher anaerobic threshold and VO_{2peak} than patients with a higher rate of postoperative complications (anaerobic threshold: 11.1 $ml \cdot kg^{-1}$·min-1 vs 9.9 $ml \cdot kg^{-1} \cdot min^{-1}$; VO_{2peak}: 15.9 $ml \cdot kg^{-1} \cdot min^{-1}$ vs 14.6 $ml \cdot kg^{-1} \cdot min^{-1}$) [59]. In turn, another study conducted in bariatric patients found that patients with a VO_{2peak} below than 15.8 $ml \cdot kg^{-1} \cdot min^{-1}$ had a postoperative complication rate of 16.7%, while those patients with a VO_{2peak} above than 15.8 $ml \cdot kg^{-1} \cdot min^{-1}$ had a postoperative complication rate of 2.8% [60].

In addition to this effect on operative complications, cardiorespiratory fitness has shown important against the prevention of obesity-related comorbidities. Sometimes, there are subjects who have obesity, and yet do not have associated pathologies, which is known as "fatness." Several studies have shown that this is due to physical fitness, and it has been reported that overweight or obese type I subjects with optimal cardiorespiratory fitness have the same risk of mortality as subjects with normal weight [61]. However, in subjects with the same type of obesity, the risk of mortality is higher in those with low cardiorespiratory fitness (Hazard Ratio of 1.38) than in individuals with adequate cardiorespiratory fitness (Hazard Ratio 0.65) [62]. In another interesting study in this regard, obese subjects were divided into two subgroups (metabolically healthy and metabolically abnormal). Participants who had one or no comorbidity associated with obesity were defined as metabolically healthy, while those patient with two or more comorbidities were defined as metabolically abnormal. The study found that those subjects who were obese but metabolically healthy had greater cardiorespiratory fitness [63].

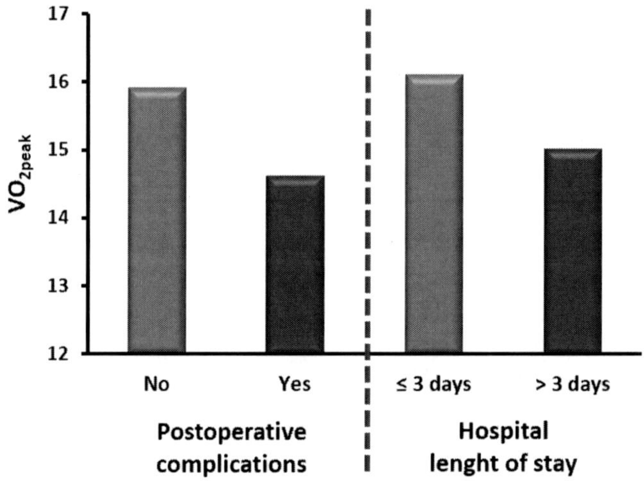

Figure 2. Relationship between peak oxygen uptake, postoperative complications and hospital length of stay [59].

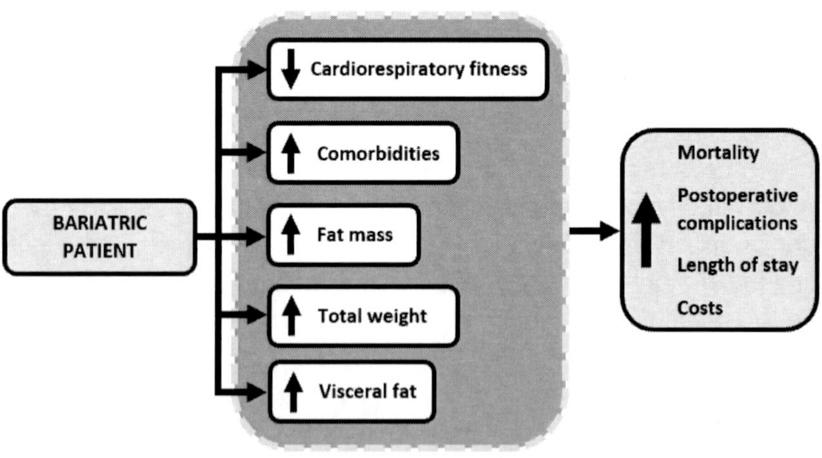

Figure 3. Main causes of complications in bariatric patients.

Therefore, by improving cardiorespiratory capacity has several advantages. On the one hand, it provides a greater cardiorespiratory reserve, preparing the patient for a potential increase in oxygen demand due to surgery. On the other hand, the improvement of aerobic capacity can contribute to reduce the number of postoperative complications and obesity-related comorbidities, which could contribute to reduce postoperative complications.

2.2. Patient's Recoverys

Currently, there is little information in the scientific literature on the effects of physical activity on postoperative recovery in patients awaiting bariatric surgery. As previously reported, it has been determined that patients with a longer hospital stay (greater than 3 days) have lower cardiorespiratory fitness (15.0 $ml \cdot kg^{-1} \cdot min^{-1}$) than patients who have a hospital length stay of 3 days or less (16.1 $ml \cdot kg^{-1} \cdot min^{-1}$). In turn, patients with a VO_{2peak} of 13.7 $ml \cdot kg^{-1} \cdot min^{-1}$ have a mean of 3.8 hospital length of stay, while in patients with a VO_{2peak} of 21.3 $ml \cdot kg^{-1} \cdot min^{-1}$ the mean length of stay is 2.8 days [60].

As there is little information on the effects of exercise in patients awaiting surgery on their postoperative recovery, the results found in the scientific literature about major abdominal surgeries will be shown. Usually, after major surgery, it takes a while for the body to recover, as it has been submitted to great surgical stress and a few days of bed rest. This will have negative consequences on the functional capacity of individuals. For example, 3 weeks after surgery, only 41% of patients undergoing colon resection surgery have a functional capacity equal to or greater than what they had prior to surgery [64]. However, patients who increase their functional capacity before surgery, have an early recovery of their functional capacity [64]. In this regard, it has been shown that 81% of patients who underwent a prehabilitation protocol (which included physical activity guidelines) completely recovered their preoperative physical function levels two months after surgery, while the subjects who did not participate in a prehabilitation program, only 40% presented physical function levels equal to those prior to surgery [65].

In bariatric patients, it has been shown a decrease in strength levels after surgery, both in the lower and upper body [66, 67], which is possibly due to a decrease in fat-free mass. At this point, the importance of muscle mass should be highlighted. Due to the stress caused by surgery (surgical stress), protein degradation is accelerated and protein synthesis is low, leading to a negative protein balance and so causing the breakdown of muscle tissue [68]. On the other hand, the loss of muscle mass can be aggravated, especially if there has been any complication that may increase the hospital lenght of stay and bed rest. For example, it has been reported that the increase in days of bed rest is associated with a greater loss of muscle mass [69]. Equally, another study showed that fat free mass and muscle strength of the lower extremities were reduced by 6.3% and 15.6% respectively with only 10 days of bed rest [70]. Similarly, it has been also reported that the bed rest also reduces cardiorespiratory fitness between 7.1 and 15.3% respectively in only two weeks [71]. In fact, different studies show reductions in maximum oxygen consumption in absolute values after surgery, although these studies were carried out 3, 6 and 12 months after surgery [72, 73].

These arguments show the need to perform an exercise programme before surgery, with the aim of increasing levels of physical fitness and improving the functional capacity of patients, with the aim of achieving an earlier recovery after surgery.

3. Bariatric Surgery Candidates Profile

Once the aspects that may hinder the surgical process in bariatric patients have been described, it is necessary to analyse the profile of the patients awaiting bariatric surgery.

3.1. Cardivovasular Risk Factors

Patients awaiting bariatric surgery have a high number of obesity-related comorbidities such as diabetes, obstructive sleep apnea, or non-alcoholic fatty liver disease. In addition, hypertension is one of the comorbidities that usually occurs to a greater extent in these patients, and studies show that it is present in 34-54.9% of these patients [74–76]. In turn, bariatric patients suffer from other cardiometabolic diseases that can complicate the surgical process, and it has been shown that between 7.4 and 50.2% suffer from dyslipidemia, while between 18 and 33.7% have type II diabetes mellitus [74–76]. On the other hand, it has been reported that these patients suffer from other comorbidities, and between 22 and 44.8% present obstructive sleep apnea [74–76]. Finally, one of the comorbidities that can greatly hinder the surgical process, liver disease, is one of the most prevalent in patients awaiting bariatric surgery, and it has been shown that non-alcoholic fatty liver disease is present in 52-91% of candidates for bariatric surgery, while non-alcoholic steatohepatitis is found in 35-88.6% of these patients [77–81].

3.2. Physical Fitness

In addition to these obesity-related comorbidities, patients awaiting bariatric surgery have a very low physical fitness. Regarding cardiorespiratory fitness, which is associated with surgical complications, these patients show deficient values, showing a peak oxygen consumption of between 15.8 and 16.0 $ml \cdot kg^{-1} \cdot min^{-1}$ [82–85]. These values are really low, especially when compared to the population mean. For instance, it has been seen that, in men aged between 40 and 49 years old, an acceptable level of cardiorespiratory capacity is between 42.4-45.4 $ml \cdot kg^{-1} \cdot min^{-1}$, while it has been defined as a cut-off point for a low cardiorespiratory fitness at a value lower than 25.1 $ml \cdot kg^{-1} \cdot min^{-1}$. Therefore, we can observe that patients awaiting surgery have a mean oxygen consumption between 27 and 30 units below an appropriate level [86].

3.3. Physical Activity Levels in Patients Awaiting Bariatric Surgery

However, despite the benefits that physical activity and exercise can generate to patients awaiting bariatric surgery, they show very low physical activity levels. On the one hand, these patients present an average of 31.1 minutes of moderate-to- vigorous physical activity per day [87], showing that up to 68% of patients do not accumulate any moderate-to-vigorous physical activity in bouts ≥ 10 minutes, while this figure drops to 13% in individuals with normal weight [88]. Other studies have evaluated the daily steps. Theses studies has been determined that 45.1% of the patients performed less than 5000 steps a day, which is considered a low level of physical activity [89]. As a result, these patients spend a great part of the day performing sedentary activities. As a result, these patients are a big part of the day doing sedentary activities. In fact, watching television is one of the activities that candidates for bariatric surgery perform to a greater extent, with an average of 2.7 hours per day [90]. Likewise, different studies that have evaluated the physical activity in these patients have concluded that this population remains between 70 and 80% of its daily time performing sedentary activities [91, 92], while other studies have classified 90% of patients awaiting surgery as sedentary subjects [93].

Therefore, physical activity levels in this population are extremely low. Only between 4.5 and 6.2% of patients awaiting surgery can be considered physically active [88, 89]. In turn, it is necessary to analyse the type of physical activity that these patients perform. On the one hand, bariatric surgery candidates only dedicate an average of 9.7 minutes a day to exercise [87]. In addition, walking most usual physical activity performed by patients awaiting bariatric surgery, being the main physical activity for 44-95% of them [94, 95]. While other studies have concluded that other activities such as housework are the most performed [87]. These types of activities are performed at low intensity and, furthermore, do not include strength training, factors that can be essential to optimize weight loss and achieve improvements in physical fitness prior to surgery.

Therefore, it is necessary to perform several functions before surgery. First, it is necessary to assess the levels of physical activity of candidates for bariatric surgery to determine the patients who need to increase them. In turn, due to its close relationship with perioperative complications and postoperative recovery, we must analyse the levels of physical fitness of bariatric patients. In this way, it is possible to recognize the operative risk of the patients, and determine which factors of the physical fitness should be improved in each patient. On the other hand, an exercise intervention must be performed in these patients, with the aim that they are in the best possible conditions to the surgical procedure.

4. Assessments in Bariatric Patients

Prior to surgery, it is necessary to perform different types of evaluations in order, on the one hand, to know the variables by which patients should improve to reduce postoperative complications, and, on the other hand, to be able to obtain the maximum possible benefits of surgery. Although it is necessary to know the comorbidities associated with obesity in order to act on them, this chapter will focus on assessments related to physical activity. In the first place, several tools will be described to assess levels of physical activity. Second, strategies will be defined to assess the physical condition in these patients.

4.1. Assessment of Physical Activity Levels

These assessments can be of great importance in bariatric patients, since knowing the levels of physical activity will allow us to identify patients who have increased their levels of physical activity and thus proposing them for surgery. Physical activity levels can be assessed using objective methods (motion sensors such as accelerometry or pedometers) or through subjective methods (questionnaires). Then, the tools that have been used to a greater extent to assess the levels of physical activity in these patients will be shown, defining their advantages and disadvantages.

4.1.1. Objective Measures

4.1.1.1. Accelerometry

Accelerometry is the gold standard method for evaluating levels of physical activity. The accelerometer is an electronic device that measures the acceleration and deceleration of the body in one or more directions. When this acceleration is generated, an electrical current proportional to the rate of acceleration is produced in the device, which allows the physical activity of a subject to be obtained [96, 97]. This device expresses its results in a unit called “counts,” which is the sum of all the absolute values of the acceleration changes produced during a specific period, that varies from 1 to 60 seconds (which is known as EPOCH). Usually, the EPOCH is expressed in 60 seconds, that is, in "counts per minute" [97]. Once the data are available, from these “counts per minute,” the intensities at which the various activities have been carried out during the recording can be obtained using various classifications. In this case, the intensity classification used by Freedson [98] will be shown, in which it differentiates between light, moderate and vigorous (vigorous) activity based on the following values:

- Light activity < 1952 count□min^{-1}.
- Moderate activity between 1952 and 5724 count□min^{-1}.
- Vigorous activity > 5724 count□min^{-1}.
- In turn, they have been defined as sedentary activities (sedentary behaviour) activity counts values < 100 count□min^{-1} [99].

Although it is a method that have a high cost and a longer time for its evaluation, it is highly recommended, due to its high degree of reliability. Currently, it is the most reliable method for measuring physical activity levels. For the evaluation used by accelerometry to be correct, some important aspects must be taken into consideration. On the one hand, the “body location” of the accelerometer must be considered. Some studies are currently recommending the placement of accelerometers on the wrist, since it is considered that in this way the individual evaluated does not remove the accelerometer during the evaluation, ensuring a complete record, especially in children. However it is still to be determined that placing the accelerometer on the wrist is more effective than placing it in other areas [100, 101]. Therefore, it is currently recommended placing the accelerometer as close as possible to the centre of mass of the body, so it is usually placed on the waist or on the right side of the hip [97, 102]. On the other hand, you must decide how many days of registration are carried out. When accelerometry is applied, it is intended to record physical activity habits in the population, so making a record of a few days can lead to an erroneous perception. Then, it is recommended to carry out long registrations, and most studies perform registrations of approximately 7 days, with a minimum of 10 hours per day [99, 103].

4.1.1.2. Pedometers

Pedometers are motion sensors that have a horizontal spring-suspended movement that moves due to the vertical acceleration generated by the hips during movement, which allows determining the steps that a person performs daily [104]. This motion sensor has certain limitations. On the one hand, it is a more limited tool than accelerometers, since it does not allow differentiating between intensities, frequency, duration or type of exercise. In addition, some pedometers only record 24 hours, so it is the individual who should record their steps, generating a significant bias in the research to be carried out [104]. In turn, pedometers are not effective in assessing physical activity in various activities (cycling, for example), and their reliability decreases when speeds are maintained below 3 km/h [104]. Finally, some studies have tried to calculate the distance travelled and energy expenditure using different formulas from the data obtained by the pedometer, however, these have not been shown to be effective in achieving these objectives, and, for example, only moderate associations have been obtained with energy expenditure ($r = 0.68$) [105].

However, it is a very interesting option to assess levels of physical activity, since it evaluates physical activity objectively and is a much cheaper alternative than accelerometry, in addition to being a reliable tool to determine the steps that a subject performs daily. The reliability of this tool has been shown in several studies, and it has been shown to have levels of agreement with accelerometry of 97% for the step count [106]. In turn, other studies have shown high correlations between pedometers and accelerometry ($r = 0.86$), while high correlations with time in observed activity have also been found, indicating that it is a reliable tool to evaluate levels of physical activity [105].

Therefore, the use of pedometers is a valid method to assess levels of physical activity, especially in ambulatory activities such as running or walking. One of the great advantages of this tool is that there are cut-off points to classify the level of physical activity of the subjects based on the steps that have been carried out [107]:

- Sedentary lifestyle < 5000 steps/day.
- Low active between 5000 and 7499 steps/day.
- Somewhat active between 7500 and 9999 steps/day.
- Active ≥ 10000 steps/day.
- Highly active > 12500 steps/day.

Finally, there is an important factor that must be considered in the use of pedometers, since it must be decided for how many days to carry out the registration. Some studies indicate that, to know the weekly physical activity levels of an adult, a single day of recording is not reliable, but that 3 days of recording would be sufficient, showing a high correlation with weekly physical activity ($r = 0.94$) [108]. On the other hand, other authors have analysed how many days of registration would be necessary to know the levels of monthly physical activity in adults, and have determined that 7 days of registration is achieved the best results [109]. These authors defend the importance of using 7 days with the main objective of including Sundays, a day in which physical activity levels are usually lower, so its registration is considered necessary [109]. Therefore, it should be to perform a 7-day registration whenever possible, while if you do not have the necessary time, a 3-day registration could be made, although it is not the most recommended.

4.1.2. Subjective Measures

4.1.2.1. Cuestionnaires

Physical activity levels can also be assessed using questionnaires. However, these present several limitations, since these assess physical activity subjectively, and various studies have shown that physical activity levels tend to be overestimated using theses methods [87, 110]. However, in bariatric patients, these differences mainly occur after surgery, especially in the long-term [111], and certain studies show that questionnaires can be useful in patients awaiting bariatric surgery [112].

Therefore, the management of certain questionnaires can be an adequate and reliable alternative for patients awaiting bariatric surgery when motion sensors are not available to determine physical activity levels. In this regard, various questionnaires have been used in bariatric patients, such as the Short Questionnaire to Assess Health Enhancing Physical Activity, The Godin Leisure Time Questionnaire, The second version of the Global Physical Activity Questionnaire or Baecke Physical Activity Questionnaire, however, the International Physical Activity Questionnaire (IPAQ) has been widely used [113].

The IPAQ is a questionnaire created in Geneva in 1998 by an international consensus group [114]. This questionnaire assesses physical activity in the 7 days prior to the test in young and middle-aged adults (18-65 years). It has two versions: a) IPAQ-long form; b) IPAQ-short form. The IPAQ-long form has a great advantage, since it allows obtaining the levels of physical activity in different domains (work, household, leisure and transportation), which provides very valuable information, but has the disadvantage that this questionnaire tends to overestimate levels of physical activity. Therefore, it is recommended to use the IPAQ in its short version, since it presents a high reliability, in addition to being a shorter questionnaire (it only has 7 questions), so it can be completed easily [115]. Moreover, the IPAQ presents a great advantage over other questionnaires. It allows obtaining physical activity at different levels (walking, moderate and vigorous), being able to provide levels of physical activity in MET-min□week^{-1}. In addition, it allows obtaining the time that a subject remains seated provides a classification of the physical activity levels of the subjects based on the results obtained [116]:

- Low <600 MET-min□week^{-1}.
- Moderate between 600 and 2999 MET-min□week^{-1}.
- High ≥ 3000 MET-min□week^{-1}.

4.2. Assessment of Physical Fitness

As previously described, physical fitness is based on two main components: skill-related components and health-related components.

This chapter will focus on health-related components, specifically on body composition, cardiorespiratory fitness and muscle strength, due to the benefits that its management can bring in bariatric patients. The different methods by which the physical fitness of bariatric patients can be assessed will be described.

4.2.1. Body Composition

In the last decades, different ways of evaluating body composition have been developed: direct methods (isotope dilution, total body counting or isotope dilution), criterion methods (densitometry, Computed Tomography and Magnetic Resonance Imaging or Dual-Energy X-ray Absorptiometry) and indirect methods (anthropometry or bioelectrical impedance analysis) [117]. The gold standard method to assess body composition is computed tomography, however, it has certain limitations that make its use difficult. On the one hand, it has a high cost, needs to be carried out by qualified personnel (technicians) and presents radiation exposure [118]. Furthermore, it has a weight limit of approximately 230 kg, which makes it difficult to use in bariatric patients [118]. For these reasons, it is not usually used in bariatric patients, and, at present, the most used methods in this population are bioelectrical impedance analysis and Dual-Energy X-ray Absorptiometry (DEXA), this latter being the best alternative to computed tomography [118]. DEXA allows obtaining fat mass, bone mass and lean mass values by means of emission of tissue specific energy by X-rays, and presenting good precision, with a 1% coefficient of variation for bone mineral density and between 2 and 3% for fat mass [119]. In turn, several studies have determined that, although it presents a certain error, it can be a valid tool to assess body composition in obese subjects [118, 120]. However, this technique also has different limitations, since it has a relatively high cost, and the machines usually have a weight limit, often being 120 kg [121].

Therefore, it is necessary to find other options for methods such as computed tomography or DEXA, since characteristics such as its high cost, the need for qualified personnel and the application time make it difficult to use. A suitable alternative to these techniques is bioelectrical impedance analysis, mainly because it is a reliable, cheap, fast and simple method. This technique is based on the principle that different body tissues have different resistance to an electrical signal. For example, fat mass is a poor conductor of electricity, due to its low amount of water. Therefore, this technique measures the impedance by applying a small electric current through the body, and depending on different formulas, it is capable of providing total fat mass, fat free mass and total body water [119, 122]. Another aspect to highlight regarding this technique is that it has been validated in bariatric patients, both to determine the levels of fat mass before surgery and to determine the changes produced by it [121, 123]. In turn, it has been observed that electrical bioimpedance has a Pearson's correlation prior to surgery, and at 6 and 12 months of 0.98, 0.94 and 0.99, respectively, to determine fat mass, while that these correlations were 0.87, 0.82 and 0.99 for the calculation of the fat free mass [124].

Therefore, the bioelectrical impedance analysis is an adequate alternative in these patients. In this regard, it should be noted that a series of considerations should be taken into account when performing the evaluation through this technique [125]:

- It must be done after, at least, 8 hours of fasting.
- Alcohol should not have been consumed at least 8 hours before the assessment.
- Do not perform physical activity at least 8 hours before.
- Carry out the assessment with an empty bladder.

4.2.2. Cardiorespiratory Fitness

There are different ways to determine cardiorespiratory fitness. This can be determined in "laboratory" or in "filed" based [126]. The incremental tests carried out in the laboratory are considered the "gold standard" method to obtain the maximum oxygen consumption (VO_{2max}). This VO_{2max} is defined as the mean of the VO_2 values of the last 15 seconds of a maximal test [53]. However, there is a consideration here that should be taken into account in bariatric patients. To determine the VO_{2max}, the test must be maximal, and for this it is necessary that at the end of the evaluation three of the following four requirements have been fulfilled [53]:

- At the end of the test, the VO_2 consumption must remain stable despite increases in intensity.

- Capillary lactic acid concentrations greater than 8 $mmol \cdot L^{-1}$ must be obtained.
- A respiratory quotient (VCO_2/VO_2) ≥ 1.15 must be reached.
- Reach the subject's theoretical maximum heart rate.

It is usual that, for different reasons, when performing a test of this type in bariatric patients, three of the requirements provided are not met, so that in bariatric patients, usually the peak oxygen consumption (VO_{2peak}) is actually obtained. In these patients, both valuations in ergometer and stationary ergometer bike have been used to calculate VO_{2peak} in the laboratory. Typically, these assessments begin with a brief warm-up (between 4 and 15 minutes [72, 127]), then continuing with gradual increases in intensity every 2 minutes until volitional fatigue [72, 127].

Although laboratory tests are the most suitable methods to obtain the aerobic capacity of patients, these tests have a relatively high cost, since a gas analyser is required and is not always available. For this reason, usually these evaluations cannot be performed, and other types of tests must be used, so different "field" tests are frequently used in bariatric patients. To date, the most "field" test used in bariatric patients, due to its ease of application, has been the 6-min-walk test (6MWT). This test measures the distance that a patient is able to travel in a 6-minute period on a hard and flat surface [128]. In addition, it should be noted that formulas have now emerged to estimate VO_{2max} from the test results. In this regard, two equations will be shown, one for the general population and one for women with obesity:

- General population: VO_{2peak} ($ml \cdot kg \cdot min^{-1}$) = 4.948 + 0.023 + mean 6MWT (in meters) [129].
- Women with obesity: VO_{2peak} ($l \cdot min^{-1}$) = (body mass index x 0.0150065) - (waist-to-hip-ratio x 0.8595088) + (fat-free-mass (in kg) x 0.0295478) + (6-min walk test (in meters) x 0.0020672) - 0.5853372 [130].

It should be noted that the 6MWT evaluates the functional capacity and not aerobic capacity. For example, many patients improve the distance travelled on the 6MWT after surgery. However, this is mainly due to the great weight reduction that occurs after the surgical procedure, which facilitates walking, and not to an improvement in aerobic capacity. So if it is intended to assess cardiorespiratory fitness, other types of test should be used. In this regard, the Astrand-Rhyming cycle ergometer test has been used in bariatric patients. This test lasts 6 minutes and is performed with a cadence of 50 revolutions per minute and with a power of between 50 and 150 W, depending on the subject's gender and physical fitness. To estimate VO_{2max}, the mean of the heart rate of the fifth and sixth minute of the test must be calculated and the monogram of this test must be used. In addition, it allows applying a correction factor based on age [86].

On the other hand, a test that can be used in this population is the Young Men's Christian Association (YMCA) test. This test lasts between 6 and 12 minutes, and consists of a 3-minute warm-up with a cadence of 50 revolutions per minute and a power of 25 W. Then, depending on the heart rate at which the patient has finished this stage, a 2nd stage of 3 minutes begins in which the power can vary between 50 and 125 W, it will depend on the heart rate at which the subject has finished the 1st stage. From here on, 25 W will be increased on each stage. The test ends when 75-85% of the theoretical maximum heart rate is reached [131]. To calculate VO_{2max}, the power and heart rate of the third minute of the last two stages performed must be recorded, and a linear regression is performed to estimate the power that would have been required to reach maximum heart rate. Then, the following formula can be applied: VO_{2max} $(ml \cdot Kg^{-1} \cdot min^{-1}) = 1.8 * (6.12 * W_{peak}) / BW + 3.5 + 3.5$ (in which "BW" is body mass in kilograms and "W_{peak}" is the power output in watts) [132].

4.2.3. Muscular Strength

Strength levels have been little studied in bariatric patients; however, it has been reported that they decrease after bariatric surgery [66, 67, 133]. In this regard, different types of measurements have been used in bariatric patients. The "gold standard" method for the evaluation of strength is carried out using an isokynthetic dynamometer. Nevertheless, this is a relatively high-cost and difficult-to-access method, so there are other tools that can be used to assess strength. On the one hand, "load cells" can be used [67], since it has a low cost, although it requires a certain organization. Another viable and economical alternative is to assess handgrip strength by hydraulic hand dynamometer. This option is quite inexpensive, and it also provides reference values that indicate muscle function [134], so it is an alternative that has been used frequently in bariatric patients.[135–137].

Finally, another alternative that has been used in this population is the calculation of one repetition maximum, which is defined as the maximum weight that can be lifted in a single repetition of a given exercise. To avoid risks, this value is usually obtained indirectly, and after a specific warm-up, the subject is asked to perform as many repetitions as possible of a given exercise until the failure, trying to adjust the weight so that they are only performed between 6-10 repetitions. The weight used and the repetitions performed must be recorded and the following formula must be applied to determine the maximum repetition: one maximum repetition = w (in kg)/[102.78-2.78 (repetitions performed)]/100, where "w" is the weight that has been moved [138].

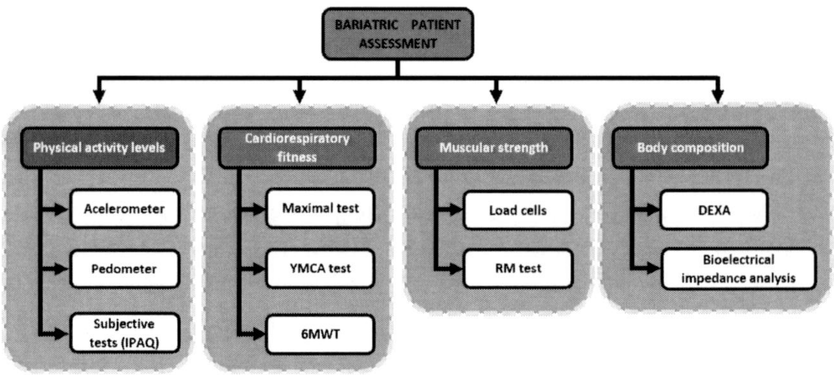

Figure 4 Recommended assessments in patients awaiting bariatric surgery. IPAQ, International Physical Activity Questionnaire; YMCA, Young Men's Christian Association; RM, maximum repetition; DEXA, Dual-Energy X-ray Absorptiometry.

5. Exercise before Bariatric Surgery

Once the characteristics of the patients awaiting bariatric surgery and the disadvantages that these may cause have been analysed, the main that must be achieved through exercise before the surgical intervention can be defined. These are the following: 1) achieve weight loss of between 5-10%; 2) maintain fat-free mass in these weight losses; 3) reduce comorbidities associated with obesity; 4) improve fitness levels, especially cardiorespiratory capacity and improve functional capacity.

Usually, prior to surgery, interventions aimed at weight loss are performed through nutritional protocols. However, adding a structured exercise program to these nutritional interventions can contribute to achieve these goals. On the one hand, adding an exercise programme to a nutritional intervention can generate greater weight loss compared to a nutritional intervention performed in isolation. Furtehermore, exercise contributes to maintain fat free mass during weight loss phases. It has been reported that when there is a weight loss achieved only through diet occurs, besides reductions in fat mass, reductions in fat-free mass. Exercise can help maintain fat-free mass in these cases. In turn, exercising will contribute greatly to the reduction of obesity-related comorbidities, and will generate improvements in the physical fitness of patients, especially in cardiorespiratory capacity.

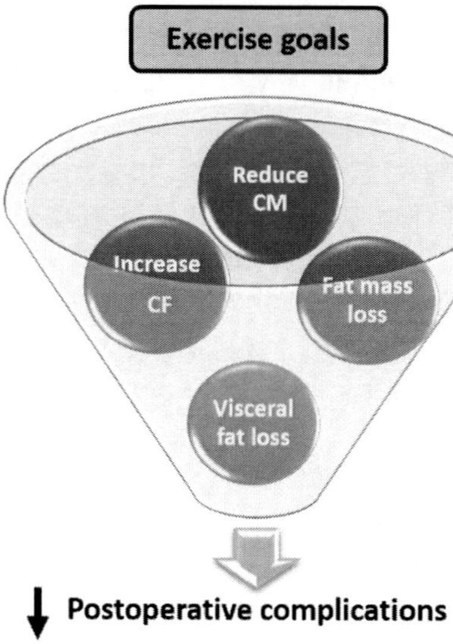

Figure 5. Exercise goals before bariatric surgery. CF, cardiorespiratory fitness; CM, comorbidities.

5.1. Exercise Programs Performed in Patients Awaiting Bariatric Surgery

Although the information in the scientific literature on the effects of exercise programmes in patients awaiting bariatric surgery is scarce, different studies are currently emerging that have addressed this issue. First, these studies show that participation in an exercise program, regardless of the type of exercise performed (endurance or resistance training), generates improvements in different parameters.

On the one hand, most of the studies carried out have shown improvements in the physical fitness of patients [84, 139–145]. Usually, the assessment that has been performed to a greater extent has been the 6MWT, and improvements have been obtained both in 2-month programs and in 6-month programmess, by using both endurance training in isolation and combined training (endurance and resistance training) [142, 146]. In another study, the VO_{2peak} of the patients was evaluated after a 3-month combined training programme in which high intensities were used, obtaining an increase of 12.1% VO_{2peak}. In turn, other studies have shown that a training programme also produces improvements in strength levels. For example, endurance training (intensity between 55-85% of the heart rate reserve) combined with resistance training for 8 weeks (3 weekly exercise sessions), produced improvements in strength levels, both in the lower and upper body [143].

In reference to body composition, the programmes performed before surgery have also obtained positive results, and large reductions have been obtained in total weight (decreases between 1.41 and 7.5%), in fat mass (reductions between 5.3 and 12.5%), in waist circumference (reductions between 3.86 and 7.8%) and in visceral fat (reductions of approximately 11%) in programmes lasting between 8 and 16 weeks [84, 139–141, 147]. Moreover, it is important to note that the exercise programmes introducing resistance training have achieved weight reductions mainly due to the reduction of fat mass, avoiding fat-free mass loss [84, 143]. For instance, in a 12-week exercise programme in which resistance and endurance training were combined, there was a reduction of 7 kg of fat mass, without there being a decrease in fat-free mass and or basal metabolic rate [84].

On the other hand, positive effects of exercise programmes prior to surgery have been evidenced on cardiovascular risk factors. For example, by performing a 6-month endurance training programmed resulted in reductions from 127.8 mg/dl to 110.6 mg/dl in blood glucose, from 132.1 mg/dl to 107.8 mg/dl of LDL cholesterol, and from 147.3 mmHg to 123.5 mmHg of systolic blood pressure, generating a 4.4-unit reduction in cardiovascular risk [146]. In turn, in another 4-month study, in which 2 weekly sessions of endurance exercise, was found significant reductions in glucose, total cholesterol, LDL cholesterol and blood pressure (systolic and diastolic) levels, while HDL cholesterol increased. In this regard, programmes between 12 and 16 weeks training, with 3 weekly sessions of strength training, (3 series of 60 seconds per exercise to muscle failure) have also been shown to be an effective alternative in improving cardiometabolic parameters, generating reductions in triglyceride levels, total cholesterol and LDL cholesterol, and a reduction of approximately 10% in blood glucose [140, 141]. Finally, in a 3-month exercise programme involving endurance training at an intensity between 60 and 80% of VO_{2peak} and resistance training at an intensity between 50 and 65% of one maximum repetition demonstrated: reductions of 17.7 mg/dl in glucose, 10.5 mmHg in systolic blood pressure, 3.9 mmHg in diastolic blood pressure and a significant reduction in glycosylated hemoglobin, and increases of 5 mg/dl in HDL cholesterol [84].

Therefore, studies that have applied an exercise programme in patients awaiting surgery have obtained improvements both in levels of physical fitness, in functional capacity, in body composition and in obesity-related comorbidities. Some guidelines for the application of a physical activity programme in patients awaiting bariatric surgery, based on the studies that have been carried out on them, and on the latest updates on exercise and weight loss, will be provided below.

5.2. Proposed Exercise Guidelines in Patients Awaiting Bariatric Surgery

Exercise programmess in patients awaiting bariatric surgery must be aimed at achieving the objectives previously shown. On the one hand, an improvement in cardiorespiratory fitness must be achieved, a factor of great relevance in the prevention of perioperative complications, while resistance training must also be performed, to prevent the loss of muscle mass and improve functional capacity, thus favouring the patient recovery. Moreover, exercising will contribute to a reduction in fat mass, visceral fat and obesity-related comorbidities, which will decrease the risk of surgical complications.

To achieve these objectives, different factors must be addressed. First, the type of training, since both endurance training and resistance training will provide different advantages. Second, endurance training will allow generating losses in fat mass and an improvement in the maximum oxygen consumption of patients. In this regard, the American College of Sports Medicine has published in its consensus document that between 150 and 250 minutes of exercise per week generates moderate weight losses, while performing more than 250 minutes of exercise per week, greater reductions are achieved in total weight [148]. Therefore, the volume of aerobic exercise is relevant to generate weight loss, and it has been shown that in 12-month programmes with less than 150 minutes per week of aerobic exercise, there was a weight reduction of 4.7%, while that when aerobic exercise is between 150 and 200 minutes per week or greater than 200 minutes per week, these reductions are 9.5% and 13.6% [149]. In addition, through endurance training are achieved improvements in cardiorespiratory fitness, which is in turn associated with less operative complications.

On the other hand, it should be considered to introduce strength training in the exercise program for bariatric patients. At present, it is well known that when there is a loss of weight, besides reductions in fat-free mass, there are also decreases in fat-free mass. It is widely accepted that, when there are weight reductions, approximately 25% of the weight lost is fat-free mass, although some studies have determined that these figures may be higher, and can reach up to 40% in men and 33% in women [150]. It should be highlighted that this can lead to a decrease in the basal metabolic rate, functional capacity and an increase in insulin resistance [41, 42, 151]. These drawbacks should be avoided, and resistance training is a suitable tool for it. Several studies have shown that implementing resistance training to a weight loss programme can prevent this loss of fat-free mass and even increase it, resulting losses exclusively due to decreases in fat mass [152–156].

Therefore, combining endurance training and resistance training is a key factor of obtaining the maximum benefits from an exercise programme in patients awaiting surgery. However, there are other factors of great importance such as training intensity. It has been reported that for resistance training to be effective in maintaining fat-free mass, it is necessary to training at appropriate intensities. For example, in studies where significant losses in fat mass and fat-free mass gains have been achieved, resistance training has been performed at intensities between 70 and 80% of one maximum repetition [152–154]. On the other hand, an interesting meta-analysis concluded that the intensities that generated the most favourable changes in body composition (loss of fat mass and maintenance of fat-free mass) were used in resistance training intensities of between 75- 80% of one maximum repetition [44]. Similar results have been obtained in endurance training, and this same meta-analysis, concluded that to maximize the effects of endurance training on the loss of fat mass, it is necessary prescribing such training at intensities greater than 75% of maximum oxygen consumption [44].

An appropriate strategy to perform endurance training at high intensities is the High Intensity Interval Training (HIIT). This type of training consists of alternating short periods of high and low intensities in the same training session, which allows the training time at high intensities to be higher than during continuous aerobic training [157]. This high intensity training leads to an increase in consumption of post-exercise oxygen [158], which has been associated with a greater mobilization of fatty acids [159]. In turn, nowadays it has been shown that HIIT is a training method as effective as continuous aerobic training to achieve losses of fat mass [160] and can generate greater increases in cardiorespiratory fitness than continuous aerobic training [161]. In addition, HIIT also achieves great improvements in the decrease of glycaemia [162], blood pressure [163, 164] and cholesterolemia [163, 165, 166]. Finally, it should be noted that HIIT achieves all these effects with a 40% less training time than if continuous training was used [160], allowing more time in a session to perform resistance training.

The type of training and the intensities that should be used have already been described, however, it must be determined how long the exercise programme should last. In this point, certain factors must be considered. On the one hand, to work at high intensities, it is necessary for the patient to progressively adapt to the training, with the aim of reducing the risk of injury and favouring adherence to the exercise programme, for which it takes time relatively long. In turn, there are already improvements in physical fitness levels in this population with only 2 months of intervention. However, when using a period of more than 3 months, in addition to improvements in physical fitness, there are improvements in cardiovascular risk factors [84, 146, 167], while a longer duration of the exercise programme can produce greater weight reductions.

Likewise, the following factor that must be considered, the patients awaiting for surgery usually have a very long waiting time. In fact, some studies have determined that it is one of the surgeries with the longest waiting time [168]. In Canada, it has been concluded that patients are on an average of 5 years on the waiting list. In turn, other countries such as Spain conclude that patients are waiting an average of approximately one year to receive bariatric surgery, and that by 68% of patients are more than 6 months awaiting for surgery [169]. This, although it is a point that must be improved, it can be an advantage in the prehabilitation of patients, since it allows enough time to apply an exercise program in which significant improvements can be achieved. For these reasons, it is recommended that the exercise programme has a minimum duration of 3 months, and that it lasts up to 6 months if possible. Finally, it seems that home-based exercise programs are not as effective in generating adherence in patients, so it is important that exercise is supervised, since it has been shown to be more effective than home-based exercise [170, 171].

General recommendations for the exercise programme in patients awaiting surgery based on existing studies on the subject and the latest updates on exercise aimed at weight loss are described below:

- The exercise programme must have a medium-long duration, between 3 and 6 months.

- Start the exercise programme with 2-3 days of training a week to progress up to 4 weekly sessions.
- Resistance training and endurance training must be combined.
- The use of HIIT allows performing resistance and endurance training in the same session.
- Endurance training should be performed at high intensities (> 75% VO_{2max}) to obtain the maximum benefits on body composition. It should start at a low-moderate intensity (40-60% VO_{2peak}) and progress to high intensities (70-80% Vo_{2peak}), when the patient is ready. Perform a minimum volume of 150 minutes per week of moderate exercise, 75 minutes per week of vigorous exercise, or a combination of both. The greater volume of endurance training, the higher loss of fat mass.
- Resistance training should be started at an intensity of 50% of one maximum repetition, performing 4 sets per muscle group and 15-20 repetitions per exercise. It should progress up to 70-80% of the maximum repetition, performing 4 series per muscle group and 8-12 repetitions. Work the large muscle groups.
- Intake a minimum of 1.5 grams per kg of body mass per day, trying to reach 1.8-1.9 grams per kg of body mass per day.

REFERENCES

[1] Church TS, Thomas DM, Tudor-locke C, et al. Trends over 5 Decades in U . S . Occupation-Related Physical Activity and Their Associations with Obesity. *PLoS One*. 2011; 6: 1–7.

[2] Frank LD, Andresen MA, Schmid TL. Obesity Relationships with Community Design, Physical Activity, and Time Spent in Cars. *Am J Prev Med*. 2004; 27: 87–96.

[3] Archer E, Shook RP, Thomas DM, et al. 45-Year Trends in Women ' s Use of Time and Household Management Energy Expenditure. *PLoS One*. 2013; 8: e56620.

[4] Blüher M. Obesity: global epidemiology and pathogenesis. *Nat Rev Endocrinol*. 2019; 15: 288–298.

[5] Juul F, Hemmingsson E. Trends in consumption of ultra-processed foods and obesity in Sweden between 1960 and 2010. *Public Health Nutr.* 2015; 18: 3096–107.

[6] Guyenet SJ, Schwartz MW. Regulation of food intake, energy balance, and body fat mass: Implications for the pathogenesis and treatment of obesity. *J Clin Endocrinol Metab.* 2012; 97: 745–755.

[7] Vasileska A, Rechkoska G. Global and Regional Food Consumption Patterns and Trends. *Procedia-Social Behav Sci.* 2012; 44: 363–369.

[8] Sellen D. Physical status: the use and interpretation of anthropometry. Report of a WHO Expert Committee. *WHO Technical Report* 1995; 854: 1–452.

[9] Bentham J, Di Cesare M, Bilano V, et al. Worldwide trends in body-mass index, underweight, overweight, and obesity from 1975 to 2016: a pooled analysis of 2416 population-based measurement studies in 128□9 million children, adolescents, and adults. *Lancet.* 2017; 390: 2627–2642.

[10] Chooi YC, Ding C, Magkos F. The epidemiology of obesity. *Metabolism.* 2019; 92: 6–10.

[11] Kelly T, Yang W, Chen CS, et al. Global burden of obesity in 2005 and projections to 2030. *Int J Obes.* 2008; 32: 1431–7.

[12] Thomas DM, Weedermann M, Fuemmeler BF, et al. Dynamic model predicting overweight, obesity, and extreme obesity prevalence trends. *Obesity.* 2014; 22: 590–597.

[13] Ng SW, Popkin BM. Time use and physical activity: A shift away from movement across the globe. *Obes Rev.* 2012; 13: 659–680.

[14] FAOSTAT, http://www.fao.org/faostat/en/#data/CC (accessed 29 April 2017).

[15] Caspersen C, Powell K, Christenson G. Physical Activity, Exercise, and Physical Fitness: Definitions and Distinctions for Health-Related Research. *Public Heal Rep.* 1985; 100: 126–131.

[16] Tremblay MS, Aubert S, Barnes JD, et al. Sedentary Behavior Research Network (SBRN) - Terminology Consensus Project process and outcome. *Int J Behav Nutr Phys Act.* 2017; 14: 1–17.

[17] Udo T, Grilo CM. Physical activity levels and correlates in nationally representative sample of U.S. adults with healthy

weight, obesity, and binge-eating disorder. *Int J Eat Disord.* 2020; 53: 85–95.

[18] Carr MM, Lydecker JA, White MA, et al. Examining physical activity and correlates in adults with healthy weight, overweight/obesity, or binge-eating disorder. *Int J Eat Disord.* 2019; 52: 159–165.

[19] Kyle UG, Morabia A, Schutz Y, et al. Sedentarism affects body fat mass index and fat-free mass index in adults aged 18 to 98 years. *Nutrition.* 2004; 20: 255–260.

[20] Ryder JR, Gross AC, Fox CK, et al. Factors associated with long-term weight-loss maintenance following bariatric surgery in adolescents with severe obesity. *Int J Obes.* 2018; 42: 102–107.

[21] Freire RH, Borges MC, Alvarez-Leite JI, et al. Food quality, physical activity, and nutritional follow-up as determinant of weight regain after Roux-en-Y gastric bypass. *Nutrition.* 2012; 28: 53–8.

[22] Chang S, Stoll CRT, Song J, et al. The Effectiveness and Risks of Bariatric Surgery An Updated Systematic Review and Meta-analysis, 2003-2012. *JAMA Surg.* 2014; 149: 275–287.

[23] Angrisani L, Santonicola A, Iovino P, et al. IFSO Worldwide Survey 2016: Primary, Endoluminal, and Revisional Procedures. *Obes Surg.* 2018; 28: 3783–3794.

[24] Livingston EH, Huerta S, Arthur D, et al. Male Gender is a Predictor of Morbidity and Age a Predictor of Mortality for Patients Undergoing Gastric Bypass Surgery. *Ann Surg.* 2002; 236: 576–582.

[25] Nguyen NT, Nguyen B, Smith B, et al. Proposal for a bariatric mortality risk classification system for patients undergoing bariatric surgery. *Surg Obes Relat Dis.* 2013; 9: 239–246.

[26] Perugini R, Mason R, Czerniach D, et al. Predictors of Complication and Suboptimal Weight Loss After Laparoscopic Roux-en-Y Gastric Bypass. *Arch Surg.* 2003; 138: 541–545.

[27] Benotti P, Wood GC, Winegar DA, et al. Risk Factors Associated With Mortality After Roux-en-Y Gastric Bypass Surgery. *Ann Surg.* 2014; 259: 123–30.

[28] Fernandez AZ, Demaria EJ, Tichansky DS, et al. Experience with over 3,000 open and laparoscopic bariatric procedures. *Surg Endosc.* 2004; 18: 193–197.

[29] Quilliot D, Sirveaux MA, Nomine-Criqui C, et al. Evaluation of risk factors for complications after bariatric surgery. *J Visc Surg.* 2018; 155: 201–210.

[30] Martins-filho ED, Ferraz B, Ferraz EM. Evaluation Of Risk Factors In Superobese Patients Submitted To Conventional Fobi-Capella Surgery. *Arq Gastroenterol.* 2008; 45: 3–10.

[31] Sanni A, Perez S, Medbery R, et al. Postoperative complications in bariatric surgery using age and BMI stratification: a study using ACS-NSQIP data. *Surg Endosc.* 2014; 28: 3302–3309.

[32] Martins-Filho ED, Câmara-Neto JB, Ferraz ÁAB, et al. Evaluation of risk factors in superobese patients submitted to conventional Fobi-Capella surgery. *Arq Gastroenterol.* 2008; 45: 3–10.

[33] Coblijn UK, Karres J, Raaff CAL De, et al. Predicting postoperative complications after bariatric surgery : the Bariatric Surgery Index for Complications, BASIC. *Surg Endosc.* 2017; 31: 4438–4445.

[34] Asad M, Roman K, Johnson S, et al. Perioperative risk factors for 30-day mortality after bariatric surgery: is functional status important? *Surg Endosc.* 2013; 27: 1772–1777.

[35] Pate RR. The evolving definition of physical fitness. *Quest.* 1988; 40: 174–179.

[36] Caspersen CJ, Powell KE, Christenson GM. Physical Activity, Exercise, and Physical Fitness: Definitions and Distinctions for Health-Related Research. *Public Heal Rep.* 1985; 100: 126–131.

[37] Husain F, Jeong IH, Spight D, et al. Risk factors for early postoperative complications after bariatric surgery. *Ann Surg Treat Res.* 2018; 95: 94–99.

[38] Benotti PN, Still CD, Wood C, et al. Preoperative Weight Loss Before Bariatric Surgery. *Arch Surg.* 2009; 144: 1150–1155.

[39] Hutcheon DA, Hale AL, Ewing JA, et al. Short-Term Preoperative Weight Loss and Postoperative Outcomes in Bariatric Surgery. *J Am Coll Surg.* 2018; 226: 514–524.

[40] Prado CMM, Wells JCK, Smith SR, et al. Sarcopenic obesity: A Critical appraisal of the current evidence. *Clin Nutr.* 2012; 31: 583–601.

[41] Curvello-silva K, Barreto-medeiros JM. Association between sarcopenic obesity and cardiovascular risk : where are we ? *Nutr Hosp.* 2016; 33: 1245–1255.

[42] Srikanthan P, Hevener AL, Karlamangla AS. Sarcopenia exacerbates obesity-associated insulin resistance and dysglycemia: Findings from the national health and nutrition examination survey III. *PLoS One.*; 5. Epub ahead of print 2010. doi: 10.1371/journal.pone.0010805.

[43] Parr EB, Coffey VG, Hawley JA. 'Sarcobesity': A metabolic conundrum. *Maturitas.* 2013; 74: 109–113.

[44] Clark JE. Diet, exercise or diet with exercise: comparing the effectiveness of treatment options for weight-loss and changes in fitness for adults (18–65 years old) who are overfat, or obese; systematic review and meta-analysis. *J Diabetes Metab Disord.* 2015; 14: 31.

[45] Stiegler P, Cunliffe A. The role of diet and exercise for the maintenance of fat-free mass and resting metabolic rate during weight loss. *Sport Med.* 2006; 36: 239–262.

[46] Wissen J Van, Bakker N, Doodeman HJ. Preoperative Methods to Reduce Liver Volume in Bariatric Surgery : a Systematic Review. *Obes Surg.* 2016; 26: 251–256.

[47] Fris RJ. Preoperative Low Energy Diet Diminishes Liver Size. *Obes Surg.* 2004; 14: 1165–1170.

[48] Martínez-Ramos D, Salvador-Sanchis JL, Escrig-Ros J. Pérdida de peso preoperatoria en pacientes candidatos a cirugía bariátrica. Recomendaciones basadas en la evidencia. *Cir Esp.* 2012; 90: 147–155.

[49] Schwartz ML, Drew RL, Chazin-Caldie M. Laparoscopic Roux-en-Y Gastric Bypass : Preoperative Determinants of Prolonged Operative Times, Conversion to Open Gastric Bypasses, and Postoperative Complications. *Obes Surg.* 2003; 13: 734–738.

[50] Schwartz ML, Drew RL, Chazin- M. Factors Determining Conversion from Laparoscopic to Open Roux-en-Y Gastric Bypass. *Obes Surg.* 2004; 14: 1193–1197.

[51] Farnsworth D, Cannon M. Exercise prescription. In: *The Sports Medicine Resource Manual.* Elsevier Inc., pp. 497–506.

[52] Weisman IM. Clinical Exercise Testing. *Clin Chest Med.* 2001; 22: 366–378.

[53] Pallarés J, Morán-Navarro R. Methodological approach to the Cardiorespiratory Endurance Training. *J Sport Heal Res.* 2012; 4: 119–136.

[54] Moran J, Wilson F, Guinan E, et al. Role of cardiopulmonary exercise testing as a risk-assessment method in patients undergoing intra-abdominal surgery: A systematic review. *Br J Anaesth.* 2016; 116: 177–191.

[55] Agnew N. Preoperative cardiopulmonary exercise testing. *Contin Educ Anaesthesia, Crit Care Pain.* 2010; 10: 33–37.

[56] Piazza O, Miccichè V, Esposito C, et al. Individualised prediction of postoperative cardiorespiratory complications after upper abdominal surgery. *Trends Anaesth Crit Care.* 2016; 6: 11–19.

[57] Shoemaker W, Appel P, Kram H. Role of oxygen debt in the development of organ failure sepsis, and death in high-risk surgical patients. *Chest.* 1992; 102: 208–215.

[58] Smith TB, Stonell C, Purkayastha S, et al. Cardiopulmonary exercise testing as a risk assessment method in non cardio-pulmonary surgery: a systematic review. *Anaesthesia.* 2009; 64: 883–893.

[59] Hennis PJ, Meale PM, Hurst RA, et al. Cardiopulmonary exercise testing predicts postoperative outcome in patients undergoing gastric bypass surgery. *Br J Anaesth.* 2012; 109: 566–571.

[60] McCullough PA, Gallagher MJ, DeJong AT, et al. Cardiorespiratory fitness and short-term complications after bariatric surgery. *Chest.* 2006; 130: 517–525.

[61] Barry VW, Baruth M, Beets MW, et al. Fitness vs. Fatness on All-Cause Mortality: A Meta-Analysis. *Prog Cardiovasc Dis.* 2014; 56: 382–390.

[62] Lavie CJ, McAuley PA, Church TS, et al. Obesity and cardiovascular diseases: Implications regarding fitness, fatness, and severity in the obesity paradox. *J Am Coll Cardiol.* 2014; 63: 1345–1354.

[63] Ortega FB, Lee DC, Katzmarzyk PT, et al. The intriguing metabolically healthy but obese phenotype: Cardiovascular prognosis and role of fitness. *Eur Heart J.* 2013; 34: 389–397.

[64] Moriello C, Mayo NE, Feldman L, et al. Validating the Six-Minute Walk Test as a Measure of Recovery After Elective Colon

Resection Surgery. *Arch Phys Med Rehabil.* 2008; 89: 1083–1089.

[65] Li C, Carli F, Lee L, et al. Impact of a trimodal prehabilitation program on functional recovery after colorectal cancer surgery: A pilot study. *Surg Endosc Other Interv Tech.* 2013; 27: 1072–1082.

[66] Hue O, Berrigan F, Simoneau M, et al. Muscle force and force control after weight loss in obese and morbidly obese men. *Obes Surg.* 2008; 18: 1112–1118.

[67] Handrigan G, Hue O, Simoneau M, et al. Weight loss and muscular strength affect static balance control. *Int J Obes (Lond).* 2010; 34: 936–942.

[68] Gillis C, Carli F. Promoting Perioperative Metabolic and Nutritional Care. *Anesthesiology.* 2015; 123: 1455–1472.

[69] Puthucheary ZA, Rawal J, McPhail M, et al. Acute skeletal muscle wasting in critical illness. *JAMA - J Am Med Assoc.* 2013; 310: 1591–1600.

[70] Kortebein P, Ferrando A, Lombeida J, et al. Effect of 10 Days of Bed Rest on Skeletal Muscle in Healthy Older Adults. *JAMA.* 2007; 297: 1772–1774.

[71] Pišot R, Marusic U, Biolo G, et al. Greater loss in muscle mass and function but smaller metabolic alterations in older compared with younger men following 2 wk of bed rest and recovery. *J Appl Physiol.* 2016; 120: 922–929.

[72] Browning MG, Franco RL, Herrick JE, et al. Assessment of Cardiopulmonary Responses to Treadmill Walking Following Gastric Bypass Surgery. *Obes Surg.* 2017; 27: 96–101.

[73] Sere L, Rodriguez O, Vila J, et al. Increased Exercise Capacity after Surgically Induced Weight Loss in Morbid Obesity.

[74] Livingston EH. Procedure incidence and in-hospital complication rates of bariatric surgery in the United States. *Am J Surg.* 2004; 188: 105–110.

[75] Goergen M, Arapis K, Limgba A, et al. Laparoscopic Roux-en-Y gastric bypass versus laparoscopic vertical banded gastroplasty : results of a 2-year follow-up study. *Surg Endosc.* 2007; 21: 659–664.

[76] Jonathan F, Kole KL, Yenumula PR, et al. Predicting Risk for Serious Complications With Bariatric Surgery Results from the

Michigan Bariatric Surgery Collaborative. *Ann Surg.* 2011; 254: 633–640.

[77] Caiazzo R, Lassailly G, Leteurtre E, et al. Roux-en-Y Gastric Bypass Versus Adjustable Gastric Banding to Reduce Nonalcoholic Fatty Liver Disease. *Ann Surg.* 2014; 260: 893–899.

[78] Machado M, Marques-vidal P, Cortez-pinto H. Hepatic histology in obese patients undergoing bariatric surgery. *J Hepatol.* 2006; 45: 600–606.

[79] Losekann A, Weston AC, Carli LA De, et al. Nonalcoholic fatty liver disease in severe obese patients, subjected to bariatric surgery. *Arq Gastroenterol.* 2013; 50: 285–289.

[80] Reha J, Lee S, Hofmann LJ. Prevalence and predictors of nonalcoholic steatohepatitis in obese patients undergoing bariatric surgery: a Department of Defense experience. *Am Surg.* 2014; 80: 595–599.

[81] Cordeiro L, Campos J, de Paula P, et al. Nonalcoholic steatohepatitis on preoperative period of gastric bypass: lack of correlation with degree of obesity. *Arq Bras Cir Dig.* 2013; 26: 39–42.

[82] Wilms B, Ernst B, Thurnheer M, et al. Differential changes in exercise performance after massive weight loss induced by bariatric surgery. *Obes Surg.* 2013; 23: 365–71.

[83] Seres L, Lopez-Ayerbe J, Coll R, et al. Increased exercise capacity after surgically induced weight loss in morbid obesity. *Obes (Silver Spring).* 2006; 14: 273–279.

[84] Marc-Hernández A, Ruiz-Tovar J, Aracil A, et al. Impact of Exercise on Body Composition and Cardiometabolic Risk Factors in Patients Awaiting Bariatric Surgery. *Obes Surg.* 2019; 1–10.

[85] De Souza SA, Faintuch J, Sant'anna AF. Effect of weight loss on aerobic capacity in patients with severe obesity before and after bariatric surgery. *Obes Surg.* 2010; 20: 871–875.

[86] Fallis A. *Guidelines for Exercise Testing.* Eight. 2013. Epub ahead of print 2013. doi: 10.1017/CBO9781107415324.004.

[87] Berglind D, Willmer M, Tynelius P, et al. Accelerometer-Measured Versus Self-Reported Physical Activity Levels and Sedentary Behavior in Women Before and 9 Months After Roux-en-Y Gastric Bypass. *Obes Surg.* 2016; 26: 1463–1470.

[88] Bond D, Jakicic J, Vithiananthan S, et al. Objective Quantification of Physical Activity in Bariatric Surgery Candidates and Normal-Weight Controls. *Surg Obes Relat Dis.* 2010; 6: 72–78.
[89] Galioto R, King WC, Bond DS, et al. Physical activity and cognitive function in bariatric surgery candidates. *Int J Neurosci.* 2014; 124: 912–918.
[90] Bond DS, Thomas JG, Unick JL, et al. Self-reported and objectively measured sedentary behavior in bariatric surgery candidates. *Surg Obes Relat Dis.* 2013; 9: 123–128.
[91] Bond DS, Unick JL, Jakicic JM, et al. Objective assessment of time spent being sedentary in bariatric surgery candidates. *Obes Surg.* 2011; 21: 811–814.
[92] Rioux B V., Sénéchal M, Kwok K, et al. Association Between Physical Activity Intensity and Physical Capacity Among Individuals Awaiting Bariatric Surgery. *Obes Surg.* Epub ahead of print 2016. doi: 10.1007/s11695-016-2448-x.
[93] Ruiz-Tovar J, Zubiaga L, Llavero C, et al. Serum cholesterol by morbidly obese patients after laparoscopic sleeve gastrectomy and additional physical activity. *Obes Surg.* 2014; 24: 385–9.
[94] King WC, Belle SH, Eid GM, et al. Physical activity levels of patients undergoing bariatric surgery in the Longitudinal Assessment of Bariatric Surgery study. *Surg Obes Relat Dis.* 2008; 4: 721–8.
[95] Freire RH, Borges MC, Alvarez-Leite JI, et al. Food quality, physical activity, and nutritional follow-up as determinant of weight regain after Roux-en-Y gastric bypass. *Nutrition.* 2012; 28: 53–8.
[96] Martínez AS, Martínez-romillo PD, Tarrío FR. Valoración del gasto energético en los niños. Implicaciones fisiológicas y clínicas. Métodos de medición. 2008; 68: 165–180.
[97] Cañada FC, Torres-Luque G, López-Fernández I, et al. Actividad física y acelerometría; orientaciones metodológicas, recomendaciones y patrones. *Nutr Hosp.* 2015; 31: 115–125.
[98] Freedson PS, Melanson E, Sirard J. Calibration of the Computer Science and Applications, Inc. accelerometer. *Medicine and Science in Sports and Exercise* 1998; 30: 777–781.

[99] Hagströmer M, Oja P, Sjöström M. Physical activity and inactivity in an adult population assessed by accelerometry. *Med Sci Sports Exerc.* 2007; 39: 1502–1508.

[100] Doherty A, Jackson D, Hammerla N, et al. Large scale population assessment of physical activity using wrist worn accelerometers: The UK biobank study. *PLoS One.* 2017; 12: 1–14.

[101] Troiano RP, McClain JJ, Brychta RJ, et al. Evolution of accelerometer methods for physical activity research. *Br J Sports Med.* 2014; 48: 1019–1023.

[102] Arvidsson D, Fridolfsson J, Börjesson M. Measurement of physical activity in clinical practice using accelerometers. *J Intern Med.* 2019; 286: 137–153.

[103] Trost SG, Pate RR, Freedson PS, et al. Using objective physical activity measures with youth: How many days of monitoring are needed? *Med Sci Sports Exerc.* 2000; 32: 426–431.

[104] Corder K, Brage S, Ekelund U. Accelerometers and pedometers: Methodology and clinical application. *Curr Opin Clin Nutr Metab Care.* 2007; 10: 597–603.

[105] Tudor-Locke C, Williams JE, Reis JP, et al. Utility of pedometers for assessing physical activity: Construct validity. *Sport Med.* 2004; 34: 281–291.

[106] O'Neill B, McDonough SM, Wilson JJ, et al. Comparing accelerometer, pedometer and a questionnaire for measuring physical activity in bronchiectasis: A validity and feasibility study? *Respir Res.* 2017; 18: 1–10.

[107] Tudor-Locke C, Bassett DR. How Many Steps/Day Are Enough? *Sport Med.* 2004; 34: 1–8.

[108] Tudor-Locke C, Burkett L, Reis JP, et al. How many days of pedometer monitoring predict weekly physical activity in adults? *Prev Med (Baltim).* 2005; 40: 293–298.

[109] Clemes SA, Griffiths PL. How many days of pedometer monitoring predict monthly ambulatory activity in adults? *Med Sci Sports Exerc.* 2008; 40: 1589–1595.

[110] Bond DS, Jakicic JM, Unick JL, et al. Pre- to postoperative physical activity changes in bariatric surgery patients: self report vs. objective measures. *Obesity (Silver Spring).* 2010; 18: 2395–7.

[111] Possmark S, Sellberg F, Willmer M, et al. Accelerometer-measured versus self-reported physical activity levels in women before and up to 48 months after Roux-en-Y Gastric Bypass. *BMC Surg.* 2020; 20: 1–10.
[112] Afshar S, Seymour K, Kelly SB, et al. Changes in physical activity after bariatric surgery: using objective and self-reported measures. *Surg Obes Relat Dis.* 2017; 13: 474–483.
[113] Moya M, Hernández A, Sarabia JM, et al. Bariatric surgery, weight loss and the role of physical activity: a systematic review. *European Journal of Human Movement* 2014; 32: 145–160.
[114] Helou K, El Helou N, Mahfouz M, et al. Validity and reliability of an adapted Arabic version of the long international physical activity questionnaire. *BMC Public Health.* 2017; 18: 1–8.
[115] Craig CL, Marshall AL, Sjöström M, et al. International physical activity questionnaire: 12-Country reliability and validity. *Med Sci Sports Exerc.* 2003; 35: 1381–1395.
[116] Chaudhary S, Kumar S, Kaur B, et al. Guidelines for Data Processing and Analysis of the International Physical Activity Questionnaire (IPAQ). *RSC Adv.* 2016; 6: 90526–90536.
[117] Duren DL, Sherwood RJ, Czerwinski SA, et al. Body composition methods: Comparisons and interpretation. *J Diabetes Sci Technol.* 2008; 2: 1139–1146.
[118] Sizoo D, de Heide LJM, Emous M, et al. Measuring Muscle Mass and Strength in Obesity: a Review of Various Methods. *Obes Surg.* Epub ahead of print 2020. doi: 10.1007/s11695-020-05082-2.
[119] Ayvaz G, Çimen AR. Methods for body composition analysis in adults. *Open Obes J.* 2011; 3: 62–69.
[120] He M, Li ETS, Kung AWC. Dual-energy X-ray absorptiometry for body composition estimation in Chinese women. *Eur J Clin Nutr.* 1999; 53: 933–937.
[121] Faria SL, Faria OP, Cardeal MDA, et al. Validation study of multi-frequency bioelectrical impedance with dual-energy X-ray absorptiometry among obese patients. *Obes Surg.* 2014; 24: 1476–1480.
[122] Alvero Cruz JR, Diego Acosta ÁM, Fernández Pastor VJ, et al. Métodos de evaluación de la composición corporal: tendencias actuales (II). *Arch Med del Deport.* 2005; 105: 45–49.

[123] Widen EM, Strain G, King WC, et al. Validity of Bioelectrical Impedance Analysis for Measuring Changes in Body Water and Percent Fat After Bariatric Surgery. *Obes Surg.* 2014; 24: 847–54.

[124] Savastano S, Belfiore A, Di Somma C, et al. Validity of bioelectrical impedance analysis to estimate body composition changes after bariatric surgery in premenopausal morbidly women. *Obes Surg.* 2010; 20: 332–339.

[125] Kyle UG, Bosaeus I, De Lorenzo AD, et al. Bioelectrical impedance analysis - Part II: Utilization in clinical practice. *Clin Nutr.* 2004; 23: 1430–1453.

[126] Adil MT, Jain V, Rashid F, et al. Meta-analysis of the effect of bariatric surgery on physical function. *Br J Surg.* 2018; 105: 1107–1118.

[127] Lund MT, Hansen M, Wimmelmann CL, et al. Increased post-operative cardiopulmonary fitness in gastric bypass patients is explained by weight loss. *Scand J Med Sci Sports.* 2015; 26: 1428–1434.

[128] Crapo RO, Casaburi R, Coates AL, et al. ATS statement: Guidelines for the six-minute walk test. *Am J Respir Crit Care Med.* 2002; 166: 111–117.

[129] Ross RM, Murthy JN, Wollak ID, et al. The six minute walk test accurately estimates mean peak oxygen uptake. *BMC Pulm Med.*; 10. Epub ahead of print 2010. doi: 10.1186/1471-2466-10-31.

[130] Metz L, Thivel D, Peirrera B, et al. A new equation based on the 6-min walking test to predict VO2peak in women with obesity. *Disabil Rehabil.* 2018; 40: 1702–1707.

[131] Golding L, Sinning W. Y ' s Way to Physical Fitness: The Complete Guide to Fitness Testing and Instruction: YMCA of the USA. *Champaign, Hum Kinet Publ.* 1989; 89–106.

[132] Medicine AC of S. *ACSM's Guidelines for Exercise Testing and Prescription*, http://books.google.com/books?hl=es&lr=&id=hhosAwAAQBAJ&pgis=1 (2013, accessed 16 January 2015).

[133] Miller GD, Nicklas BJ, You T, et al. Physical function improvements after laparoscopic Roux-en-Y gastric bypass surgery. *Surg Obes Relat Dis.* 2009; 5: 530–537.

[134] Norman K, Stobäus N, Gonzalez MC, et al. Hand grip strength: Outcome predictor and marker of nutritional status. *Clin Nutr.* 2011; 30: 135–142.
[135] Otto M, Kautt S, Kremer M, et al. Handgrip Strength as a Predictor for Post Bariatric Body Composition. *Obes Surg.* 2014; 24: 2082–2088.
[136] Smelt HJM, Pouwels S, Celik A, et al. Assessment of physical fitness after bariatric surgery and its association with protein intake and type of cholecalciferol supplementation. *Med.* 2019; 55: 1–9.
[137] Soriano-Maldonado A, Martínez-Forte S, Ferrer-Márquez M, et al. Physical Exercise following bariatric surgery in women with Morbid obesity. *Medicine (Baltimore).* 2020; 99: e19427.
[138] Brzycki M. Strength Testing—Predicting a One-Rep Max from Reps-to-Fatigue. *J Phys Educ Recreat Danc.* 1993; 64: 88–90.
[139] Delgado Floody P, Caamaño Navarrete F, Jerez Mayorga D, et al. Efectos de un programa de tratamiento multidisciplinar en obesos mórbidos y obesos con comorbilidades candidatos a cirugía bariátrica. *Nutr Hosp.* 2015; 31: 2011–2016.
[140] Delgado Floody P, Cofré Lizama A, Alarcón Hormazábal M, et al. Evaluación de un programa integral de cuatro meses de duración sobre las condiciones preoperatorias de pacientes obesos candidatos a cirugía bariátrica. *Nutr Hosp.* 2015; 32: 1022–1027.
[141] Delgado Floody P, Jerez Mayorga D, Caamano Navarrete F, et al. [Effectiveness of Comprehensive Treatment on the Preoperative Conditions of Obese Women Candidates for Bariatric Surgery]. *Nutr Hosp.* 2015; 32: 2570–2575.
[142] Ortega LS, Juan CS, García AA. Valoración de un programa de ejercicio físico estructurado en pacientes con obesidad mórbida pendientes de cirugía bariátrica. *Nutr Hosp.* 2014; 29: 64–72.
[143] Baillot A, Mampuya WM, Comeau E, et al. Feasibility and impacts of supervised exercise training in subjects with obesity awaiting bariatric surgery: A pilot study. *Obes Surg.* 2013; 23: 882–891.
[144] Adair JD, Wollner SB, DaCosta ME, et al. Progressive Resistance Training for Patients with Class III Obesity. *Obes Weight Manag.* 2010; 6: 115–118.
[145] Marcon ER, Baglioni S, Bittencourt L, et al. What Is the Best Treatment before Bariatric Surgery? Exercise, Exercise and

Group Therapy, or Conventional Waiting: a Randomized Controlled Trial. *Obes Surg.* 2016; 27: 763–773.

[146] Marcon ER, Gus I, Neumann CR. Impacto de um programa mínimo de exercícios físicos supervisionados no risco cardiometabólico de pacientes com obesidade mórbida. *Arq Bras Endocrinol Metabol.* 2011; 55: 331–338.

[147] Delgado Floody P, Jerez Mayorga D, Caamaño Navarrete F, et al. Doce semanas de ejercicio físico intervalado con sobrecarga mejora las variables antropométricas de obesos mórbidos y obesos con comorbilidades postulantes a cirugía bariátrica. *Nutr Hosp.* 2015; 32: 2007–2011.

[148] Donnelly JE, Blair SN, Jakicic JM, et al. Appropriate Physical Activity Intervention Strategies for Weight Loss and Prevention of Weight Regain for Adults. *Medicine and Science in Sports and Exercise* 2009; 41: 459–471.

[149] Jakicic J, Marcus B, Gallagher K, et al. Effect of Exercise Duration and Intensity on Weight Loss in Overweight, Sedentary Women. A Randomized Tria. *JAMA.* 2003; 290: 1323–30.

[150] Dixon JB, Lambert EA, Grima M, et al. Fat-free mass loss generated with weight loss in overweight and obese adults: What may we expect? *Diabetes, Obes Metab.* 2015; 17: 91–93.

[151] Cauley JA. An Overview of Sarcopenic Obesity. *J Clin Densitom.* 2015; 18: 499–505.

[152] Willis LH, Slentz CA, Bateman LA, et al. Effects of aerobic and/or resistance training on body mass and fat mass in overweight or obese adults. *J Appl Physiol.* 2012; 113: 1831–7.

[153] Sanal E, Ardic F, Kirac S. Effects of aerobic or combined aerobic resistance exercise on body composition in overweight and obese adults: Gender differences. A randomized intervention study. *Eur J Phys Rehabil Med.* 2013; 49: 1–11.

[154] Park SK, Park JH, Kwon YC, et al. The effect of combined aerobic and resistance exercise training on abdominal fat in obese middle-aged women. *J Physiol Anthropol Appl Human Sci.* 2003; 22: 129–35.

[155] Stiegler P, Cunliffe A. The Role of Diet and Exercise for the Maintenance of Fat-Free Mass and Weight Loss. *Sport Med.* 2006; 36: 239–262.

[156] Campbell W, Haub M, Wolfe R, et al. Resistance Training Preserves Fat-free Mass Without Impacting Changes in Protein Metabolism After Weight Loss in Older Women. *Bone*. 2011; 23: 1–7.

[157] Buchheit M, Laursen PB. High-intensity interval training, solutions to the programming puzzle: Part I: cardiopulmonary emphasis. *Sports Med.* 2013; 43: 313–38.

[158] Laforgia J, Withers RT, Gore CJ. Effects of exercise intensity and duration on the excess post-exercise oxygen consumption. *J Sports Sci.* 2006; 24: 1247–1264.

[159] Børsheim E, Bahr R. Effect of exercise intensity, duration and mode on post-exercise oxygen consumption. *Sport Med.* 2003; 33: 1037–1060.

[160] Wewege M, van den Berg R, Ward RE, et al. The effects of high-intensity interval training vs. moderate-intensity continuous training on body composition in overweight and obese adults: a systematic review and meta-analysis. *Obes Rev.* Epub ahead of print 2017. doi: 10.1111/obr.12532.

[161] Milanović Z, Sporiš G, Weston M. Effectiveness of High-Intensity Interval Training (HIT) and Continuous Endurance Training for VO2max Improvements: A Systematic Review and Meta-Analysis of Controlled Trials. *Sport Med.* 2015; 45: 1469–1481.

[162] Jelleyman C, Yates T, O'Donovan G, et al. The effects of high-intensity interval training on glucose regulation and insulin resistance: A meta-analysis. *Obes Rev.* 2015; 16: 942–961.

[163] Paoli A, Pacelli QF, Moro T, et al. Effects of high-intensity circuit training, low-intensity circuit training and endurance training on blood pressure and lipoproteins in middle-aged overweight men. *Lipids Health Dis.* 2013; 12: 131.

[164] Batacan RB, Duncan MJ, Dalbo VJ, et al. Effects of high-intensity interval training on cardiometabolic health: a systematic review and meta-analysis of intervention studies. *Br J Sports Med.* 2016; 51: 494–503.

[165] Alvarez L, Ramírez-Campillo R, Flores O, et al. Metabolic response to high intensity exercise training in sedentary hyper-glycemic and hypercholesterolemic women. *Rev Med Chil.* 2013; 141: 1293–1299.

[166] Racil G, Ben Ounis O, Hammouda O, et al. Effects of high vs. moderate exercise intensity during interval training on lipids and adiponectin levels in obese young females. *Eur J Appl Physiol.* 2013; 113: 2531–40.

[167] Marcon ER, Baglioni S, Bittencourt L, et al. What Is the Best Treatment before Bariatric Surgery? Exercise, Exercise and Group Therapy, or Conventional Waiting: a Randomized Controlled Trial. *Obes Surg.* 2017; 27: 763–773.

[168] Christou NV., Efthimiou E. Bariatric surgery waiting times in Canada. *Can J Surg.* 2009; 52: 229–234.

[169] Arteaga-González IJ, Martín-Malagón AI, Ruiz de Adana JC, et al. Bariatric Surgery Waiting Lists in Spain. *Obes Surg.* 2018; 28: 3992–3996.

[170] van den Houten MML, Hageman D, Gommans LNM, et al. The Effect of Supervised Exercise, Home Based Exercise and Endovascular Revascularisation on Physical Activity in Patients With Intermittent Claudication: A Network Meta-analysis. *Eur J Vasc Endovasc Surg.* 2019; 58: 383–392.

[171] Hageman D, Fokkenrood HJ, Gommans LN, et al. Supervised exercise therapy versus home-based exercise therapy versus walking advice for intermittent claudication (Review). *Cochrane Database Syst Rev.* 2018; 2018: 88.

In: Enhanced Recovery after Surgery ... ISBN: 978-1-53619-976-5
Editor: Jaime Ruiz-Tovar

Chapter 6

IMMEDIATE PREOPERATIVE ASSESSMENT

Pablo Royo Dachary*[*], *MD, PhD
and Helen Almeida Ponce, MD
Department of Surgery, University of Zaragoza, Zaragoza, Spain

ABSTRACT

An Inmediate Preoperative Assesment could be defined as the set of measures to be taken in the hours prior to any surgical procedure designed to ensure patiens safety as well as comfort. In the singular contex of bariatric patients the urge to take special considerations may deviate this measures from what´s actually the correct evidence-based pathway.

In this chapter we will review two of the available strategies, within health-caregivers control, in the immediate preoperative period: Preoperative fasting, and anxiolytic premedication, analysing why are the wrong decisions taken and stating the correct conducts based on evidence within ERAS protocols frame.

Keywords: preoperative, fasting, ansyolitics

---

* Corresponding Author's Email: prdachary@hotmail.es.

INTRODUCTION

The ultimate goals of preoperative assessment are to reduce the patient´s surgical and anesthetic perioperative morbidity and/or mortality. A preanesthetic evaluation, focusing on risk factors, specially on cardiac and pulmonary condition, is mandatory and should be done before scheduling surgery.

Once the patient has been admitted to the hospital, time for optimization is limited, but it´s still important to ensure that the patient reaches the surgical theatre in the best conditions. In this chapter we will review two of the available strategies, within health-caregivers control, in the immediate preoperative period: Preoperative fasting, and anxiolytic premedication.

PREOPERATIVE FASTING

A Brief History Review… How did We Reach this Point?

Medical breakthroughs are hard to implement, as it usually takes more than ten years since something is statistically demonstrated until it reaches the general practice. The history of preoperative fasting pushes this topic to the limit, as it is taking many years to accept the statistical evidence on preoperative fasting, and it´s hard to predict when updated guidelines recommendations will become a general practice all around the world.

J Roger Maltby (J. Roger Maltby 2006) perfectly captures the essence of how a wrong interpretation became a dogma for anesthesiologist all around the world, creating a stone hard to break for ERAS protocols, despite the wide evidence that can be found in the literature. We recommend Maltby´s paper if the reader wants to expand the knowledge of this subject.

The first book of anaesthesia, published in 1847, did not mention preoperative fasting. The unpleasantness of vomiting during surgery was translated in the advice of carryng it out before breakfast or about the time the patient would be ready for another meal.

Chloroform was first used as anesthetic in 1847 by the Scottish Obstetrician James Young Simpson, but it wasn´t popularized until 1853, when the English physician Sir John Snow used it to assist the eight childbirth of the queen Victoria, during this year, a British soldier in the second Anglo-Burmese war had vomited during surgery, he died soon afterwards and autopsy showed that the trachea was "filled with vomited matters". In 1862 a "new cause of death under chloroform" was first reported in a medical meeting in Edinburgh (Balfour 1862).

In 1883 Sir Joseph Lister, the British surgeon, published in fasting guidelines: "While it is desirable that there should be no solid matter in the stomach when chloroform is administered, it will be found very salutary to give a cup of tea or beef-tea about two hours previously"(Lister 1883). He was the first to distinguish clear fluids from solid food, and this became the standard recommendations for most textbooks until 1960s.

John Alfred Lee wrote in the 4th edition of *A Synopsis of Anaesthesia* that "apart from sweets, food should not be taken during the six hours preceding operation". In the 5th edition, in 1964, he wrote that food and drink should be withheld for 6 hours and added that it was "often wise to order nothing on the day of operation". This recommendation, that ignores the distinction between liquids and solids without a scientific basis, reflects the beginning of a paradigm that still survive nowadays. (Lee)

Some facts could explain the paradigm origins:

Investigations on volume and acidity of gastric remnant resulted in what was known as triple prophylaxis. Magnesium trisilicate or sodium citrate was used routinely to raise gastric fluid pH; H2-receptors blockers such as cimetidine or ranitidine to block gastric acid secretion; and gastrokinetic drugs to stimulate gastric emptying.

In 1977 Hester and Heath (Hester & Heath 1977) incidentally found than fasting for >4h did not influence the volume or pH of gastric fluid at induction of anesthesia. Miller (M. Miller, Wishart, y Nimmo 1983), in 1983, found that a light breakfast <4h before surgery made no significant difference compared with an overnight fast. A new era had begun. There were reasons to doubt the stablished tradition, and the first drinking versus fasting randomized clinical trials were developed in 1985 (J. R. Maltby et al. 1986).

Year	Clinical milestone
1946	Mendelson (Mendelson 1946), obstetrician, New York. Described the Mendelson´s syndrome as the pulmonary damage due to aspirated gastric content during general anaesthesia. Stomach content was found in the lungs of 66 patients in the records of 44.016 pregnancies at the New York Lying-In Hospital from 1932 to 1945. The incidence of Mendelson Syndrome, in a high risk of delayed gastric emptying group, was 0.15%. "*There was a higher incidence of prolonged labor and more than half of the cases required longer administration and greater depth of anesthesia*". Two deaths (0.0045%) occurred in this group because of suffocation from solid food aspiration. The remaining 64 patients experienced aspiration of solid or liquid material but were fully recovered in ten days. Mendelson promoted the "nothing by mouth" and alkalinization and emptying of stomach contents before general anesthesia.
1950s	Multiple anesthetic induction techniques for high-risk patients were developed, differentiating the active vomiting that requires voluntary contraction of muscles, and the passive regurgitation as a gravitational process due to esophageal sphincters relaxation during general anesthesia
1951	Morton and Wylie (Morton y Wylie 1951) studied 43 cases of death resulted from regurgitation or vomiting, although they didn´t mention from how many general anesthesia records. "(...) *in many of the reports there was evidence of inexperience on the part of the anesthetist, inasmuch as precautionary measures were either inadequate, or had not been taken even when clearly indicated*"
1974	The belief that many healthy patients with no risk factors are also at high risk of acid aspiration may have started with the statement by Roberts and Shirley (Roberts y Shirley 1974): "*Our preliminary work in the Rhesus monkeys suggest that 0.4mL/Kg is the maximum acid aspirate that does not produce significant changes in the lung. As this translate to approximately 25ml in the adult human female, we have arbitrarily defined the patient at risk as that patient with at least 25mL of gastric juice of pH below 2.5 in the stomach at the time of delivery*". This affirmation, with important clinical implications, was based on previous research that showed that acid instilled directly on monkey´s bronchus caused pneumonitis (Roberts y Shirley 1980). Investigators didn´t take into account that pH of gastric content can vary considerably based on many factors and, in case of regurgitation, not all the gastric content goes straight into de trachea.

At least twelve clinical trials from 1985 to 1993, showed similar conclusions. Clear liquids are safe until 2 hours before surgery, and even the remnant gastric volume was lower compared to fasting from midnight. Although small milk volume (10ml) behaves as clear liquid and passed unimpeded through pylorus, higher volumes (150ml) produced a solid mass similar to yoghurt, confirming that a glass of milk should not be considered clear liquid. Clinical trials in several countries using similar protocols and gastric aspiration techniques between 1985 and 1993 are summarized in Table 1.

Table 1. "NPO after midnight" versus preoperative clear liquid: residual gastric fluid volume (RGV) and pH. (J. Roger Maltby 2006)

Author and year	Oral intake	Drink on day of surgery		NPO from midnight	
		Fast	RGV (mL)	Fast	RGV mL
Maltby et al. (Canada) 1986	Water 150 mL	2½ hr	18 (0-56)	16½ hr	27 (0-80)
Sutherland et al. (Canada) 1987	Water 150 mL	2½ hr	21 (0-50)	13½ hr	30 (2-75)
Hutchinson et al. (Canada) 1988	Coffee/juice 150 mL	2½ hr	24 (0-96)	14½ hr	23 (0-75)
McGrady and Macdonald (UK) 1988	Water 100 mL	2 hr	17 (4-52)	12 hr	35 (0-58)
Agarwal et al. (India) 1989	Water 150 mL	2½ hr	21 (0-50)	12 hr	30 (0-75)
Scarr et al. (Canada) 1989	Coffee/juice 150 mL	2-3 hr	25 (0-90)	>8 hr	26 (0-120)
Read and Vaughan (UK) 1991	Water no limit	2 hr			
Maltby et al. (Canada) 1991	Coffee/juice No limit	2-3 hr	22 (3-70)	>8 hr	25 (0-107)
Mahiou et al. (France) 1991	Clear liquid 1000 mL	2 hr	38 ±18	11 hr	35 ±15
Lam et al. (Hong Kong) 1993	Water 150 mL	2-3 hr	26 (3-66)	11½ hr	22 (1-78)
Phillips et al. (UK) 1993	Clear liquid, no limit	2¼ hr	21 (0-80)	13 hr	19 (0-63)
Søreide et al. (Norway) 1993	Water 300-450 mL	1½ hr	23 ±20	13 hr	31 ± 30

Values are mean (range) or mean ±SD.

All those Clinical trials didn´t have the desired impact in the daily clinical practice. It was not until 1990 when the first editorials call for a change in the inherited clinical paradigm. The idea of allowing certain liquids before surgery has the purpose of avoiding thirst and patient discomfort, and headache due to abstinence in coffee drinkers. In 1986,

Plourde and Hardy (Plourde y Hardy 1986) demonstrated that the gastric remnant required to produce regurgitation was 21ml/Kg, 20 times higher than the volume estimated by Roberts and Shirley twelve years before.

110 years later, the circle was closed, and the recommendations Lister gave in 1883 were the same that scientific societies began to share in editorials and guides, although with a scientific baseline. Textbooks were slow to change their recommendations, although more extensive sections on gastric physiology were included and results of preoperative oral liquid studies were discussed. The 1990 3rd edition of Miller's Anesthesia mentioned the rapid emptying of clear liquids, and that it did not seem logical to forbid small volumes of liquids before elective surgery in low-risk patients, but concluded that 'NPO for 6-8 h' should probably still apply(Lichtor 1990). Since then, the guides and anesthesia textbooks include all these general recommendations for healthy adults undergoing elective surgery:

- light meal (dry toast and clear liquid) not less than 6 hr before surgery.
- unrestricted clear liquid (water, fruit juice without pulp, carbonated beverages, clear tea, black coffee) until 2 hr before surgery.
- no routine use of gastrointestinal stimulants, gastric acid secretion blockers or oral antacids for healthy patients undergoing elective surgery

However, changes in daily practice are harder to achieve, and after almost 20 years these recommendations are still not followed by a majority of anesthesiologist, maybe due to the defensive medicine overspread during the last century.

Physiology

The stomach is a complex organ that plays an important role in digestion and nutrition, due to its motor, secretory and neuroendocrine function. Saliva production is 1ml/Kg/h and HCl 0.6 ml/Kg/h (Søreide et al. 2005). During fasting period, stomach constantly produces 5-15ml/h of gastric secretion, which results in 40-120ml of acid gastric content after 8 fasting hours.

Fasting

Fasting for 8 hours results in metabolic and hydroelectrolytic alterations, which worsen the preoperative status of the patient and extend hospital stay. This effect is especially important in patients with medical comorbidities, and could ease severe hypotension episodes during anesthetic induction (Henriksen et al. 2003).

Basal glucose consumption during fasting is 2mg/Kg/min, of which brain consumes half (Soop et al. 2001; Soto Moreno y García Luna 2000). A standard 70Kg patient consumes 140mgr/min of glucose, which is what hepatic glycogenolysis could produce. Once hepatic reserves are depleted, some defense mechanisms are activated, which results in insulin resistance, dehydration and hypovolemia.

Insulin Resistance

Stress hormones (glucagon, cortisol and catecholamines) and inflammatory mediators (cytokines, TNF and interleukins 1-6) are released during stress situations, as fasting or surgery. These hormones generate a catabolic response destined to maintain adequate glycemic levels to preserve vital functions. After 12 hours the hepatic glycogen, first and fast glucose reserve of organism, runs out, and other metabolic substrates are consumed (skeletal muscle glycogen, fat free acids, ketone bodies...) which difficult postoperative recovery and extend hospital stay.

To ensure the glucose supply to brain, periphery glucose consumption is deactivated. This is regulated by glucose transporter protein (GLUT). GLUT-1 (brain and erythrocytes) and GLUT-3 (brain) is not regulated by insulin, while GLUT-4 (adipose tissues and striated muscle) needs insulin for its activation. During fasting, GLUT-4 is deactivated to favor the glucose supply to brain, which results in an insulin resistance and a compensatory increase in insulin secretion; same as in type 2 diabetes.

Another GLUT-4 stimulus is muscle contraction, so physical activity improves the use of glucose by skeletal muscle. Insulin and muscle contraction have additive effects on GLUT-4 expression, that´s why bed rest during the postoperative period worsens insulin resistance.

Soop (Soop et al. 2001) demonstrated the importance of adding sugar to clear liquids given preoperatively, not just for the patients well-being (prevention of thirst) but also for the metabolic effect of avoidign insulin resistance. Henriksen (Henriksen et al. 2003) demonstrated that catabolism in patients receiving preoperative polisacarids is diminished, which is evidenced by a lower inhibition of the glycogen synthetase and less loss of quadriceps strength. These benefits were maintained a week and a month after the intervention. Nygren (Nygren, Thorell, y Ljungqvist 2001) observed that hospital stay was reduced by 20%.

Dehydration

Fasting can quickly result in dehydration. Daily water loss for a healthy sedentary man is approximately 2.6 liters; These losses are due to urinary excretion (1.5l), respiratory tract (0.4l), faecium excretion (0.2l) and sudation (0.5l).

Glucagon increase generates natriuresis and polyuria. A 12 hours fasting may generate a deficit of almost 1 liter, which results in dehydration and the need for fluid replacement during anesthesia in addition to increasing the potential for replacing blood lost during the surgical procedure. Dehydration and blood loss during the surgical procedure reduces blood volume and alters drug kinetics, which can lead to more side effects.

Different procedures, as colonic preparation used before colonoscopies or some surgeries, can even worsen the dehydration. Osmotic laxatives used for the preparation (polyethylene-glycol or sodium phosphate) can produce at least 3l of water loss. In those cases, it´s especially important to ingest at least 4 liters of water until 2 hours before the procedure, and it´s important to add carbohydrates to avoid hypoglycemia and insulin resistance.

Dehydration can cause irritability, drowsiness, vertigo, lightheadedness, and hypotension, especially in children and elderly patients. All this, together with the stress generated by a situation and an environment that the patient feels hostile, makes the preoperative period a traumatic situation for the patient, which is, obviously, a bad way to start a postoperative recovery.

Gastric Emptying

The stomach plays many different roles. It functions as food reservoir, expanding 10-15 times its empty state volume without a significant increase in intragastric pressure. The distal corpus and proximal antrum constitute the peristaltic pump that primarily serves as a mixer. The terminal antrum and the pyloric sphincter works as grinder for solid food, and as a filter to allow a controlled delivery of chime into the duodenum (Goyal, Guo, y Mashimo 2019).

Liquids may leave the stomach promptly using the Magenstrasse tunnel, a functional tunnel along the lesser curvature, but solids are little by little released from the corpus to the pyloric region, where the pyloric complex act as a grinder to form the chime. The pylorus only allows the passage to the duodenum of particles smaller than 2-3mm. Liquids and digestible solids are emptied 2-3 hours after a meal. However, large food particles that escape mincing during the digestive period, can be retained in the stomach for long periods, and are force-fully dumped into the small bowel during the inter-digestive period. Figure 1 shows gastric empty rates.

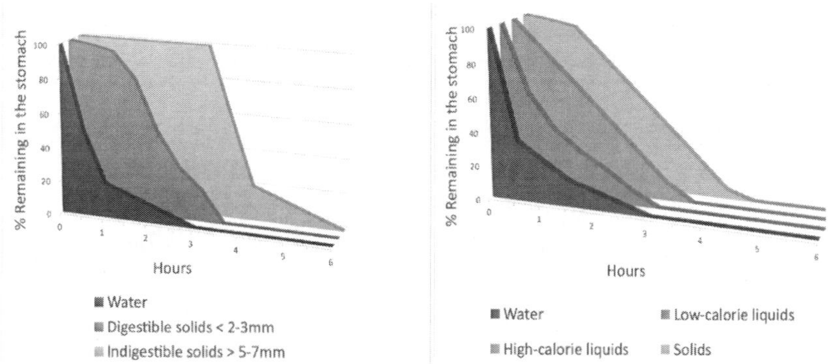

Figure 1. Gastric emptying rates according to physical characteristics and caloric density of food. (a) Effect of physical characteristics on the rate of gastric emptying. Water or 5% glucose leave the stomach at a fast rate. Digestible solids begin to leave after a lag period and leave the stomach slowly. Large pieces of indigestible solids are retained in the stomach during the digestive period and are then rapidly emptied. (b) Effect of caloric density of the liquid meal. Water leaves the stomach very fast and only 50% remains in the stomach at 10 min. Hig-hcalorie liquids empty at a slower rate with 50% remaining in the stomach at 2 h. Low-calorie liquids empty at an intermediate rate so the 50% leave the stomach by 1 h.

Solid gastric emptying depends on several factors: gastric motility, volume ingested, physical characteristic and caloric density of food. Gastric motility can be diminished because of fear, pain, infections, intestinal obstruction, diabetes, etc. Also, the higher the volume or the caloric density, the longer the time for gastric emptying. Regarding food composition, those with high fat content delay their evacuation by duodenal regulation through different hormones: secretin, gastric inhibitory peptide (GIP) and cholecystokinin.

A complete meal, consisting of carbohydrates, proteins, fats, and waste, is completely evacuated from the stomach in about 8 hours. Candies and lollipops are also considered solid, so they must be suspended 8 hours before surgery (Smith et al. 2011). Milk is a liquid food, consisting in proteins and fats in a complex colloidal dispersion, that destabilizes in acid environment, as it occurs in the stomach, forming curds. Gastric emptying times depend on the type of milk considered. Cow's milk and formula are evacuated from the stomach in 6 hours, but breast milk does so in just 4 hours. A light breakfast composed only of carbohydrates and milk is eliminated from the stomach in 6 hours, for example: two cookies, milk, jelly or honey and strained juice. Polysaccharides are emptied from the stomach in 90 minutes, for this reason the addition of sugar, honey or jelly does not alter the established fasting time of 2 hours for clear liquids.

Clear liquids, by definition, is a liquid not containing proteins or fats, such as water, infusions (tea, coffee, mate), synthetic juices and strained fruits (raw and cooked), isotonic drinks (Gatorade, Powerade), gelatin and broth defatted and strained. The emptying of clear liquids is passive, does not require gastric motility and is completed in less than 60 minutes. Clear liquids have a washing effect and drag the gastric content (hydrochloric acid and saliva) towards the duodenum, decreasing its volume and acidity. Lower volumes and gastric acidity were found in patients who did a 2-hour fast of clear liquids than in those who did a complete 8-hour fast, confirming the safety of just 2 hours fasting for clear liquids before a general anesthesia procedure. Volume of clear liquids ingested has no impact on residual gastric volume after 2 hours.

Particularities of Obese Patient

Different situations can cause the gastric emptying to be delayed: obesity, diabetes, gastroesophageal reflux, dysphagia, pancreatic cancer, pregnancy…; but except for achalasia, current fasting guidelines recommendations are fully applicable in all these pathologies.

Obesity and diabetes are generally related, so that the conjunction of both comorbidities is very frequent in the bariatric patient. The rate of gastric emptying is a critical determinant of postprandial glycaemia, and is itself modulated by acute changes in glycaemia (Phillips et al. 2015). Disordered gastric emptying occurs frequently in patients with longstanding diabetes, and gastroparesis, defined as abnormally delayed gastric emptying in the absence of mechanical obstruction, is thought to affect 30–50% of patients with either longstanding type 1 diabetes mellitus (T1DM) or type 2 diabetes mellitus (T2DM). In patients with severe diabetic gastroparesis, pathological changes are highly variable and are characterized by loss of interstitial cells of Cajal and an immune infiltrate.

Diabetic gastroparesis can be classified according to symptom severity. Grade 1 is characterized by intermittent symptoms with no abnormality in nutrition status and can be managed by dietary measures. Patients with moderate changes (grade 2) can be treated with antiemetics and prokinetics. Patients with severe gastroparesis (grade 3) have compromised nutritional state, often require inpatient and emergency care, and endoscopic or operative approaches could be considered as therapy.

Metoclopramide, domperidone, cisapride and erythromicine are some prokinetics available for treatment of gastroparesis (Abell et al. 2006). Most of prokinetics, with also antiemetic effect, have shown some kind of tolerance or tachyphylaxis to the prokinetic effect, but not for antiemetic effect. There should be taken into account that some prokinetics, as erythromicine or cisapride have shown attenuated effect in the setting of hyperglycemia (Jones et al. 1999; Horowitz et al. 2002). Table 2 shows hormones that can affect the gastric emptying.

Table 2. Hormone that causes slow gastric emptying and that cause fast gastric emptying

Slow gastric emptying	Fast gastric emptying
Cholecystokinin	Ghrelin
Leptin	Motilin
Glucagon-like peptide-1	
Glucagon	
Oxynomodulin	
Peptide YY	
Gastric-releasing peptide	
Enterostatin	
Pancreaqtic amylin	
Pancreatic polypeptide	

RECOMMENDATIONS

According to last evidence, recommendations have remained unchanged since last 20 years, despite the lack of adhesion of majority of anesthesiologist and surgeons. In Spain, the RICA guideline in 2007 recommended a preoperative fasting of 2 hours for clear liquids and 6 hours for light meals. The update carried out in 2020, didn´t found changes in bibliographic evidence, and keeps the same recommendations.

> "Regarding preoperative carbohydrate drinks, they improve patient perception and decrease stay, without increasing complications or worsening safety (regurgitation, ...)"

These recommendations can be fully applicable to most bariatric patients, despite the high incidence of diabetic gastroparesis. However, selected cases, with history of clinical symptomatic gastroparesis, should be assessed individually.

ANSYOLITIC PREMEDICATION

Preoperative benzodiazepines are frequently prescribed the night before surgery to relieve preoperative anxiety, although the effect of benzodiazepines on reducing preoperative anxiety remains controversial (Jeon et al. 2018). Some anaesthesiologists might also use benzodiazepine premedication for prevention of intraoperative awareness, induction of sedation, haemodynamic stabilisation, and analgesia. This prescription is frequently due to protocols based on historic tradition, with no distinction of patient characteristics. Recent data in younger patients showed that there is an urge to reconsider the purpose of midazolam premedication (Jeon et al. 2018). Respiratory depression and decreased blood pressure are dose-dependant unwanted effects, but also paradox reactions and anterograde amnesia have been described as unpleasant effects experienced by some patients. Also, incidence of pneumonia with an increased mortality was associated with the intake of benzodiazepines (Chen et al. 2018; Obiora et al. 2013; Sanders et al. 2013). Postoperative delirium (POD) in elderly patients (> 65 years) coud be a serious complication with lethal consequences. Overall, 13–50% of non-cardiac surgical patients experience POD (Inouye, Westendorp, y Saczynski 2014).

In contrast, preoperative anxiety in elderly patients (> 65 years) is not associated with an increased risk for POD. A non-pharmacological treatment of preoperative sleeping disorders and anxiety is recommended in these patients. This is underlined in the American Geriatrics Society guideline for POD in elderly patients, which advises to avoid delirium-causing drugs including benzodiazepines (The American Geriatrics Society Expert Panel on Postoperative Delirium in Older Adults 2015).

A Cochrane analysis showed similar discharge time between patients with premedication compared to placebo in day case surgery, although this analysis failed to report efficacy (Walker y Smith 2009). A randomized controlled trial is actually trying to justify the waiving of indiscriminate premedication with benzodiazepines in elderly patients (Kowark et al. 2019), but we still have to wait until first results are published.

Premedication of surgical patients with benzodiazepines has become questionable regarding risk-benefit ratio and lack of evidence. Though preoperative benzodiazepines might alleviate preoperative anxiety, a higher risk for adverse events is described, particularly for elderly patients (≥ 65 years).

Recently, Goretti et al. (Goretti et al. 2020) published the implementation of ERAS recommendations, associated to Value-Based Healthcare strategy (VBHC), in a high-volume bariatric center in Italy. The Standardized anesthetic protocol included dexmedetomidine infusion for premedication, with no other anxiolytic medication prior to surgery, concluding that "*building a caring relationship by a multidisciplinary team, adding patient wellness in a VBHC framework on top of ERAS as a patient-centered approach, increases patients' adherence to the pathway of care, resulting in better health outcomes*"

Actual Guidelines

Spanish RICA guideline points that use of long duration sedatives as opioids or benzodiazepines, preoperatively, prevents an early recovery, causing a delay in mobilization and oral tolerance, and increasing hospital stay. Short duration anxiolytics could interfere in recovery, but with no interference in hospital stay, so they are a valid alternative to ease the performance of regional anesthesia techniques.

Last review of ERAS protocols also recommend to avoid sedative medications as premedication, prioritizing the patient education as measure to diminish the stress of the patient.

This recommendation has been unchanged during last years due to lack of new evidence or quality studies.

References

Abell, T. L., Bernstein, R. K., Cutts, T., Farrugia, G., Forster, J., Hasler, W. L., McCallum, R. W., et al. (2006). "Treatment of Gastroparesis: A Multidisciplinary Clinical Review". *Neurogastroenterology and Motility: The Official Journal of the European Gastrointestinal Motility*

Society, *18* (4), 263-83. https://doi.org/10.1111/j.1365-2982.2006.00760.x.

Balfour, G. (1862). *"New cause of death by chloroform"*, *8*, 194-95.

Chen, Tien-Yu, John W. Winkelman, Wei-Chung Mao, Chia-Lin Liu, Chung-Yao Hsu. & y Chi-Shin Wu. (2018). "The Use of Benzodiazepine Receptor Agonists and the Risk of Hospitalization for Pneumonia: A Nationwide Population-Based Nested Case-Control Study". *Chest*, *153* (1), 161-71. https://doi.org/10.1016/j.chest.2017.07.030.

Goretti, Giulia, Giuseppe M. Marinari, Elena Vanni. & y Chiara Ferrari. (2020). "Value-Based Healthcare and Enhanced Recovery After Surgery Implementation in a High-Volume Bariatric Center in Italy". *Obesity Surgery*, *30* (7), 2519-27. https://doi.org/10.1007/s11695-020-04464-w.

Goyal, Raj K., Yanmei Guo. & y Hiroshi Mashimo. (2019). "Advances in the Physiology of Gastric Emptying". *Neurogastroenterology & Motility*, *31* (4), e13546. https://doi.org/10.1111/nmo.13546.

Henriksen, M. G., Hessov, I., Dela, F., Vind Hansen, H., Haraldsted, V. & Rodt, y. S. Å. (2003). "Effects of Preoperative Oral Carbohydrates and Peptides on Postoperative Endocrine Response, Mobilization, Nutrition and Muscle Function in Abdominal Surgery: Effects of Preoperative Oral Carbohydrates". *Acta Anaesthesiologica Scandinavica*, *47* (2), 191-99. https://doi.org/10.1034/j.1399-6576.2003.00047.x.

Hester, J. B. & Heath, y. M. L. (1977). "Pulmonary Acid Aspiration Syndrome: Should Prophylaxis Be Routine?" *British Journal of Anaesthesia*, *49* (6), 595-99. https://doi.org/10.1093/bja/49.6.595.

Horowitz, Michael, Karen L. Jones, Philip E. Harding. & y Judith M. Wishart. (2002). "Relationship between the Effects of Cisapride on Gastric Emptying and Plasma Glucose Concentrations in Diabetic Gastroparesis". *Digestion*, *65* (1), 41-46. https://doi.org/10.1159/000051930.

Inouye, Sharon K., Rudi G. J. Westendorp. & y Jane S. Saczynski. (2014). "Delirium in Elderly People". *Lancet* (London, England), *383*, (9920), 911-22. https://doi.org/10.1016/S0140-6736(13)60688-1.

Jeon, Soeun, Hyeon-Jeong Lee, Wangseok Do, Hae-Kyu Kim, Jae-Young Kwon, Boo Young Hwang. & y Jihwan Yun. (2018).

"Randomized Controlled Trial Assessing the Effectiveness of Midazolam Premedication as an Anxiolytic, Analgesic, Sedative, and Hemodynamic Stabilizer". *Medicine*, *97* (35), e12187. https://doi.org/10.1097/MD.0000000000012187.

Jones, K. L., Berry, M., Kong, M. F., Kwiatek, M. A., Samsom, M., Horowitz, y. M. (1999). "Hyperglycemia Attenuates the Gastrokinetic Effect of Erythromycin and Affects the Perception of Postprandial Hunger in Normal Subjects". *Diabetes Care*, *22* (2), 339-44. https://doi.org/10.2337/diacare.22.2.339.

Kowark, Ana, Rolf Rossaint, András P. Keszei, Petra Bischoff, Michael Czaplik, Berthold Drexler, Peter Kienbaum., et al. (2019). "Impact of PReOperative Midazolam on OuTcome of Elderly Patients (I-PROMOTE): Study Protocol for a Multicentre Randomised Controlled Trial". *Trials*, *20* (1), 430. https://doi.org/10.1186/s13063-019-3512-3.

Lichtor, J. L. (1990). "Psychological Preparation and Preoperative Medication". En *Miller´s anesthesia*, de RD Miller, 3rd ed., 895-928. Philadelphia: Churchill Livingstone.

Lister, J. (1883). "A system of surgery". En *Anaesthetics*, de T Holmes. London: Longmans Green and Co.

Maltby, J. R., Sutherland, A. D., Sale, J. P. & Shaffer, y E. A. (1986). "Preoperative Oral Fluids: Is a Five-Hour Fast Justified Prior to Elective Surgery?" *Anesthesia and Analgesia*, *65* (11), 1112-16.

Maltby, J. Roger. (2006). "Fasting from Midnight--the History behind the Dogma". *Best Practice & Research. Clinical Anaesthesiology*, *20* (3), 363-78. https://doi.org/10.1016/j.bpa.2006.02.001.

Mendelson, C. L. (1946). "The Aspiration of Stomach Contents into the Lungs during Obstetric Anesthesia". *American Journal of Obstetrics and Gynecology*, *52* (agosto), 191-205. https://doi.org/10.1016/s0002-9378(16)39829-5.

Miller, M., Wishart, H. Y. & Nimmo, y. W. S. (1983). "Gastric Contents at Induction of Anaesthesia. Is a 4-Hour Fast Necessary?" *British Journal of Anaesthesia*, *55* (12), 1185-88. https://doi.org/10.1093/bja/55.12.1185.

Morton, H. J. V. & Wylie, y. W. D. (1951). "Anaesthetic Deaths Due to Regurgitation or Vomiting". *Anaesthesia*, *6* (4), 190-201; passim. https://doi.org/10.1111/j.1365-2044.1951.tb01388.x.

Nygren, J., Thorell, A. & Ljungqvist, y. O. (2001). "Preoperative Oral Carbohydrate Nutrition: An Update". *Current Opinion in Clinical Nutrition and Metabolic Care, 4* (4), 255-59. https://doi.org/10.1097/00075197-200107000-00002.

Obiora, Eneanya, Richard Hubbard, Robert D. Sanders. & y Puja R. Myles. (2013). "The Impact of Benzodiazepines on Occurrence of Pneumonia and Mortality from Pneumonia: A Nested Case-Control and Survival Analysis in a Population-Based Cohort". *Thorax, 68* (2), 163-70. https://doi.org/10.1136/thoraxjnl-2012-202374.

Phillips, Liza K., Adam M. Deane, Karen L. Jones, Chris K. Rayner. & y Michael Horowitz. (2015). "Gastric Emptying and Glycaemia in Health and Diabetes Mellitus". *Nature Reviews. Endocrinology, 11* (2), 112-28. https://doi.org/10.1038/nrendo.2014.202.

Plourde, G. & Hardy, y. J. F. (1986). "Aspiration Pneumonia: Assessing the Risk of Regurgitation in the Cat". *Canadian Anaesthetists' Society Journal, 33* (3 Pt 1), 345-48. https://doi.org/10.1007/BF03010748.

Roberts, R. B. & Shirley, y. M. A. (1974). "Reducing the Risk of Acid Aspiration during Cesarean Section". *Anesthesia and Analgesia, 53* (6), 859-68. https://doi.org/10.1213/00000539-197453060-00010.

Roberts, R. B. & Shirley, y. M. A. (1980). "Antacid Therapy in Obstetrics". *Anesthesiology, 53* (1), 83. https://doi.org/10.1097/00000542-198007000-00025.

Sanders, Robert D., Alexandra Godlee, Toshifumi Fujimori, John Goulding, Gang Xin, Samira Salek-Ardakani, Robert J. Snelgrove, Daqing Ma, Mervyn Maze. & y Tracy Hussell. (2013). "Benzodiazepine Augmented γ-Amino-Butyric Acid Signaling Increases Mortality From Pneumonia in Mice*": *Critical Care Medicine, 41* (7), 1627-36. https://doi.org/10.1097/CCM.0b013e31827c0c8d.

Smith, Ian, Peter Kranke, Isabelle Murat, Andrew Smith, Geraldine O'Sullivan, Eldar Søreide, Claudia Spies, Bas in't Veld. & y European Society of Anaesthesiology. (2011). "Perioperative Fasting in Adults and Children: Guidelines from the European Society of Anaesthesiology". *European Journal of Anaesthesiology, 28* (8), 556-69. https://doi.org/10.1097/EJA.0b013e3283495ba1.

Soop, M., Nygren, J., Myrenfors, P., Thorell, A. & Ljungqvist, y. O. (2001). "Preoperative Oral Carbohydrate Treatment Attenuates Immediate Postoperative Insulin Resistance". *American Journal of Physiology. Endocrinology and Metabolism, 280* (4), E576-583. https://doi.org/10.1152/ajpendo.2001.280.4.E576.

Søreide, E., Eriksson, L. I., Hirlekar, G., Eriksson, H., Henneberg, S. W., Sandin, R. & Raeder, J. y. (2005). (Task Force on Scandinavian Pre-operative Fasting Guidelines, Clinical Practice Committee Scandinavian Society of Anaesthesiology and Intensive Care Medicine). "Pre-Operative Fasting Guidelines: An Update". *Acta Anaesthesiologica Scandinavica, 49* (8), 1041-47. https://doi.org/10.1111/j.1399-6576.2005.00781.x.

Soto Moreno, A. M. & García Luna, y. P. P. (2000). "Respuesta endocrino-metabólica en el ayuno prolongado". En *Nutrición CLínica. Bases y fundamentos*, de A Miján de la Torre, 67-71. Madrid: Doyma.

The American Geriatrics Society Expert Panel on Postoperative Delirium in Older Adults. (2015). "American Geriatrics Society Abstracted Clinical Practice Guideline for Postoperative Delirium in Older Adults". *Journal of the American Geriatrics Society, 63* (1), 142-50. https://doi.org/10.1111/jgs.13281.

Walker, Kevin J. & y Andrew F. Smith. (2009). "Premedication for Anxiety in Adult Day Surgery". *The Cochrane Database of Systematic Reviews*, n.º 4 (octubre), CD002192. https://doi.org/10.1002/14651858.CD002192.pub2.

In: Enhanced Recovery after Surgery ... ISBN: 978-1-53619-976-5
Editor: Jaime Ruiz-Tovar

Chapter 7

ANTIBIOTIC AND ANTITHROMBOTIC PROPHYLAXIS IN BARIATRIC SURGERY

Andrés García-Marín[1,2,*], MD, PhD and Mercedes Pérez-López[3]

[1]Department of Surgery, Hospital de Hellín, Albacete, Spain
[2]Medicine, University Alfonso X El Sabio, Madrid, Spain
[3]Department of Nursery, Hospital San Vicente del Raspeig, Alicante, Spain

ABSTRACT

Obesity is a significant risk factor for surgical site infection. Antibiotic prophylaxis in bariatric procedures has not been adequately evaluated. Obesity is associated with an increased risk of thromboembolic events. Venous thromboembolisms are the most common postoperative medical complications after bariatric surgery. Moreover, most bariatric procedures actually are performed by laparoscopic approach, implying an increased intraabdominal pressure during the surgical procedure that may favor the development of thrombus. The chapter summarizes the recent evidence about microbiology, recommended antibiotics, dosages and other routes of administration in obese and morbidly

[*] Corresponding Author's Email: agmarin1980@gmail.com.

obese patients undergoing bariatric procedures, as well as the recommendations about primary prophylaxis of thromboembolic events.

Keywords: bariatric surgery, surgical site infection, antibiotic prophylaxis, thromboembolic prophylaxis

INTRODUCTION

According to the World Health Organization, there are 1.6 billion overweight and 400 million obese people worldwide. Bariatric surgery has demonstrated to be the most effective and sustainable method for the regulation of morbid obesity, superior to both pharmaceutical interventions and combinations of diet and lifestyle regimens. Therefore, the number of bariatric procedures performed, mainly in developed countries, is increasing every year. Obesity is associated with an increased risk of surgical site infection and thromboembolic events [1, 2].

ANTIBIOTIC PROPHYLAXIS

Obesity is considered a risk factor for surgical site infection independently of other comorbidities and, specifically in clean and clean-contaminated abdominal procedures, so antibiotic prophylaxis is always needed in laparoscopic and open bariatric procedures [1-6]. The goal of antimicrobial prophylaxis is to control bacterial burden maintaining antibiotic levels above the minimum inhibitory concentration of the bacteria throughout the procedure.

General principles are: A) Intravenous administration. B) Antibiotic: narrower-spectrum agents to cover the typical microorganisms, bactericidal activity, extended half life, good tissue distribution and low adverse effects. C) Posology: maximum dose, 30 - 60 minutes before the start of the procedure with special attention to intraoperative redosing [1, 3]. The main involved microorganisms in bariatric procedures are gram-positive cocci (*Staphylococcus spp.*, *Streptococcus spp.* and, less frequently, *Enterococcus spp.*) and, in the case of gastrointestinal anastomosis, gram-negative bacilli (*Escherichia coli, Proteus spp., Klebsiella spp.*) and anaerobes (*Bacteroides spp.*) are included [3, 7].

Antibiotic and Dosages

The recommended antibiotic depends on the bariatric procedure. For surgeries above the duodenum, cefazolin and, in patients with β-lactam allergies, vancomycin and gentamicin, clindamycin and gentamicin or levofloxacin are preferred. For surgeries below the duodenum, amoxicillin-clavulanic and, in patients with β-lactam allergies, moxifloxacin, levofloxacin and metronidazole or gentamicin and metronidazole are preferred [1, 3, 8].

The alteration in body composition in obese patients involves a higher risk of erroneous dosing and, therefore, a possible therapeutic failure or toxicity. There is a little pharmacokinetic and pharmacodynamic evidence related to the optimal dose in bariatric procedures [3, 9]. The main parameters for doses calculation are:

a) Body mass index (BMI): weight (kg)/height (meters)^2.
b) Ideal weight: Men: 50 + 0.9 x [height (centimeters) – 152]. Women: 45.5 + 0.9 x [height (centimeters) – 152].
c) Adjusted weight: corrective factor x (total weight – ideal weight) + ideal weight. Corrective factor represents the percentage of excess of weight in which antibiotic is estimated to be distributed and varies between 0.25 – 0.4 [3].

Suggested initial dose and time to redosing for recommended antibiotics would be:

a) Cefazolin and amoxicillin-clavulanic: 2gr., with dose repetition if the surgery lasts more than 3 - 4 hours. There are different studies related to the assessment of the adequate antibiotic prophylaxis. Anlicoara et al. described a higher concentration of cefazolin in adipose tissue with 2gr preoperative followed by continuous infusion of 1gr diluted in 250ml of saline solution, above the minimum inhibitory concentration of the main causal agents of the SSI [10], whereas Chen et al. have reported cefazolin protective levels in serum and adipose tissue with a 2gr., and they concluded that neither high dose of cefazolin (3 - 4gr.) nor intraoperative redosing are necessary [11].

b) Gentamicin: 5 - 7mg/kg of adjusted weight with a corrective factor of 0.47. Dose repetition is not required [3].
c) Vancomycin: 15mg/kg of total weight (maximum dose 2gr.). Dose repetition is not required [3, 12].
d) Clindamycin: 900 - 1200 (BMI ≥ 50)mg., with dose repetition if the surgery lasts more than 6 hours [1, 2].
e) Quinolones: maximum doses, levofloxacin 500 - 750 (BMI ≥ 50)mg. and moxifloxacin 800mg [1, 3].
f) Metronidazole: 15mg/kg of total weight. Dose repetition is not required.
g) Cefoxitin. Brunetti et al. evaluated plasma and adipose tissue concentrations of cefoxitin after preoperative standard dose (2gr.) in 6 patients undergoing sleeve gastrectomy and they described subtherapeutic concentrations in subcutaneous tissue at the time of closure so they recommend more studies to define the appropriate dosage [13]. Moine et al. described that weight-based dosing regimen (40mg/kg of total weight) was better than fixed dose, although the desired pharmacodynamic targets were suboptimal in serum and subcutaneous tissue, so more studies are needed [14].
h) Ertapenem. Borracci et al. evaluated the standard dose of 1gr of ertapenem in 10 female patients undergoing bariatric surgery and they concluded that it may not provide optimal clinical levels to prevent surgical site infection [15].

Other Routes of Administration

The application of topical, subcutaneous and intraperitoneal antibiotics has also been studied. Peritoneal lavage with antibiotic solution has been used by many surgeons in abdominal surgery to reduce the bacterial load and possibly minimize the risk of surgical site infection [16]. Ruiz-Tovar et al. performed a randomized clinical trial comparing peritoneal lavage with antibiotic solution (gentamicin 240mg. – clindamycin 600mg. dissolved in 500ml. of physiologic saline) versus physiologic saline after laparoscopic sleeve gastrectomy and they described a significant reduction in peritoneal contamination, inflammatory markers, post-operative pain and a shorter length of hospital stay in the group of antibiotic solution. More studies with a higher sample size are needed to obtain significant conclusions about SSI with peritoneal lavage with antibiotic solution [17]. Alexander et al. evaluated the infusion of kanamycin solution 0.1% into the subcutaneous at the time of closure in 837 patients undergoing open bariatric procedures in addition to standard intravenous prophylaxis. Surgical site infection developed in subcutaneous tissues of 0.72% of patients and they concluded that prolonged contact with kanamycin solution reduced surgical site infection in the deep subcutaneous space. However, no control group was included in the study, so more studies are needed to evaluate the use of topical solutions and the surgical site infection [18].

ANTITHROMBOTIC PROPHYLAXIS

Venous thromboembolism is the most common postoperative medical complication after bariatric surgery. The incidence of deep vein thrombosis after laparoscopic bariatric surgery is about 3% and that of pulmonary embolism is less than 1%. However, mortality associated with PE is estimated to be between 50% and 75% [19-21].

Obesity itself is associated with an increased risk of thromboembolic events. It has been determined that obesity is associated with a hypercoagulability status. Morbidly obese patients present increased fibrinogen levels that may reach twofold the normal value. It has been proved that venous circulation flow is slower in the infradiaphragmatic territory and especially in the lower limbs. Both facts, associated with disorders in several coagulation factors, favor the appearance of venous thrombosis, thrombophlebitis, and thromboembolic events, mainly pulmonary thromboembolisms, which are the first cause of mortality in obese patients. Venous stasis and hypercoagulability improve with weight loss, mostly after bariatric surgery. This improvement is achieved several months after the surgical procedure, when an important weight reduction has been obtained. More than 90% of patients undergoing any bariatric procedure present a relevant reduction of their hypercoagulability [21-25].

Moreover, most bariatric procedures are actually performed by a laparoscopic approach, implying an increased intraabdominal pressure during the surgical procedure that may favor the development of thrombus. In laparoscopic abdominal surgery, the increase of intraabdominal pressure by the pneumoperitoneum, the prolonged operation time, and the anti-Trendelenburg position are considered risk factors for venous thromboembolisms. Moreover, hypercapnia induces vasoconstriction.

It has been also demonstrated that surgical dissection induces the release of procoagulant cytokines. Other causes of venous thromboembolism after bariatric surgery is dehydration, especially after restrictive procedures, when patients hardly drink [26].

Primary Prophylaxis

Venous thromboembolisms are life-threatening conditions. Several measures, including prophylactic low molecular weight heparins and compressive stockings, are adopted to reduce their incidence.

Up to the present there is no consensus about the optimal dosage of low molecular weight heparins in the antithromboembolic prophylaxis for patients undergoing bariatric surgery. The dosage must be adjusted according to the weight of the patient, implying the need of administration of high preoperative doses. Intra- and postoperative bleeding is one of the main complications of bariatric surgery. Many surgeons fear these complications and administer lower doses of lower molecular weight heparins than that recommended by most groups (Enoxaparin 0.5mg/kg/day or Bemiparin 5000UI/day or Dalteparin 50UI/kg/day or Nadroparin 4100UI/day) [27-29]. However, other authors report that this dose is insufficient because these patients are at high risk of developing thrombotic events [30-36].

The postoperative prolongation of prophylaxis is also a debated issue as some authors defend that a prolongation of 5 – 7 days is enough, whereas others report the need for maintaining it during 1 month, considering laparoscopic bariatric surgery as a high-risk procedure performed in high-risk patients [37-39]. In our opinion, a preoperative dose of 0.5mg/kg/day administered 12h before surgery and maintained postoperatively for 1 month is an adequate scheme for pharmacological antithromboembolic prophylaxis. We also fear intraoperative bleeding, but at these doses, it is not especially relevant in our experience. However, a postoperative thromboembolic event is a life-threatening condition for us that, once established, could be very difficult to manage.

Compression stockings must be maintained during the surgical event and postoperatively until the patient is able to make a proper ambulation [40, 41].

Secondary Prophylaxis: Screening for Asymptomatic Venous Thromboembolism

As has already been mentioned, venous thromboembolisms are asymptomatic in many cases. In deep vein thrombosis it is especially important to achieve an early diagnosis to avoid the development of life-threatening conditions, such as pulmonary embolism. With this aim, our group performed a prospective observational study of 100 consecutive patients undergoing laparoscopic sleeve gastrectomy as a bariatric procedure. Deep vein thrombosis and porto-spleno-mesenteric vein thrombosis were investigated 3 months after surgery with Doppler ultrasound and contrast-enhanced abdominal computed tomography scan.

The results of this study revealed that 2% presented unnoticed deep vein thrombosis and 1% unnoticed porto-spleno-mesenteric vein thrombosis.

All these patients were asymptomatic. According to these results, we concluded that a routine postoperative screening with Doppler ultrasound or contrast-enhanced computed tomography seems to be unnecessary [42].

REFERENCES

[1] Chopra, T., Zhao, J., Alangaden, G., Wood, M., Kaye, K. Preventing surgical site infections after bariatric surgery: Value of perioperative antibiotics regimens. *Expert Rev. Pharmacoecon. Outcomes Res.,* 2010; 10:317 - 28.

[2] Winfield, R. D., Reese, S., Bochicchio, K., Mazuski, J. E., Bochicchio, G. V. Obesity and the risk for surgical site infection in abdominal surgery. *Am. Surg.,* 2016; 82:331 - 6.

[3] Badía Pérez, J. M., Arroyo García, N., Guirao Garriga, X. Profilaxis antibiótica en cirugía [Antibiotic prophylaxis in surgery]. En: Badía Pérez, J. M., Guirao Garriga, X. *Infecciones quirúrgicas.* 2ª ed. Madrid: Arán Ediciones SL; 2016. p. 179 - 205.

[4] Sauerland, S., Angrisani, L., Belachew, M., Chevallier, J. M., Favretti, F., Finner, N. et al. Obesity surgery: Evidence-based guidelines of the European Association for Endoscopic Surgery (EAES). *Surg. Endosc.,* 2005; 19:200 - 21.

[5] Aktas, A., Kayaalp, C., Gunes, O., Kirkil, C., Tardu, A., Can Aydin, M. et al. Surgical site infections after laparoscopic bariatric surgery: Is routine antibiotic prophylaxis required? *Surg. Infect.,* (Larchmt). 2021; [epub ahead of print].

[6] Dang, J., Szeto, V., Elnahas, A., Ellsmere, J., Okrainec, A., Neville, A. et al. Canadian consensus statement: Enhanced recovery after surgery in bariatric surgery. *Surg. Endosc.,* 2020; 34:1366 - 75.

[7] Martín García-Almenta, E., Ruiz-Tovar Polo, J., Sánchez Santos, R. Vía clínica en cirugía bariátrica [Clinical pathway in bariatric surgery]. Albacete: Asociación Española de Cirujanos; 2017.

[8] Fischer, M. I., Dias, C., Stein, A., Meinhardt, N. G., Heineck, I. Antibiotic prophylaxis in obese patients submitted to bariatric surgery. A systematic review. *Acta Cir. Bras.,* 2014; 29:209 - 17.

[9] Freeman, J. T., Anderson, D. J., Hartwig, M. G., Sexton, D. J. Surgical site infections following bariatric surgery in community hospitals: A weighty concern? *Obes. Surg.,* 2011; 21:836 - 40.

[10] Anlicoara, R., Ferraz, A. A., da P. Coelho, K., de Lima Filho, J. L., Siqueira, L. T., de Araujo, J. G. et al. Antibiotic prophylaxis in bariatric surgery with continuous infusion of cefazolin:

Determination of concentration in adipose tissue. *Obes. Surg.,* 2014; 24:1487 - 91.

[11] Chen, X., Brathwaite, C. E., Barkan, A., Hall, K., Chu, G., Cherasard, P. et al. Optimal cefazolin prophylactic dosing for bariatric surgery: No need for higher doses or intraoperative redosing. *Obes. Surg.,* 2017; 27:626 - 9.

[12] Rybak, M. J., Lomaestro, B. M., Rotschafer, J. C., Moellering, R. C., Craig, W. A., Billeter, M. et al. Vancomycin therapeutic guidelines: a summary of consensus recommendations from the infectious diseases Society of America, the American Society of Health-System Pharmacists and the Society of Infectious Diseases Pharmacists. *Clinc. Infect. Dis.,* 2009; 49:325 - 7.

[13] Brunetti, L., Kagan, L., Forrester, G., Aleksunes, L. M., Lin, H., Buyske, S., Nahass, R. G. Cefoxitin plasma and subcutaneous adipose tissue concentration in patients undergoing sleeve gastrectomy. *Clin. Ther.,* 2016; 38:204 - 10.

[14] Moine, P., Mueller, S. W., Schoen, J. A., Rothchild, K. B., Fish, D. N. Pharmacokinectic and pharmacodynamic evaluation of a weightbased dosing regimen of cefoxitin for perioperative surgical prophylaxis in obese and morbidly obese patients. *Antimicrob. Agents Chemother.,* 2016; 60:5885 - 93.

[15] Borracci, T., Adembri, C., Accetta, G., Berti, J., Cappellini, I., Lucchese, M. et al. Use of the parenteral antibiotic ertapenem as short term prophylaxis in bariatric surgery: a pharmaco-kinetic-pharmacodynamic study in class III obese female patients. *Minerva Anestesiol.*, 2014; 80:1005 - 11.

[16] Williams, M. D., Champion, J. K. Experience with routine intraabdominal cultures during laparoscopic gastric bypass with implications for antibiotic prophylaxis. *Surg. Endosc.,* 2004; 18: 755 - 6.

[17] Ruiz-Tovar, J., Llavero, C., Muñoz, J. L., Zubiaga, L., Díez, M. Obelche Group. Effect of peritoneal lavage with clindamycin-gentamicin solution on postoperative pain and analytic acute-phase reactants after laparoscopic sleeve gastrectomy. *Surg. Infect.*, (Larchmt), 2016; 17:357 - 62.

[18] Alexander, J. W., Rahn, R., Goodman, H. R. Prevention of surgical site infections by an infusion of topical antibiotics in morbidly obese patients. *Surg. Infect.,* (Larchmt), 2009; 10:53 - 7.

[19] Stroh, C., Birk, D., Flade-Kuthe, R., Frenken, M., Herbig, B., Höhne, S. et al. Evidence of thromboembolism prophylaxis in bariatric surgery: Results of a quality assurance trial in bariatric surgery in Germany from 2007 to 2007 and review of literature. *Obes. Surg.,* 2009; 19:928 - 36.

[20] Melinek, J., Livingston, E., Cortina, G., Fishbein, M. C. Autopsy findings following gastric bypass surgery for morbid obesity. *Arch. Pathol. Lab. Med.,* 2002; 126:1091 - 95.

[21] Chan, M. M., Hamza, N., Ammori, B. J. Duration of surgery independently influences risk of venous thromboembolism after laparoscopic bariatric surgery. *Surg. Obes. Relat. Dis.,* 2013; 9: 88 - 93.

[22] Avenell, A., Brown, T. J., McGee, M. A., Campbell, M. K., Grant, A. M., Broom, J. et al. What are the long-term benefits of weight reducing diet in adults? A systematic review of randomized controlled trials. *J. Hum. Nutr. Diet.,* 2004; 17: 317 - 35.

[23] Solomon, H., Liu, G. Y., Alami, R., Morton, J., Curet, M. J. Benefits to patients choosing preoperative weight loss in gastric bypass surgery: New results of a randomized trial. *J. Am. Coll. Surg.,* 2009; 2008:241 - 5.

[24] Mhuircheartaigh, J., Abedin, S., Bennett, A. E. Imaging features of bariatric surgery and its complications. *Semin. Ultrasound CT MR.,* 2013; 34: 311 - 24.

[25] Switzer, N. J., Mangat, H. S., Karmali, S. Current trends in obesity: Body composition assessment, weight regulation and emerging techniques in managing severe obesity. *J. Interv. Gastroenterol.,* 2013; 3: 34 - 6.

[26] Cottam, D. R., Mattar, S. G., Barinas-Mitchell, E., Eid, G., Kuller, L., Kelley, D. E. et al. The chronic inflammatory hypothesis for the morbidity associated with morbid obesity: Implications and effects of weight loss. *Obes. Surg.,* 2004; 14: 589 - 600.

[27] Brotman, D. J., Shihab, H. M., Prakasa, K. R., Kebede, S., Haut, E. R., Sharma, R. et al. Pharmacologic and mechanical strategies for preventing venous thromboembolism after bariatric surgery: A

systematic review and meta-analysis. *JAMA Surg.,* 2013; 148: 675 - 86.

[28] Ikesaka, R., Delluc, A., Le Gal, G., Carrier, M. Efficacy and safety of weight-adjusted heparin prophylaxis for the prevention of acute venous thromboembolism aong obese patients undergoing bariatric surgery: A systematic review and meta-analysis. *Thromb. Res.,* 2014; 133:682 - 7.

[29] Becattini, C., Agnelli, G., Manina, G., Noya, G., Rondelli, F. Venous thromboembolism after laparoscopic bariatric surgery for morbid obesity: Clinical burden and prevention. *Surg. Obes. Relat. Dis.,* 2012; 8: 108 - 15.

[30] Gómez-Ambrosi, J., Salvador, J., Rotellar, F., Silva, C., Catalán, V., Rodríguez, A. et al. Increased serum amyloid A concentrations in morbid obesity decrease after gastric by-pass. *Obes. Surg.,* 2006; 16: 262 - 9.

[31] O'Brien, K. D., Brehm, B. J., Seeley, R. J., Bean, J., Wener, M. H., Daniels, S. et al. Diet induced weight los sis associated with decreases in plasma serum amyloid A and C-reactive protein independent of dietary macronutrient composition in obese subjects. *J. Clin. Endocrinol. Metab.,* 2005; 90:2244 - 9.

[32] Ruiz-Tovar, J., Oller, I., Tomas, A., Llavero, C., Arroyo, A., Calero, A. et al. Midterm impact of sleeve gastrectomy, calibrated with a 50-Fr bougie, on weight loss, glucose hemostasis, lipid profiles and comorbidities in morbidly obese patients. *Am. Surg.,* 2012; 78:969 - 74.

[33] Hamadi, R., Marlow, C., Nassereddine, S., Taher, A., Finianos, A. Bariatric venous thromboembolism prophylaxis: an update on the literature. *Expert Rev. Hematol.,* 2019; 12: 763 - 71.

[34] Abyoglu, H., Tolga, M. A., Odabasi, M. A new protocol for venous thromboembolism prophylaxis in bariatric surgery. *Obes. Surg.,* 2019; 29:729 - 34.

[35] Venclauskas, L., Maleckas, A., Arcelus, J. ESA VTE Guidelines Task Force. European guidelines on perioperative venous thromboembolism prophylaxis: Surgery in the obese patients. *Eur. J. Anaesthesiol.,* 2018; 35:147 - 153.

[36] Almarshad, F., Almegren, M., Alshuaibi, T., Alobaodi, N., Almutawa, A., Basunbl, H. et al. Thromboprophylaxis after bariatric surgery. *Blood Res.,* 2020; 55:44 - 48.
[37] Chivot, C., Robert, B., Lafaye, N., Fuks, D., Dhahri, A., Verhaeghe, P. et al. Laparoscopic sleeve gastrectomy: Imaging of normal anatomic features and postoperative gastrointestinal complications. *Diagn. Interv. Imagin.,* 2013; 94:823 - 34.
[38] Langer, F. B., Reza Hoda, M. A., Bohdjalian, A., Felberbauer, F. X., Zacherl, J., Wenzl, E. et al. Sleeve gastrectomy and gastric banding: Effects on plasma ghrelin levels. *Obes. Surg.,* 2005; 15:1024 - 29.
[39] Rosenberg, J. M., Tedesco, M., Yao, D. C., Eisenberg, D. Portal vein thrombosis following laparoscopic sleeve gastrectomy for morbid obesity. *JSLS.,* 2012; 16:639 - 43.
[40] Singh, P., Sharma, M., Ghandhi, K., Nelson, J., Kaul, A. Acute mesenteric vein thrombosis after laparoscopic gastric sleeve. *Surg. Obes. Relat. Dis.,* 2010; 6: 107 - 8.
[41] Huerta, S., Li, Z., Livingston, E. H. Outcome of portal injuries following bariatric operations. *Obes. Surg.,* 2006; 16:105 - 9.
[42] Alsina, E., Ruiz-Tovar, J., Alpera, M. R., Ruiz-García, J. G., López-Perez, M. E., Ramón-Sánchez, J. F. et al. Incidence of deep vein thrombosis and thrombosis of the portal-mesenteric axis after laparoscopic sleeve gastrectomy. *J. Laparoendosc. Adv. Surg. Tech. A.*, 2014; 24:601 - 5.

In: Enhanced Recovery after Surgery ... ISBN: 978-1-53619-976-5
Editor: Jaime Ruiz-Tovar

Chapter 8

INTRAOPERATIVE ANESTHETIC MEASURES

Carmen Vallejo Lantero**, MD
and Esther García Villabona, MD
Anesthesiology Department,
Hospital Universitario de La Princesa, Madrid, Spain

ABSTRACT

Obesity is a worldwide issue and its prevalence is growing every year. Bariatric surgery as a method of treatment has become an established and renowned therapy for the management of patients with morbid obesity. The expanding popularity of surgical therapy for morbid obesity has led to an increase in the awareness of the peculiar challenges that bariatric patients pose both to anaesthesiologists and surgeons. Enhanced recovery after surgery (ERAS) protocol is well established in many surgical disciplines and leads to a decrease in the length of hospital stay and morbidity [1]. Multimodal protocols have also been introduced to bariatric surgery. In this way, we will pay special attencion to intraoperative interventions in this chapter, especially to intraperative anesthesic measures for bariatric surgery.

* Corresponding Author's Email: c.vallejo_26@hotmail.com.

Keywords: bariatric surgery, anesthesia, Enhanced recovery after surgery (ERAS)

Introduction

Obesity is a global health problem, presenting as a complex disease affecting, along with overweight, over a third of the world's population. Compared with nonsurgical modalities, bariatric surgery represents the most effective treatment for morbid obesity, contributing to significant and long-lasting weight loss as well as reduced obesity-related comorbidities. At present, the most widely used surgical procedures for morbid obesity are laparoscopic sleeve gastrectomy and laparoscopic Roux-en-Y gastric bypass, whereas laparoscopic one-anastomosis gastric bypass represents an emerging procedure. However, as with any major surgery, bariatric procedures pose potential health risks both in the short- and in the long-term.

Enhanced recovery after surgery (ERAS) pathways involve a series of perioperative evidence-based interventions that have been shown to improve postoperative outcomes by reducing morbidity and length of hospital stay in various

surgical specialties. Although increasingly investigated, its application in bariatric surgery still lacks definition and major concerns refer to the presence of complex high-risk medical comorbidities that may possibly require specialist perioperative care [2].

In this chapter we will focused in the intraoperative period, paying special attention to intraoperative anesthesic measures required in obese patients.

Intraoperative Anesthesic Measures

Tromboprophylaxis

In many studies, thromboembolic complications represent the main cause of morbidity and 50% of mortality after bariatric surgery. Risk factors, in addition to obesity itself, include history of venous thromboembolism, increased age, smoking, varicose veins, heart or respiratory failure, obstructive sleep apnoea, thrombophilia and oestrogen oral contraception [3].

Although not shown to reduce the incidence of fatal pulmonary embolism, mechanical methods such as intermittent pneumatic compression or graduated compression stockings should be used. Moreover, early mobilisation and the use of calf-length compression stockings were associated, with a low incidence of deep venous thromboembolism [4].

Bariatric surgery patients are at least at moderate risk of thromboembolism and, therefore, mechanical methods should be combined with pharmacological prophylaxis (preferably low molecular weight heparins administered 8-12h after surgery) [5].

Monitoring

Although obese patients are recommended to have a standard monitorization including blood pressure, ECG, oxygen saturation, EtCO2, oxygen-inspired fraction, temperature and glycemia; there may not be a suitable size of head for blood pressure measurement. Blood pressure measurements may be inaccurate if the used cuff has a wrong size. It can be falsely increased, if the cuff is too small for the arm. In this case, hand or ankle may be used as a measuring site or invasive artery monitoring may be preferred.

Temperature monitoring must be central with a high level of evidence, just as the anesthetic depth will be monitored using the bispectral index (BIS). In addition, recovery from the effect of muscle relaxants should be monitored by train of four (TOF) monitoring [6].

Glycemia will be monitored, since intraoperative hyperglycemia can lead to increased complications in the postoperative period, although the use of intensive insulin therapy should be avoided, due to the risk of hypoglycemia.

There is only a low level of evidence that the control of hourly, peroperative urinary output has clinical value and its sustained use may increase morbidity. The urinary catheterization can be maintained in case of needs derived from surgical or pathophysiological complications. When a bladder catheter is placed, it will be done with the appropriate aseptic measures, and, if possible, it will be removed 24 hours after surgery [6].

Non-Routine Monitoring

- Invasive monitoring is not routinely indicated, but invasive arterial cannulation is useful in selected patients. Especially indicated in those patients who present serious cardiorespiratory alterations and who may present problems in the postoperative period.
- Central venous catheter (CVC) insertion is not routinely indicated. It will be assessed in selected cases. The use of central venous catheters is limited to patients with respiratory diseases in whom it is anticipated that they may need administration of vasopressors or inotropics in continuous infusion [7].

Airway Management

Possibility of a difficult intubation and potential airway management problems must be considered and preparation should be made for it. Anaesthetists should pay close attention to airway management in obese patients undergoing bariatric surgeries, as difficult or unsuccessful intubation attempts are more common in these patients than in non-obese individuals (up to 15% of patients with higher Body Mass Index). Obesity is an independent risk factor for difficult intubation; therefore, preoperative airway assessment is important [8]. Large neck circumference and high Mallampati score are some of the most important parameters of the preoperative assessment and reliable predictors of problematic intubation in morbidly obese patients.

The supine position is not well-tolerated by a morbidly obese patient. Proper positioning can be obtained by the elevation of the head, neck, and shoulders with a towel or folded blankets under the shoulders and head. In this position, known as "stacked" or "ramped" position, the tip of the chin is placed at a higher level than the chest and the patient's ear is placed at the same level with his sternum to facilitate laryngoscopy and intubation. The patients should be with 30-40 degrees elevated trunk (half-sitting) during induction, preferably be a special pillow or by adjusting the operation table. This position has three functions: it will prevent regurgitation, improve lung function (compared to supine) and also facilitate mask ventilation and laryngoscopy for intubation.

It is necessary to preoxygenate the patients in the reverse Trendelenburg position until their SpO2 reaches to 100% and remains for several minutes. As functional residual capacity is reduced and O2 reserves are limited in the obese patients with apnea, hemoglobin will quickly desaturate. A rapid IV induction in addition to cricoid pressure is the best way to establish airway for most of the patients [9]. The experience and skills of anaesthesiologists are probably the most important factors for securing the airway in this patient group.

Ventilation Strategies

In the presence of obesity, mechanical ventilation management must be conducted with special attention, due to the inflammatory and mechanical alterations observed in these patients. Several ventilatory strategies have been proposed to improve gas exchange patients with morbid obesity. A 2012 systematic review and meta-analysis on ventilation in bariatric patients did not identify any benefit between volume control and pressure control modes of mandatory ventilation [10]. Atelectasis is common after induction of anesthesia of morbidly obese patients and use of high positive end-expiratory pressure (PEEP) may theoretically be beneficial for its improvement. However, PEEP combined with a large tidal volume (Vt) can decrease cardiac output and O2 delivery to the tissues, and thereforeworsen hypoxemia. Concurrent use of PEEP and recruitment improved intraoperative oxygenation and pulmonary mechanics. In a wider surgical population, adoption of the other elements of lung protective ventilation (LPV) was associated with significant reduction in postoperative complications [4].

In this line, the following ventilation strategies may be considered [11]:

1) Recruitment maneuvers associated with PEEP may work better than application of PEEP only. Furthermore, PEEP should be titrated according to best respiratory system dynamic compliance.
2) Stepwise increase in airway pressure, compared to other recruitment maneuvers aiming to open up atelectatic alveoli and increase end-expiratory lung volume, may lead to less deleterious effects.
3) Vt titration according to predicted body weight (PBW) may lead to high Vt, which, in combination with low end-expiratory lung volume, increases strain. On the other hand, tidal volume titration according to actual body weight may result in low Vt, which may aggravate atelectatic areas and hypoxemia. Thus, we suggest titrating Vt according to inspiratory capacity.
4) High inspired oxygen may prevent wound infection, even though recent studies were not able to demonstrate beneficial effects.

Neuromuscular Blockade

As non-depolarising muscle relaxants are polarised drugs with a hydrophilic structure, their distributions are unaltered in obese patients. Therefore, these drugs should be dose-adjusted according to lean body weight (LBW). There is no evidence of the superiority of these non-depolarising muscle relaxants and there is no evidence to show the preferably of any nondepolarizing muscle relaxants in bariatric surgery. Neuromuscular recovery time is not different between obese and nonobese patients with atracurium, rocuronium, or vecuronium. Succinylcholine dosages are increased and calculated based on total body wieght (TBW), because plasma cholinesterase levels and activity increases in obesity [9]. Rocuronium, a muscle relaxant used in this study, may be preferred because of its very low volume of distribution, absence of active metabolites and rapid recovery with sugammadex [8].

Benefits of deep Block: Higher pressure pneumoperitoneum, to facilitate laparoscopic surgery, can have deleterious cardiovascular effects and increased depth of neuromuscular blockade may improve surgical conditions, without the need to increase insufflation pressure.

Data from small trials in non-bariatric surgery suggest that deep blockade may facilitate manoeuvrability during laparoscopic procedures. Although this may be extrapolated to bariatric procedures, results from prospective trials have yet to be reported [4].

Obese patients have a high risk of developing postoperative respiratory complications, such as airway obstruction, hypoventilation, hypercapnia, hypoxia and acute respiratory failure. The presence of post-operative residual block can increase the risk of developing these complications. Postoperative residual block is more frequent in obese than in non-obese individuals (33% vs. 26%) [12]. There is evidence to suggest that a nerve-stimulated TOF ratio of 0.9 translates into recovery benefits. Trials in different healthcare settings have shown an association between residual blockade and post anaesthesia care unit (PACU) pulmonary complications. Reductions in PACU discharge time associated with TOF ratio > 0.9 have been demonstrated. A higher level of neuromuscular function was also associated with patient perceived satisfaction with the quality of recovery [4].

Sugammadex is an effective reversal agent of neuromuscular block. It permanently binds to rocuronium and inhibits its effect. Acetylcholinesterase blocking agents, such as neostigmine, have a different mechanism of action. Sugammadex was used because of the lack of side effects that are observed with acetylcholinesterase-blocking agents (especially bradycardia), its superiority in preventing postoperative residual block and the rapid reversal of neuromuscular block [12].

Key Points

For bariatric surgery, the literatura supporting the use of ERAS is comparatively sparse. In these terms, ERAS Society promotes an initiative to present a consensus review of optimal perioperative care for bariatric surgery. In this chapter we have tried to summarize, based on best evidence available currently, intraoperative anesthesic measures required in obese patients.

- Importance of the use of intermittent pneumatic compression devices to reduce the risk of thromboembolic complications.
- Routine monitoring should include electrocardiogram, non-invasive blood pressure, pulse oximetry, inspired oxygen fraction, capnography, temperature and intraoperative blood glucose.
- Anesthetic depth should be monitored using BIS and recovery from the effect of muscle relaxants by TOF monitoring.
- Invasive monitoring, central venous catheter insertion, and bladder catheterization are not routinely indicated.
- It is necessary to preoxygenate the patients in the reverse Trendelenburg position until their SpO2 reaches to100%.
- Anesthetic induction in "ramped" position to facilitate laryngoscopy and intubation.
- A rapid IV induction to minimize apnea period and risk of desaturation.
- Concurrent use of lung protective ventilation, PEEP and recruitment maneuvers, was associated with significant reduction in postoperative complications.
- Use of rocuronium as a first-line neuromuscular relaxant, if sugammadex is available.

References

[1] Malczak P, Pisarska M et al. Enhanced Recovery after Bariatric Surgery: Systematic Review and Meta-Analysis. *Obes. Surg.* 2017; 27:226–235.

[2] Nagliati C, Troian M et al. Enhanced Recovery after Bariatric Surgery: 202 Consecutive Patients in an Italian Bariatric Center. *Obes. Surg.* 2019;29:3133-3141.

[3] Overby D W, Kohn G P et al. Prevalence of trombophilias in patients presenting for bariatric surgery. *Obes. Surg.* 2009;19: 1278-85.

[4] Thorell A, MacCormick A D et al. Guidelines for Perioperative Care in Bariatric Surgery: Enhanced Recovery After Surgery (ERAS) Society Recommendations. *World J. Surg.* 2016;40:2065-83.

[5] American Society for Metabolic and Bariatric Surgery Clinical Issues Commitee. ASMBS update position statement on prophylactic measures to reduce risk of venous thromboembolism in bariatric surgery patients. *Sur. Obes. Relat. Dis.* 2013;9(4):493-7.

[6] Grupo de Trabajo de la Vía Clínica de Recuperación Intensificada en Cirugía Abdominal (RICA). Vía Clínica de Recuperación Intensificada en Cirugía Abdominal (RICA). Madrid: Ministerio de Sanidad, Servicios Sociales e Igualdad;2015.

[7] Rui-Tovar J, Sánchez-Santos R et al. Rehabilitación multimodal en cirugía bariátrica. *Cir. Esp.* 2019;97(10):551-559.

[8] Kaya C, Bilgin S et al. Anaesthetic Management of Patients Undergoing Bariatric Surgery. *J. Coll. Physicians Surg. Pak.* 2019; 29(8):757-762.

[9] Soleimanpour H, Safari S et al. Anesthetic Considerations in Patients Undergoing Bariatric Surgery: A Review Article. *Anesth. Pain Med.* 2017;7(4):e57568.

[10] Aldenkortt M, Lysakowski C et al. Ventilation strategies in obese patients undergoing surgery: A quantitative systematic review and meta-analisis. *Br. J. Anaesth.* 2012;109:493-502.

[11] Leme Silva P, Pelosi P and Rocco P R M. Mechanical ventilation in obese patients. *Minerva Anestesiol.* 2012;78:1136-45.

[12] Gaszynski T, Szewczyk T et al. Randomized comparison of sugammadex and neostigmine for reversal of rocuronium-induced muscle relaxation in morbidly obese undergoing general anaesthesia. *Br. J. Anaesth.* 2012;108:236-9.

In: Enhanced Recovery after Surgery ... ISBN: 978-1-53619-976-5
Editor: Jaime Ruiz-Tovar

Chapter 9

OPIOID-FREE ANESTHESIA AND GOAL-DIRECTED FLUID THERAPY

Esther García Villabona*, MD
and Carmen Vallejo Lantero, MD
Anesthesiology Department, Hospital Universitario La Princesa, Madrid, Spain

ABSTRACT

The implementation of enhanced recovery (ERAS) pathway protocols has resulted in significant benefits to both patients and hospitals. Two emerging components and key elements for the success of these protocols are the concepts of opioid-free anesthesia and goal-directed fluid therapy (GDFT).

Keywords: multimodal analgesia, adjuvant analgesics, TAP-block, liberal vs restrictive fluid therapy, static vs dynamic hemodynamic parameters

* Corresponding Author's Email: esthergarciavillabona@gmail.com.

OPIOID FREE ANESTHESIA

In the obese patient, the goal of perioperative pain management is provision of comfort, early mobilization and improved respiratory function, without causing inadequate sedation and respiratory compromise.

Perioperative opioid overuse contributes to various complications after minimally invasive surgery including nausea and vomiting, postoperative ileus, prolonged hospital stay, and increased healthcare costs. As a consequence, the use of multimodal opioid-sparing analgesia in the perioperative period has been advocated to improve postoperative outcomes, as well as to decrease opioid use and the risk of subsequent opioid addiction [1, 2].

Intraoperative Management

Most common side effects of opioids are well known: respiratory depression, pruritus, nausea and vomiting, ileus, constipation, urinary retention, tolerance by desensitization, immediate hyperalgesia that could evolve into chronic pain syndrome, reduced cardiac output, dizziness, somnolence and short duration central muscle stiffness. Opioid induced ventilatory impairment is well known by anesthesiologists and is easily treated in the post anesthesia care unit, but this complication is still problematic, especially in the bariatric surgery population. Another side effect is pharyngeal muscle weakness, contributing to obstructing breathing patterns in every patient. This side effect should certainly be avoided in obese patients and especially in patients with obstructive sleep apnoea (OSA), given the potential for aggravation and further breathing obstruction. Accordingly, recommendations for anesthesiologists are to avoid or minimize the perioperative use of opioids in these patients.

If no opioids are used during surgery, fewer opioids are needed to achieve a pain-free recovery, as addiction has not yet destroyed the mu receptor system. Opioid induced hyperalgesia and chronic pain syndromes are more frequent when high-dose opioids are used perioperatively [3].

Multimodal Analgesia

Over the last two decades, the minimally invasive approach has been increasingly used in abdominal surgery because it is associated with reduced morbidity and improved functional recovery, without compromising surgical outcome. Adequate postoperative analgesia is, however, imperative for early recovery, timely discharge, and patient satisfaction. Currently, consensus is lacking regarding the optimal management of postoperative pain after minimally invasive surgery, with a broad range of opioid-sparing multimodal analgesia elements described in the literature [1].

Pain from surgery has three major components: tissue injury, nociceptor stimulation and activation of central pathways. Using a unimodal pain treatment method, it may be difficult to attain adequate analgesia without inhibiting normal functions (movement of gastrointestinal function), or producing other side effects (sedation or nausea).

Pre-emptive analgesia refers to the concept that blocking neuronal pathways before or during surgery, can reduce or eliminate the hyperexcitability of these pathways and pain memory during recovery. This technique improves postoperative pain relief and decreases the total opioid requirement, thus reducing undesirable side effects.

The term multimodal analgesia refers to the simultaneous use of multiple analgesic methods. These protocols are based on routine use of NSAID's and paracetamol. It should be adopted if not contraindicated in patients undergoing open or laparoscopic bariatric surgery with the aim to reduce opioid consumption and their dose-dependent side effects that impair recovery [1, 2].

Systemic Medications

a) Paracetamol and Nsaid's:
   - Paracetamol has shown to improve postoperative analgesia, have an opioid-sparing effect but do not reduce opioids side effects. Its mechanism of action is still not completely understood.
   - Ciclo-oxygenase inhibitors are the most widely used components of multimodal analgesia. Ketorolac

administered regularly postoperatively can result in lower opioid consumption in patients with morbid obesity. Perioperative use of Ketorolac alone or in combination with local anesthesia leads to significant improvement of postoperative pain control.

b) Intermediate analgesics:
   - Tramadol and Tapentadol are both intermediate potency-analgesics that may benefit surgical patients due to their multimodal mechanisms of action.

c) Adjuvant analgesics:
   - NMDA antagonists: N-methyl-D-aspartate receptor is linked to nociceptive pain transmission and central sensitization. Ketamine, magnesium, methadone and dexamethasone all have NMDA-blocking ability.
     a) High dose systemic steroids have also shown promising results, when used carefully in patients undergoing gastrointestinal surgery. Glucocorticoids may have analgesic properties possibly related to anti-inflammatory properties and should be considered as part of a multimodal perioperative pain protocol. The concern for significant hyperglycaemia (>180 mg/dL) in bariatric patients has not been confirmed.
     b) Intravenous Ketamine has been evaluated as a part of multimodal analgesia protocols. It has been found in several studies that ketamine IV infusions were associated with decreased postoperative pain medications use compared with placebo and with a decreased risk of persistent postsurgical pain. Low doses of ketamine (0.1-0.5 mg/Kg) used in morbid obese patients lead to a significant reduced opioid consumption and reduced need for rescue analgesia importantly. If administered perioperatively, Ketamine is associated with an increased risk of hallucinations and nightmares. Limiting factors for use are coexisting severe arterial hypertension and cardiac failure.
     c) Magnesium was the first agent discovered to be a NMDA channel blocker. At very high doses, perioperative

intravenous magnesium sulphate has been reported to reduce morphine consumption but not postoperative pain scores. However, as it crosses the blood-brain barrier poorly in humans, it is not clear whether the therapeutic effect is related to the NMDA antagonism in the central nervous system.

- Other adjuvants:
  a) Dexmedetomidine is a highly selective α-2 agonist with sedative and analgesic sparing properties. It is approximately 8-times more specific to α-2 adrenergic-receptors than clonidine and its elimination half-life is much shorter. This medication should be administered cautiously as several cardiovascular effects may occur. For example, Dexmedetomidine should be given over at least ten minutes, as hypertensive episodes may otherwise be provoked. Nonetheless, a generally hypotensive effect of dexmedetomidine (as well as clonidine) may be observed later as well. In addition, bradycardia may commonly occur, and even cases of asystole have been reported. Importantly, the use of Dexmedetomidine is contraindicated in patients with higher degree AV-blocks. While there are certainly many benefits associated with the use of dexmedetomidine in the perioperative setting, caution is required. Various studies in morbid obesity population have shown safety of dexmedetomidine infusion perioperatively and the capacity to minimize narcotic requirements, length of stay after laparoscopic bariatric procedures and the risk of developing PONV.
  b) Gabapentin or pregabalin should be considered as part of a multimodal analgesia protocol. They are anticonvulsants, but are also neuromodulators, as they reduce neuronal excitability by inhibiting a subunit of calcium-gated channels on presynaptic axons. Both medications are associated with reduced opioid requirements and appear effective when administer as a preoperative dose in non-obese patients. It is difficult to

determine optimal doses because higher doses might be more effective, but they might also be associated with more sedation. They are only available in oral form, potentially limiting their use in the immediate postoperative period. There is no consensus for dose, frequency or duration treatment. Their use in the perioperative period requires careful assessment of the risk: benefit in patients with morbid obesity and/or obstructive sleep apnoea.

c) In view of its antinociceptive and anti-inflammatory properties, systemic administration of lidocaine as adjuvant to systemic opioids has been shown to improve postoperative analgesia, reduce opioid consumption and speed surgical recovery. Its exact mechanism of action remains not fully explain, but bolus and continuous lidocaine infusion has clear analgesic effects. It clearly improves the postoperative outcomes with increased patient satisfaction when used in the context of an ERAS protocol. With recommended protocols, safety will be as great as efficacy. Side effects are directly related to serum levels, and are more pronounced in patients with liver dysfunction and pulmonary diseases when the predominant problem is carbon dioxide retention and congestive heart failure [4].

Regional Techniques

Recently, there has been a heightened interest in regional analgesia, notably peripheral nerve blocks. Among these, local infiltration analgesia (LIA) of the port site remains one of the most commonly used methods, with wide acceptance, perhaps due to the simplicity of the technique and low cost.

On the other hand, routine use of epidural analgesia in minimally invasive surgery is not recommended [5].

- Thoracic epidural anesthesia

Initiation of neuraxial blockade before surgery and its maintenance throughout surgery decreases the need for anesthetic agents, opioids and muscle relaxants. Compared with parenteral opioids, epidural blockade has shown to provide better postoperative static and dynamic analgesia for the first 72 hours, to accelerate the recovery of gastrointestinal function, to reduce insulin resistance and impact positively on cardiovascular and respiratory complications. But epidural anesthesia also has well-known side effects: hypotension, urinary retention, pruritus and motor blockade [1, 2].

Although it has been commonly accepted as the reference standard for analgesia in open abdominal surgery, its role in minimally invasive surgery remains controversial because of the high risk: benefit ratio and lack of superiority over other alternatives [5].

- Tap block:

Performed mostly under ultrasound guidance, transversus abdominis plane (TAP) block has emerged as an equivalent alternative to epidural analgesia and more effective than LIA in terms of pain control and opioid consumption, most notably appreciated in the setting of bariatric surgery.

Laparoscopic guided techniques for TAP block, which involve deposition of local anesthetic in the TAP under direct vision of the laparoscope, have recently been described. These methods are pragmatic, performed by surgeons and obviate the need for ultrasound skills.

There is a recent systematic review and meta-analysis, which demonstrates that L-TAP is safe and effective for pain management in minimally invasive surgery. L-TAP seems to be as effective as US-TAP, more effective than LIA with respect to early pain control, opioid use, and patient satisfaction, and a potential pragmatic and safer alternative to epidural analgesia [5].

Importantly, none of the trials included in this meta-analysis reported L-TAP or US-TAP-related adverse events, including local complications and symptoms of local anesthetic toxicity. These results are in accordance with previous meta-analyses showing a low incidence of complications for both methods of TAP block.

Additionally, the results confirm that as part of an ERAS program, L-TAP contributes to shortening of hospital stay after laparoscopic surgery, without increasing complications or readmission rates. Future studies should focus on procedure-specific outcomes, type and concentration of local anesthetic drug administered (i.e., dose-ranging studies), as well as directly comparing L-TAP with epidural analgesia [5].

Conclusions

1. Thoracic epidural analgesia (T6-T11) still remains the gold standard for postoperative pain control in patients undergoing open bariatric surgery.
2. Opioid free anesthesia protocols combine several non-opioid analgesic treatments in order to eliminate, or at least minimize opioid dosing. In the case of laparoscopic bariatric surgery this works remarkably well.
3. These regimens include drugs that can stabilize the sympathetic nervous system, including α-2 agonists (clonidine and dexmedetomidine), locoregional anesthetics given intravenously (lidocaine or procaine), magnesium, gamma-aminobutyric acid modulators (gabapentin), ketamine, paracetamol, NSAID´s and glucocorticoids.
4. A transversus abdominal plane block is an efferent block of the anterior abdominal wall that reduce pain when employed in the context of multimodal analgesia.

Goal-Directed Fluid Therapy

Introduction

Decisions regarding fluid therapy are among the most challenging and important tasks that clinicians face on a daily basis. Perioperative fluid management and accurate assessment of volume status in morbidly obese patients are a challenge. Reasons for this include physiological differences, the presence of multiple comorbidities (and associated polypharmacy), preoperative preparation (rapid weight loss diet), inaccuracies associated with the use of non-invasive monitoring and higher incidence of rhabdomyolysis postoperatively. Present fluid management paradigms are based on studies of liberal versus restrictive strategies in non-obese patients whereby fluid excess or "imbalance" resulted in worsened outcomes than maintaining 'fluid balance.' Both approaches (liberal vs restrictive) have their own benefits and risks [6].

Fluid overload leads to a decrease in muscular oxygen tension. Due to surgical trauma, a systemic inflammatory response arises, which leads to a fluid shift to the extravascular space. Following a large fluid shift, generalized oedema may occur, which decreases tissue oxygenation and impedes tissue healing. By contrast, hypovolemia leads to arterial and tissue hypoxia due to a decrease in cardiac output.

Patients with more liberal fluid management (40 mL/Kg vs 15 mL/Kg total body weight) also produced significantly higher urine output in the operating room, in the post-anesthesia care unit, and on postoperative days 0 and first. On the other hand, surgical patients whose fluid balance was managed in the more restrictive fashion (15ml/kg) demonstrated faster recovery of gastrointestinal function, better wound healing, and improvement in pulmonary function and tissue oxygenation. There were no differences in postoperative rhabdomyolysis following laparoscopic bariatric surgery compared to more liberal strategies (40 ml/kg). No differences in intraoperative urine output were noted when morbidly obese patients were randomised to intraoperative low (4 ml/kg/h) vs high (10 ml/kg/h) volumes of Ringer's lactate. In the bariatric setting, limiting intravenous fluids reduced the incidence of postoperative pulmonary dysfunction and hypoxia, and shortened hospital stay [6].

Definition

It is well established that both hypovolemia and hypervolemia are associated with postoperative morbidity. GDFT is based on the optimization of tissue perfusion by rational fluid management, guided by hemodynamic parameters. These algorithms are designed to avoid excessive fluid infusion and to maximize cardiac output by measuring hemodynamic parameters.

The historical method of predicting fluid losses is based on fasting duration and insensible losses that may occur during surgery. In addition, fluid administration was titrated based on static parameters such as urine output, heart rate (HR), and blood pressure (BP). The theory of GDFT encourages clinicians to manage fluid/volume administration based on objective goals of hemodynamic parameters that are evidence based [1, 2].

Goal-directed fluid therapy encompasses a technique involving intensive monitoring to assess fluid responsiveness and aggressive management of intraoperative hemodynamics. Fluid responsiveness is defined as an ability of the heart to increase stroke volume in response to volume expansion.

Numerous meta-analyses showed outstanding benefits of GDFT over standard fluid therapies in terms of reducing morbidity and mortality rates in high-risk surgeries. Furthermore, administration of GDFT protocols were reported to decrease length of hospital stay, incidence of respiratory failure, acute renal failure, and surgical site infections, and reduce postoperative morbidity such as nausea and vomiting [1, 2].

Guiding Parameters for Administering Fluids

Intravascular Volume Status Monitorization

Accurate intraoperative determination of intravascular volume status is challenging because of some inherent intraoperative conditions like: anesthetic drugs, surgical volume losses, preexistent preoperative hypovolemia... as well as the manifestations of the normal physiological responses to surgery. Additionally, not all patients who are fluid responders require volume expansion. The decision to administer fluid should be supported by an apparent need for hemodynamic improvement in the context of a volume deficit and by the lack of associated risk [7].

Volume status assessment can be achieved with continuous intraoperative monitoring of factors such as HR, BP, end-tidal CO_2, central venous pressure (CVP), urine output, systolic volume (SV), cardiac output (CO), and their derivatives.

The hemodynamic parameters used for GDFT are stroke volume (SV) and cardiac output (CO), or dynamic volume response parameters such pulse pressure variation (PPV) and stroke volume variation (SVV). Classic static hemodynamic indicators (such as HR, BP, urine output, or CVP) are not the best indicators to estimate the patient's hydration status and they are poor predictor markers of fluid therapy response. According to the parameters measured, GDFT algorithms are designed to maximize cardiac output while avoiding fluid excess [9].

GDFT Monitors

There are now many different monitoring systems available, and physicians may feel somewhat confused by the multiple possibilities. These systems can be easily listed in order of invasiveness, from the highly invasive pulmonary artery catheter (PAC) to the completely non-invasive bioimpedance/bioreactance technique and the transthoracic echo-Doppler. Advances in minimally and non-invasive monitoring technologies should be considered as an effort to decrease the degree of invasiveness and a possibility of increasing its frequency of application, especially in the operating room.

These techniques provide information of systemic flow and cardiac performance as well as intravascular fluid status. Classifying them according to how accurate (closeness of measured values to the 'true' value, expressed as the bias) or precise (variability of values due to random errors of measurement) they are, is more difficult, in part because of the lack of a perfect "gold" standard for comparison.

Most devices have been evaluated by comparing their results with those obtained by intermittent thermodilution from the PAC as the reference, although this technique has its own limitations and may not represent the best choice of comparator [8].

GDFT Variables

Dynamic parameters such as pulse pressure variation (PPV) and stroke volumen variation (SVV), derived from arterial waveform analysis, have been suggested as the most reliable indicators of fluid responsiveness in mechanically ventilated patients as long as sinus rhythm is maintained. A recent study by Jain and Dutta demonstrated the value of SVV in the bariatric population. PPV or SVV values greater than 13 percent indicate fluid responsiveness, while patients with PPV below 9 percent should be considered non responders. Twenty-five percent of the patients with PPV value between 9 and 13 percent represent the so called "grey zone" when fluid responsiveness cannot be reliably predicted [8].

Dynamic parameters were reported to have lower accuracy in predicting fluid responsiveness when used in patients with low pulmonary compliance, or when high tidal volume (>8 ml/kg) was administered. For increased elastic resistance of chest wall and decreased respiratory compliance in obesity, some studies reported clinical benefits of lung-protective ventilation by using low tidal volumes. Since the use of lung-protective ventilation may interfere with dynamic parameters in predicting fluid responsiveness in bariatric patients, we did not include those patients with low pulmonary compliance [9].

Conclusions

1. Optimal perioperative fluid management is an important component of the ERAS pathways and it can reduce postoperative complications.
2. Regardless of the monitoring technique, it is important for the clinician to effectively plan and implement preoperative and intraoperative fluid goals.
3. Excess crystalloid fluid administration should be avoided.
4. In some low-risk patients undergoing low-risk surgery, a "zero-balance" approach is encouraged.
5. For the majority of patients undergoing major surgery, Goal Directed Fluid Therapy (GDT) is recommended.
6. In high-risk patients with morbid obesity undergoing high-risk surgical procedures, consider the use of advanced, invasive monitoring systems.

References

[1] Thorell, A., MacCormick, A. D. et al. Guidelines for Perioperative Care in Bariatric Surgery: Enhanced Recovery after Surgery (ERAS) Society Recommendations. *World J. Surg.* 2016; Sep; 40(9): 2065-83.

[2] Ruiz-Tovar, J., Sánchez-Santos, R. et al. Grupo de Trabajo de Cirugía Bariátrica del Grupo Español de Rehabilitación Multimodal (GERM) [Bariatric Surgery Working Group of the Spanish Multimodal Rehabilitation Group (GERM)]. Enhanced recovery after bariatric surgery. *Cir. Esp.* 2019. Dec; 97(10)551-559.

[3] Mulier, J. Opioid free general anesthesia: A paradigm shift? *Rev. Esp. Anestesiol. Reanim.* 2017. Oct; 64(8):427-430.

[4] Budiansky, A. S., Margarson, M. P. Acute pain management in morbid obesity - an evidence based clinical update. *Surg. Obes. Relat. Dis.* 2017; 13:523-532.

[5] Hamid, H. K., Emile, S. H. et al. Laparoscopic-Guided Transversus Abdominis Plane Block for Postoperative Pain Management in Minimally Invasive Surgery: Systematic Review and Meta-analysis. *J. Am. Coll. Surg.* 2020 Sep;231(3):376-386.

[6] Bundgaard-Nielsen, M., Secher, N. H. et al. 'Liberal' vs. 'restrictive' perioperative fluid therapy-a critical assessment of the evidence. *Acta Anaesthesiol. Scand.* 2009; 53:843-851.

[7] Poso, T., Kesek, D. et al. Morbid obesity and optimization of preoperative fluid therapy. *Obes. Surg.* 2013; 23:1799-1805.

[8] Demirel, I., Bolat, E. et al. Efficacy of Goal-Directed Fluid Therapy via Pleth Variability Index during laparoscopic Roux-en-Y gastric bypass surgery in morbidly obese patients. *Obes. Surg.* 2018; 28:358-363.

[9] Vincet et al. Clinical review: Update on hemodynamic monitoring a consensus of 16. *Crit. Care.* 2011; 15:229.

In: Enhanced Recovery after Surgery ... ISBN: 978-1-53619-976-5
Editor: Jaime Ruiz-Tovar

Chapter 10

INTRAOPERATIVE SURGICAL MEASURES

Dennis César Lévano-Linares[1,*], MD, PhD, Patricia Sanchez-Salcedo[2] and Jaime Ruíz-Tovar[1], MD, PhD

[1]Department of Surgery, University Rey Juan Carlos, Móstoles, Madrid, Spain

[2]Surgical Nursery Department, Fundacion Jimenez Diaz, Madrid, Spain

ABSTRACT

Laparoscopic Roux-en-Y gastric bypass and sleeve gastrectomy are the two most common bariatric operations. Wittgrove and Clark performed the first laparoscopic gastric bypass in 1993, and by the turn of the century, bariatric surgery became almost exclusively performed using the laparoscopic technique. This has led to decreased length of stay, rare utilization of intensive care units for the standard bariatric operation, and a progression towards enhanced recovery methods. With the implementation of enhanced recovery protocols, surgeons tend to use less invasive methods of perioperative management. This chapter analyzes the

---

* Corresponding Author's Email: cesdenlinares@gmail.com.

different intraoperative measures adopted by surgeons to improve the recovery of patients undergoing bariatric surgery.

Keywords: laparoscopic Roux-en-Y gastric bypass, sleeve gastrectomy, enhanced recovery after surgery protocols

1. INTRODUCTION

Obesity is an endemic disease and surgery remains a consistent and successful method of managing this disease. Actually, laparoscopic sleeve gastrectomy (LSG) and laparoscopic Roux-en-Y gastric bypass (LRYGB) are the most popular bariatric surgical techniques and the growing demand for bariatric surgery has been accompanied by an increased number of procedures and the necessity to improve the quality of care [1]. Thanks to the widespread adoption of laparoscopic surgery and the implementation of perioperative care of obese patients, bariatric surgery stands out from other surgical fields as leading to lower morbidity and mortality and shorter lengths of hospital stay (LOS) [2]. Nevertheless, bariatric surgeons are still making efforts to further improve the care of bariatric patients through the application of Enhanced recovery after surgery (ERAS) programmes in bariatric surgery. ERAS has changed the approach of perioperative care towards mainly surgical procedures [3]. While in the first period of its implementation, the ERAS endpoint was focused on improvement of logistic aspects, especially to increase the number of surgical procedure as well as to achieve cost savings, recent data reported its positive impact also on clinical outcomes [4]. The objective of ERAS programmes is to incorporate evidence-based strategies into the preoperative, intraoperative and postoperative care plan with the aim of reducing patients' surgical stress response and accelerating their functional recovery in order to improve quality of care, decrease complications and shorten hospital stays [5].

The ERAS protocol started with colorectal subspecialty in an active and multimodal approach for the care of surgical patients, resulting in optimized outcomes in terms of reduced morbidity, faster recovery, and shorter LOS in reference units [6]. In bariatric and metabolic surgery,

ERAS protocol was introduced recently, and recommendations were published 5 years ago: ERAS Society guidelines for bariatric surgery date back only to 2016 [7]. The bariatric protocol contains 21 components, distributed in the three steps: pre, intra and postoperative periods. Since the publication of the ERAS protocol in bariatric surgery, data from centers using this protocol have been collected and reported.

To date, three earlier metaanalyses and several observational studies comparing the adoption of ERAS versus standard of care in bariatric surgery have suggested that ERAS is safe and capable of shortening LOS [8, 9].

The objective of this chapter is to know the intraoperative measures used in the ERAS protocol in bariatric surgery and their results in clinical practice.

1.1. Anesthesia

Anesthetic considerations are detailed in ERAS guidelines designed for gastrointestinal surgeries [10]. However, the optimal anesthetic protocol should follow the mainstay principles of reduced opioid use which will help decrease patient recovery time.

Recent guidelines for the management of postoperative nausea and vomiting (PONV) recommend a multimodal approach by reducing the baseline risk with the use of antiemetics according to patient risk factors. Recommended strategies include Propofol for induction and maintenance of anaesthesia, avoidance of volatile anaesthetics, minimisation of intra- and postoperative opioids and avoidance of fluid overload [11]. A recent RCT comparing opioid-free TIVA with volatile-opioid anaesthesia in bariatric surgery, reported a significantly lower rate and severity of PONV in the opioid-free TIVA group. In addition to this baseline risk reduction, the recommended antiemetics for PONV prophylaxis are 5-hydroxytryptamine receptor antagonists, corticosteroids, butyrophenones, neurokinin-1 receptor antagonists, antihistamines and anticholinergics. The use of a combination of antiemetics in bariatric surgery is supported by a randomised trial demonstrating the superiority of triple combination of haloperidol, dexamethasone and ondansetron over a single or double combination in laparoscopic sleeve gastrectomy [12].

Perioperative fluid management and accurate assessment of volume status in morbidly obese patients are a challenge. Patients should receive a balanced volume of IV fluids intraoperatively. In bariatric surgery, rhabdomyolysis (RML) rates of 5-77% were reported (defined by elevation of serum creatine kinase (CK) of C1000 IU/L) (although 65% of these procedures were performed by laparotomy. Of those with RML, the overall incidence of renal failure was 14% and mortality 3%. One study examined the outcomes of intraoperative fluid replacement in laparoscopic bariatric surgery and found that conservative (15 mL/kg) versus liberal (40 mL/kg) IV fluid administration did not change postoperative creatinine or CK [13]. Therefore, a conservative volume of IV fluids is recommended over a liberal approach to prevent fluid overload.

Although there has been some advocacy for combined epidural with general anesthesia for abdominal surgery, our consensus statement does not recommend epidural analgesia in primary laparoscopic bariatric surgery.

Hypothermia increases a patient's risk for wound infection and delays healing; therefore, intraoperative normotherapy with preoperative warming in the holding area is recommended [14]. The use of heated insufflation during surgery is not recommended as a Cochrane systematic review demonstrated minimal increases in core temperatures with no reduction in adverse outcomes.

To prevent postoperative ileus, it is important to avoid excessive intravenous fluids through early discontinuation of intravenous infusions and early return to oral fluid intake. Regarding prokinetic agents, a Cochrane systematic review of 39 RCTs (n = 4615) demonstrated insufficient evidence to recommend prokinetic agents for the treatment of postoperative ileus [15]. However, alvimopan, a gamma-opioid receptor antagonist, has been shown to improve recovery times in patients postoperatively compared to placebo [16]. Other agents such as bisacodyl have been found to be effective in accelerating gastrointestinal motility following elective colorectal surgery and is an option to treat postoperative ileus. Oral magnesium oxide is another intervention that has demonstrated benefit in preventing postoperative ileus [3]. The recommendation is to avoid fluid overload by initiating early enteral feeds and discontinuation of intravenous infusions when possible. Overall, no current prokinetic agent has been shown to be effective in the treatment of postoperative ileus; however, alvimopan, bisacodyl, or magnesium oxide may be considered.

1.2. Laparoscopy

Laparoscopic bariatric surgery has rapidly superseded open surgery [17]. Three RCTs including more than 50 patients, compared open with laparoscopic gastric bypass [18]. The main findings were significantly shorter LOS as well as reduced rate of incisional hernia favouring laparoscopy. Further beneficial effects like reduction in intraoperative blood loss, diminution of postoperative pain and earlier recovery were also shown [19]. None of these studies found any difference in terms of weight loss. However, due to decreased postoperative adhesions, laparoscopic approach may be associated with increased rates of internal herniation [20]. It´s important to mention that higher costs of laparoscopic surgery are compensated for by fewer postoperative complications and shorter LOS [21]. On the other hand, the use of robotic surgery has also been described in bariatric surgery: a recently published systematic review included results from 2 557 patients found similar overall major and minor complications between robotic and laparoscopic groups, but the costs for robotic gastric bypass were higher [22].

1.3. Direct Trocar Entry and Veress Needle Entry in Laparoscopic Bariatric Surgery

The injury rates due to the trocar entry may account for up to 40% of all laparoscopic surgery complications. Direct trocar insertion (DTI), Veress needle insertion (VNI), direct optical trocar insertion, and Hasson's techniques are the most common laparoscopic entry techniques.

The "blind" insertion of the Veress needle can cause vascular and visceral injuries. The angle of the Veress needle insertion should vary according to the body mass index (BMI) of the patient: approximately a 45° angle in non-obese patient to 90° in obese patient [23]. One entry site is the left subcostal margin in the midclavicular line with elevation of the linea alba. Elevating the linea alba during Veress needle insertion is safe. No movement of the Veress needle was observed after insertion. Even among the obese patients, the double-click is a safety test for correct intraperitoneal placement of the Veress needle. The abdominal pressure may be increased immediately prior to insertion of the first trocar. After CO2 is inserted into the peritoneal cavity, the laparoscope is introduced to verify location of the Veress needle. The Veress intraabdominal pressure correlates positively with the BMI [24].

Direct trocar insertion (bladeless trocar) without creating a pneumoperitoneum decreases operating time and is associated with less insufflation-related complications such as gas embolism, especially in morbidly obese patients. One alternative is to enter the abdomen with an optical trocar under direct view while transecting abdominal wall layers and with a gentle rotating motion. Optical trocar insertions are trocars that accommodate a 0 or 30° laparoscope. The optical trocar enters successively through the subcutaneous fat, anterior rectus sheath, rectus abdominis muscle, posterior rectus sheath, preperitoneal fat, and peritoneum. It's preferable to place the first trocar through the rectus abdominis (two rectus sheath) than through the linea alba (one rectus sheath). The optical trocar combines the advantages of the different entry techniques as it allows clear optical entry, reducing the force necessary for insertion (particularly in the obese patient), and minimizing the size of the entry wound. All of the above, all bariatric surgeons should be familiar with all these Laparoscopic entry techniques because the use of Veress needle is not always feasible, especially in cases of revision surgery.

1.4. Nasogastric Intubation

Historically, routine nasogastric intubation following abdominal surgery was the standard of care. However, research has shown that there is a limited role for nasogastric tubes in abdominal surgery or in bariatric surgery. A Cochrane systematic review, which included 37 studies (n = 5711), demonstrated that patients who were did not have nasogastric tubes had an earlier return of bowel function ($p < 0.001$), lower rates of respiratory complications ($p = 0.09$), and lower rates of ventral hernias ($p = 0.09$) and concluded that routine nasogastric intubation following open abdominal surgery should be abandoned in favour of selective use [25]. Despite this, nasogastric intubation may be helpful to decompress the stomach during Veress needle insertion. On the other hand, as routine postoperative nasogastric intubation has not been proven to protect against complications like leakage, and even increases pulmonary infection risk and time to recovery, nasogastric tubes placed during surgery should be removed before reversal of anaesthesia. Therefore, the current recommendation is that nasogastric intubation may be used during Veress needle access but has no role postoperatively.

1.5. Intraoperative Leak Testing

Table 1. Recommendations for intraoperative care in bariatric surgery

Element	Recommendation
Perioperative fluid management	Excessive intraoperative fluids are not needed to prevent rhabdomyolysis and maintain urine output. Functional parameters, such as stroke volume variation facilitate goal-directed fluid therapy and avoid intraoperative hypotension and excessive fluid administration. Postoperative fluid infusions should be discontinued as soon as practicable with preference given to use of the enteral route
PONV	A multimodal approach to PONV prophylaxis should be adopted in all patients
Standardised anaesthetic protocol	The current evidence does not allow recommendation of specific anaesthetic agents or techniques.
Laparoscopy	Laparoscopic surgery for bariatric surgery is recommended whenever expertise is available.
Nasogastric tube	Routine use of nasogastric tube is not recommended postoperatively.
Abdominal drainage	There is insufficient evidence to recommend routine use of abdominal drainage.

There are currently no standard guidelines and requirements to perform intraoperative leak testing in bariatric surgery. However, early recognition and treatment of anastomotic or staple line leaks are important to reducing complications and length of stay. In prospective series, 342 LRYGB cases underwent air leak testing with six positive cases, requiring reinforcement of the gastrojejunal anastomosis [26]. However, there is no evidence supporting that intraoperative leak testing reduces the incidence of postoperative leaks. The method in which intraoperative leak testing is performed varies and can be performed by air or methylene blue during intraoperative endoscopy. The use of an orogastric tube to administer air or methylene blue is not recommended as a retrospective study demonstrated a lower rate of leak detection (8 vs. 4%) than with intraoperative endoscopy [27].

1.6. Abdominal Drainage

In a systematic review on the role of drainage after Roux-en-Y gastric bypass, the sensitivity of drainage in detecting postoperative leakage varied between 0 and 94%, and the efficacy of drainage for the non-operative treatment of leakage was between 12.5 and 100% [28]. Only one study reported data about non-operative treatment of leakage without drainage, which was pursued in one out of three patients. However, there are no RCTs evaluating the role and efficacy of prophylactic abdominal drainage following bariatric sur- gery. A recent retrospective study on laparoscopic Roux-en-Y gastric bypass compared an historical group of 272 patients with routine drain and 483 without and concluded that the leakage and reoperation rates were similar [29]. In one RCT including both subtotal and total gastrectomy with D2 lymph node dissection for gastric cancer, there was no significant difference between the groups with or without drainage in the incidence of intraabdominal abscess, wound infection or pneumonia. Despite lack of evidence in bariatric surgery, systematic use of abdominal drainage might be unnecessary. However, drains may be considered for complicated or revisional cases as there are much higher leak rates in these cases.

REFERENCES

[1] Trotta M., Ferrari C., D'Alessandro G., Sarra G., Piscitelli G., Marinari G. M. Enhanced recovery after bariatric surgery (ERABS) in a high-volume bariatric center. *Surg Obes Relat Dis.* 2019;15(10):1785-92.

[2] Cardoso L., Rodrigues D., Gomes L., Carrilho F. Short- and long-term mortality after bariatric surgery: A systematic review and meta-analysis. *Diabetes Obes Metab.* 2017;19(9):1223-32.

[3] Gustafsson U. O., Scott M. J., Hubner M., Nygren J., Demartines N., Francis N., et al., Guidelines for Perioperative Care in Elective Colorectal Surgery: Enhanced Recovery After Surgery (ERAS). *World J Surg.* 2019;43(3):659-95.

[4] Spanjersberg W. R., van Sambeeck J. D., Bremers A., Rosman C., van Laarhoven C. J. Systematic review and meta-analysis for laparoscopic versus open colon surgery with or without an ERAS programme. *Surg Endosc.* 2015;29(12):3443-53.

[5] Ljungqvist O., Scott M., Fearon K. C. Enhanced Recovery After Surgery: A Review. *JAMA Surg.* 2017;152(3):292-8.

[6] Muller S., Zalunardo M. P., Hubner M., Clavien P. A., Demartines N., Group ZFTS. A fast-track program reduces complications and length of hospital stay after open colonic surgery. *Gastroenterology.* 2009;136(3):842-7.

[7] Thorell A., MacCormick A. D., Awad S., Reynolds N., Roulin D., Demartines N., et al., Guidelines for Perioperative Care in Bariatric Surgery: Enhanced Recovery After Surgery (ERAS) Society Recommendations. *World J Surg.* 2016;40(9):2065-83.

[8] Meunier H., Le Roux Y., Fiant A. L., Marion Y., Bion A. L., Gautier T., et al., Does the Implementation of Enhanced Recovery After Surgery (ERAS) Guidelines Improve Outcomes of Bariatric Surgery? A Propensity Score Analysis in 464 Patients. *Obes Surg.* 2019;29(9):2843-53.

[9] Brethauer S. A., Grieco A., Fraker T., Evans-Labok K., Smith A., McEvoy M. D., et al., Employing Enhanced Recovery Goals in Bariatric Surgery (ENERGY): a national quality improvement project using the Metabolic and Bariatric Surgery Accreditation and

Quality Improvement Program. *Surg Obes Relat Dis.* 2019;15(11):1977-89.

[10] Feldheiser A., Aziz O., Baldini G., Cox B. P., Fearon K. C., Feldman L. S., et al., Enhanced Recovery After Surgery (ERAS) for gastrointestinal surgery, part 2: consensus statement for anaesthesia practice. *Acta Anaesthesiol Scand.* 2016;60(3):289-334.

[11] Gan T. J., Belani K. G., Bergese S., Chung F., Diemunsch P., Habib A. S., et al., Fourth Consensus Guidelines for the Management of Postoperative Nausea and Vomiting. *Anesth Analg.* 2020;131(2):411-48.

[12] Benevides M. L., Oliveira S. S., de Aguilar-Nascimento J. E. The combination of haloperidol, dexamethasone, and ondansetron for prevention of postoperative nausea and vomiting in laparoscopic sleeve gastrectomy: a randomized double-blind trial. *Obes Surg.* 2013;23(9):1389-96.

[13] Wool D. B., Lemmens H. J., Brodsky J. B., Solomon H., Chong K. P., Morton J. M. Intraoperative fluid replacement and postoperative creatine phosphokinase levels in laparoscopic bariatric patients. *Obes Surg.* 2010;20(6):698-701.

[14] Kurz A., Sessler D. I., Lenhardt R. Perioperative normothermia to reduce the incidence of surgical-wound infection and shorten hospitalization. Study of Wound Infection and Temperature Group. *N Engl J Med.* 1996;334(19):1209-15.

[15] Traut U., Brügger L., Kunz R., Pauli-Magnus C., Haug K., Bucher H. C., et al., Systemic prokinetic pharmacologic treatment for postoperative adynamic ileus following abdominal surgery in adults. *Cochrane Database Syst Rev.* 2008(1):CD004930.

[16] Delaney C. P., Weese J. L., Hyman N. H., Bauer J., Techner L., Gabriel K., et al., Phase III trial of alvimopan, a novel, peripherally acting, mu opioid antagonist, for postoperative ileus after major abdominal surgery. *Dis Colon Rectum.* 2005;48(6):1114-25; discussion 25-6; author reply 27-9.

[17] Nguyen N. T., Nguyen B., Shih A., Smith B., Hohmann S. Use of laparoscopy in general surgical operations at academic centers. *Surg Obes Relat Dis.* 2013;9(1):15-20.

[18] Luján J. A., Frutos M. D., Hernández Q., Liron R., Cuenca J. R., Valero G., et al., Laparoscopic versus open gastric bypass in the treatment of morbid obesity: a randomized prospective study. *Ann Surg.* 2004;239(4):433-7.

[19] Nguyen N. T., Goldman C., Rosenquist C. J., Arango A., Cole C. J., Lee S. J., et al., Laparoscopic versus open gastric bypass: a randomized study of outcomes, quality of life, and costs. *Ann Surg.* 2001;234(3):279-89; discussion 89-91.

[20] Higa K. D., Ho T., Boone K. B. Internal hernias after laparoscopic Roux-en-Y gastric bypass: incidence, treatment and prevention. *Obes Surg.* 2003;13(3):350-4.

[21] Sussenbach S. P., Silva E. N., Pufal M. A., Casagrande D. S., Padoin A. V., Mottin C. C. Systematic review of economic evaluation of laparotomy versus laparoscopy for patients submitted to Roux-en-Y gastric bypass. *PLoS One.* 2014;9(6):e99976.

[22] Bailey J. G., Hayden J. A., Davis P. J., Liu R. Y., Haardt D., Ellsmere J. Robotic versus laparoscopic Roux-en-Y gastric bypass (RYGB) in obese adults ages 18 to 65 years: a systematic review and economic analysis. *Surg Endosc.* 2014;28(2):414-26.

[23] Vilos G. A., Ternamian A., Dempster J., Laberge P. Y. No. 193-Laparoscopic Entry: A Review of Techniques, Technologies, and Complications. *J Obstet Gynaecol Can.* 2017;39(7):e69-e84.

[24] Vilos A. G., Vilos G. A., Abu-Rafea B., Hollett-Caines J., Al-Omran M. Effect of body habitus and parity on the initial Veres intraperitoneal CO2 insufflation pressure during laparoscopic access in women. *J Minim Invasive Gynecol.* 2006;13(2):108-13.

[25] Nelson R., Edwards S., Tse B. Prophylactic nasogastric decompression after abdominal surgery. *Cochrane Database Syst Rev.* 2007(3):CD004929.

[26] Al Hadad M., Dehni N., Elamin D., Ibrahim M., Ghabra S., Nimeri A. Intraoperative Endoscopy Decreases Postoperative Complications in Laparoscopic Roux-en-Y Gastric Bypass. *Obes Surg.* 2015;25(9):1711-5.

[27] Alaedeen D., Madan A. K., Ro C. Y., Khan K. A., Martinez J. M., Tichansky D. S. Intraoperative endoscopy and leaks after laparoscopic Roux-en-Y gastric bypass. *Am Surg.* 2009;75(6):485-8; discussion 8.

[28] Liscia G., Scaringi S., Facchiano E., Quartararo G., Lucchese M. The role of drainage after Roux-en-Y gastric bypass for morbid obesity: a systematic review. *Surg Obes Relat Dis.* 2014;10(1):171-6.

[29] Kavuturu S., Rogers A. M., Haluck R. S. Routine drain placement in Roux-en-Y gastric bypass: an expanded retrospective comparative study of 755 patients and review of the literature. *Obes Surg.* 2012;22(1):177-81.

In: Enhanced Recovery after Surgery ... ISBN: 978-1-53619-976-5
Editor: Jaime Ruiz-Tovar

Chapter 11

Early Postoperative Course in Bariatric Surgery

Andrei Sarmiento[1,*], MD, Ramiro Carbajal[2], MD, Jorge Orrego[2], MD and Juan Valverde Alva[3], MD

[1]Department of Surgery,
Universidad Privada San Juan Bautista, Lima, Perú
[2]Department of Surgery,
Hospital Nacional Edgardo Rebagliati Martins, Lima, Perú
[3]Department of Surgery, Hospital Castilla -ESSALUD, Lima, Perú

Abstract

The management of early postoperative after bariatric surgery is essential and involves components of Enhanced recovery after surgery (ERAS) protocols with the aim of improving patient outcomes, reducing in-hospital stay, and lowering health-care costs. The purpose of this chapter is to summarize the recent evidence about the effect of implementation of early postoperative diet, early ambulation, multimodal analgesia, and CPAP after bariatric surgery.

---

* Corresponding Author's Email: andrei.sarmiento @upsjb.edu.pe.

Keywords: Early posteoperative diet, early ambulatión, multimodal analgesia, CPAP

Early Postoperative Diet

The ERAS protocols are designed to improve patient outcomes, improving hospital stay, and lowering health-care cost [1]. Despite the fact that ERAS protocols have been successfully applied in a variety of surgical areas, there is limited research on the utility of ERAS in bariatric surgery.

They cover several aspects of pre-operative, intra-operative, and post-operative interventions such as medical education, early post-operative feeding and ambulation, and restricted use of narcotic analgesia [2].

The main goal of initial oral tolerance following bariatric surgery is to reduce the risk of early post-surgery side effects (nausea, vomiting, abdominal pain, and so on).

It is encouraged to initiate oral tolerance to liquids in the first 6 postoperative hours [3]. Recent research has suggested that implementation of early post-operative feeding protocol was associated with a significantly shorter overall LOS among patients undergoing bariatric surgery and is safe for both primary and revision LSG and RYGB patients [4].

Early Ambulation

It is now well established that obese patients have a higher risk of deep vein thrombosis, and pulmonary embolism, however there is a current paucity of understanding about the underlying prothrombotic mechanisms.

Some evidence suggests that Obesity-driven chronic inflammation and impaired fibrinolysis, these mechanisms appear to be major effector of thrombosis in obesity, although further work is required to confirm these finding [5].

In the postoperative setting, patients who have had bariatric surgery are at a high risk of venous thromboembolic events, also one of the most common causes of death is pulmonary embolism. Early mobilization, the use of intermittent pneumatic compression systems, and pharmacological prophylaxis of low molecular-weight heparin are all routinely prescribed in all patients. In the operating room, intermittent pneumatic compression should be started and continued until the patient is fully mobile [6]. Immobility has been linked to an increase in insulin resistance, as well as a reduction in muscle strength, respiratory function, and tissue oxygenation [7].

Overall, early ambulation is linked to a faster recovery period, a shortened hospital stay, and less postoperative complications [8]. In view of all that has been mentioned so far, early ambulation would be essential. Mobilization will be indicated 4 - 6 hours after the surgery [9].

ANALGESIA IN BARIATRIC SURGERY

Postoperative pain control is critical for successful recovery because it facilitates early intake, early ambulation, and discharged with less complications [10].

Injury to tissue during surgery causes two types of changes in the nociceptive system's responsiveness: peripheral sensitization and central sensitization. Therefore, multimodal analgesia approach has become the gold standard for postoperative pain management after bariatric surgery, requiring the utilization of medications or the use of multiple analgesic or anesthetic methods to minimize the need for postoperative opioid [11].

All of these, in order to prevent opioid-related risks such as PONV, sedation, ileus, and respiratory depression. Because of the respiratory depression caused by these medications, patients with SAHS are much more at risk. When used separately, paracetamol, NSAIDs, or COX-2 antagonists, gabapentinoids, ketamine, and alpha-2 agonists have all been shown to decrease postoperative opioid use and increase pain relief [12].

Acetaminophen and NSAIDs

Paracetamol (Acetaminophen): paracetamol has central mechanism of action. The exact mechanism of paracetamol's action is still unknown. There is evidence for a range of key processes, including effects on prostaglandin synthesis as well as serotonergic, opioid, nitric oxide (NO), and cannabinoid pathways, and it is possible that a combination of linked pathways is involved.

It has been shown to reduce opioid needs and also lead to a shorter duration of stay in the perioperative setting [13].

In 2008, Bergland *et al.* demonstrated the efficacy of paracetamol in safe management of patients undergoing laparoscopic gastric bypass using it as a component of multimodal opioid-free analgesia [14].

Nonsteroidal Anti-Inflammatory Drugs (NSAIDs)

NSAIDs work by inhibiting the enzyme cyclooxygenase (COX). Non-steroidal anti-inflammatory drugs are the most widely used component of multimodal anesthesia.

In patients with morbid obesity undergoing abdominal laparoscopic procedures, Govindrajan et al, observed that perioperative ketorolac was superior to remifentanil for analgesia, early discharge, and improved intraoperative hemodynamic control.

Additionally, an intraoperative administration of ketorolac decreased pain scores while also lowering the frequency of nausea and vomiting after surgery (PONV) [15].

Opioids Analgesics

Long-acting opioids' sedative and respiratory depressant effects are particularly detrimental to obese patients. Given this fact, with the aim of minimizing opioid use, multimodal analgesia is advised for bariatric surgery.

When used separately, paracetamol, NSAIDs, or COX-2 antagonists, gabapentinoids, ketamine, and alpha-2 agonists have all been shown to decrease postoperative opioid use and increase pain relief [12].

Multimodal Analgesia

Multimodal analgesia utilizes several analgesic agents to improve pain relief, whether in combination with or without opioids. Multimodal analgesia has better efficacy and fewer complications. It was associated with better postoperative analgesia, shorter PACU duration, lower postoperative opioid requirement, less PONV, earlier postoperative oral intake, earlier ambulation and shorter hospital stay also with economic benefits [16, 17].

Adjuvants Analgesics

Using multimodal analgesia, it is possible to avoid using potent long-acting opioids in anaesthesia for bariatric surgery.

Pregabalin and Gabapentin

Pregabalin: 150mg, single preoperative administration. Resulted in improved analgesia, was opioid-sparing and reduced adverse effects such as nausea and vomiting [18].

Gabapentin: 100mg of gabapentin, preoperative administration. Pregabalin used as a single-dose premedication during the preoperative phase of bariatric surgery has been shown to significantly reduce the need for postoperative analgesics that persists into the first postoperative day [19]. However, both have been associated with increased sedation and postoperative respiratory depression.

Hence, their use in the perioperative period requires careful assessment of the risk/benefit in patients with morbidly obese and/or OSA.

Ketamine

Ketamine is a noncompetitive (uncompetitive) NMDAR antagonist. Low doses (0,1 - 0,5mg/kg) of ketamine used in morbidly obese people result in a substantial reduction in opioid utilization and, most significantly, a reduction in the need for rescue analgesia. According to Sollazzi et al. [20] pre-induction ketamine infusion was associated with early extubation and reduced postoperative analgesic requirements in patients with morbid obesity undergoing bilio-pancreatic diversion for weight loss surgery. Ketamine has been shown in several studies to reduce analgesic needs and reduce total opioid use dramatically within the first 48 hours after surgery.

Dexmedetomidine

Dexmedetomidine is an alpha 2 adrenergic receptor (RAA2) agonist used for sedation, analgesia and as an adjuvant of anesthesia. Another important finding is that dexmedetomidine delivers anesthesia without inducing apnea or decreasing airway tone, which is particularly relevant in patients with morbid obesity and OSA.

When compared to patients who do not receive any supplementary dexmedetomidine infusion, intraoperative dexmedetomidine infusion decreases both intraoperative and postoperative opioid needs [21].

Lidocaine

Systemic lidocaine may minimize analgesic utilization and reduce postoperative pain, although there are few trials available and the appropriate dosing schedule in morbidly obese patients has yet to be established [22].

Sugammadex

Sugammadex has been shown to accelerate neuromuscular recovery following rocuronium muscle relaxation and reduce postoperative pain after laparoscopic bariatric surgery. Additionally, Sugammadex decreased PONV allows a faster discharge from the Post-Anesthesia Care Unit [23].

REGIONAL TECHNIQUES

TAP Blocks

The transversus abdominal plane (TAP) block is a regional anesthesia strategy in which local anesthetic is administered into the fascial planes between the transversus abdominis muscles to provide analgesia to the anterior-lateral abdominal wall. The effectiveness of TAP blocks, like all regional procedures, is operator dependent, and TAP blocks can be more difficult to perform in patients with morbid obesity. TAP blocks can be beneficial in patients with morbid obesity who are undergoing certain forms of abdominal surgery, especially laparoscopic procedures, according to current recommendations [24].

Ruiz-Tovar et al. demonstrated in a randomized clinical trial the efficacy of laparoscopic-guided transversus abdominis plane (TAP) block in Roux-en-Y gastric bypass (RYGB) patients. This research compared laparoscopic-guided TAP block versus port-site infiltration and found that the TAP block group had significantly less postoperative pain, required less morphine rescues, had shorter hospital LOS, and have higher rates of discharge within 48 hours [25].

Neuroaxial Techniques

Numerous studies have shown that neuroaxial pain control techniques are particularly effective in reducing opioid-related complications. In addition to intravenous analgesia, Ruiz-Tovar et al. contrasted three analgesic schemes in laparoscopic sleeve gastrectomy, showing the additional advantage of epidural and local anesthetic infiltration [26].

Intraperitoneal Bupivacaine Infusions

In obese patients undergoing laparoscopic bariatric surgery, intraperitoneal lavage with bupivacaine is an effective strategy to overcome postoperative pain. On the other hand, continuous surgical wound infusion with ropivacaine improved pain relief and accelerated recovery and discharge reducing overall costs of care [27, 28].

Obstructive Sleep Apnea and CPAP

In the bariatric patient population, Obstructive Sleep Apnea (OSA) is quite common. Owing to the elevated incidence of OSA in morbidly obese subjects and the heightened likelihood of perioperative complications, mandatory OSA screening seems to be required [28]. Nocturnal polysomnography (PSG) is the gold standard for assessment. Nevertheless, ordering PSG for a bariatric patient on a regular basis is not recommended due to cost-effective issues. The number of apneic episodes can be counted during PSG. The apnea-hypopnea index (AHI) indicates the absense of sleep apnea if less than 5, mild OSA for 5 – 15, moderate OSA for >15, and severe OSA if >30. Other resources, such as the STOP-Bang and the Berlin Sleep Questionnaire, may be used to classify patients who are at high risk [29]. Patients with moderate to severe OSA should be advised to accept CPAP therapy before surgery. For patients with pre - existing OSA, anesthesiologists advise the following perioperative recommendations: use of multimodal analgesia to limit opioid use, minimize sedative use, use of supplementary oxygen, preservation of continuous positive airway pressure (CPAP) postoperatively, and continuous pulse oximetry [30]. In obese patients' early reinstatement of CPAP after surgery improves arterial blood gas and reduces the need for intubation. However, there is concern that using CPAP (continuous positive airway pressure) could raise the risk of an anastomotic leak by forcing air into the gastric pouch. However, it has been shown that when CPAP is used, there are no shifts in transmural gastric pouch pressure [31]. According to ASA (The American Society of Anesthesiologists), patients with OSA who are on CPAP therapy should keep doing it as soon as possible after surgery. Recommendations based on expert opinion and not scientific evidence suggest that patients with OSA should be observed for three hours longer than non-OSA patients before being discharged from the PACU [32].

References

[1] Thorell, A., MacCormick, A. D., Awad, S., Reynolds, N., Roulin, D., Demartines, N. et al. Guidelines for perioperative care in bariatric

surgery: Enhanced Recovery After Surgery (ERAS) society recommendations. *World J. Surg.,* 2016; 40(9):2065 - 83.

[2] Ruiz-Tovar, J., Sanchez-Santos, R., Martín-García-Almenta, E., García Villabona, E., Hernandez, A. M., Hernández-Matías, A. et al. Rehabilitación multimodal en cirugía bariátrica. *Cir. Esp.*, 2019; 97:551 - 559.

[3] Mechanick, J. I., youdim, A., Jones, D. B., Timothy Garvey, W., Hurley, D. L., Molly McMahon, M. et al. Clinical practice guidelines for the perioperative nutritional, metabolic, and nonsurgical support of the bariatric surgery patient–2013 update: Cosponsored by American Association of Clinical Endocrinologists, the Obesity Society, and American Society for Metabolic and Bariatric Surgery. *Surgery Obes. Relat. Dis.,* 2013; 9:159 - 91.

[4] Bevilacqua, L. A., Obeid, N. R., Spaniolas, K., Bates, A., Docimo, S., Jr., Pryor, A. Early postoperative diet after bariatric surgery: Impact on length of stay and 30-day events. *Surg. Endosc.,* 2019; 33(8): 2475 - 2478.

[5] Blokhin, I. O. and Lentz, S. R. Mechanisms of thrombosis in obesity. *Curr. Opinion Hematol.,* 2013; 20(5): 437 - 444.

[6] American Society for M, Bariatric Surgery Clinical Issues C. ASMBS updated position statement on prophylactic measures to reduce the risk of venous thromboembolism in bariatric surgery patients. *Surg. Obes. Relat. Dis.,* 2013; 9:493 - 7.

[7] Kehlet, H., Wilmore, D. W. Multimodal strategies to improve surgical outcome. *Am. J. Surg.,* 2002; 183(6):630 - 41.

[8] Geubbels, N., Bruin, S. C., Acherman, Y. I., van de Laar, A. W., Hoen, M. B., de Brauw, L. M. Fast track care for gastric bypass patients decreases length of stay without increasing complications in an unselected patient cohort. *Obes. Surg.,* 2014; 24(3):390 - 6.

[9] Awad, S., Carter, S., Purkayastha, S., Hakky, S., Moorthy, K., Cousins, J. et al. Enhanced Recovery After Bariatric Surgery (ERABS): Clinical Outcomes from a Tertiary Referral Bariatric Centre. *Obes. Surg.,* 2014; 24:753 - 8.

[10] Apfelbaum, J. L., Chen, C., Mehta, S. S., Gan, T. J. Postoperative pain experience: Results from a national survey suggest postoperative pain continues to be undermanaged. *Anesth. Analg.,* 2003; 97:2.

[11] Brown, E. N., Pavone, K. J. and Naranjo, M. Multimodal General Anesthesia: Theory and Practice. *Anesth. Analg.,* 2018; 127(5): 1246 - 1258.
[12] Carron, M., Safaee Fakhr, B., Ieppariello, G., Foletto, M. Perioperative care of the obese patient. *The Br. J. Surg.,* 2020; 107(2): e39 - e55.
[13] Pickering, G., Esteve, V., Loriot, M. A. et al. Acetaminophen reinforces descending inhibitory pain pathways. *Clin. Pharmacol. Ther.*, 2008; 84: 47 - 51.
[14] Bergland, A., Gislason, H., Raeder, J. Fast-track surgery for bariatric laparoscopic gastric bypass with focus on anaesthesia and peri-operative care. Experience with 500 cases. *Acta Anaesthesiol. Scand.*, 2008; 52(10):1394 - 1399.
[15] Govindarajan, R., Ghosh, B., Sathyamoorthy, M. K., Kodali, N. S., Raza, A., Aronsohn, J. et al. Efficacy of ketorolac in lieu of narcotics in the operative management of laparoscopic surgery for morbid obesity. *Surg. Obes. Relat. Dis.,* 2005; 1(6):530 - 535.
[16] Ziemann-Gimmel, P., Hensel, P., Koppman, J., Marema, R. Multimodal analgesia reduces narcotic requirements and antiemetic rescue medication in laparoscopic Roux-en-Y gastric bypass surgery. *Surg. Obes. Relat. Dis.,* 2013; 9(6):975 - 80.
[17] King, A. B., Spann, M. D., Jablonski, P. et al. An enhanced recovery program for bariatric surgical patients significantly reduces perioperative opioid consumption and postoperative nausea. *Surg. Obes. Relat. Dis.*, 2018; 14:849 - 56.
[18] Cabrera Schulmeyer, M. C., de la Maza, J., Ovalle, C., Farias, C., Vives, I. Analgesic effects of a single preoperative dose of pregabalin after laparoscopic sleeve gastrectomy. *Obes. Surg.,* 2010; 20(12):1678 - 1681.
[19] Schung, S. A., Rayman, A. Posoperative pain management of the obese patient. *Best Pract. Res. Clin. Anaesthesiol.*, 2011; 25: 73 - 81.
[20] Sollazzi, L., Modesti, C., Vitale, F., Sacco, T., Ciocchetti, P., Idra, A. S. et al. Preinductive use of clonidine and ketamine improves recovery and reduces postoperative pain after bariatric surgery. *Surg. Obes. Relat. Dis.,* 2009; 5(1):67 - 71.

[21] Bakhamees, H. S., El-Halafawy, Y. M., El-Kerdawy, H. M., Gouda, N. M., Altemyatt, S. Effects of dexmedetomidine in morbidly obese patients undergoing laparoscopic gastric bypass. *Middle East J. Anesthesiol.*, 2007; 19(3):537 - 551.

[22] De Oliveira, G. S. Jr., Duncan, K., Fitzgerald, P. et al. Systemic lidocaine to improve quality of recovery after laparoscopic bariatric surgery: A randomized double-blinded placebo-controlled trial. *Obes. Surg.,* 2014; 212:24 - 8.

[23] Castro, D. S., Leão, P., Borges, S. et al. Sugammadex reduces postoperative pain after laparoscopic bariatric surgery: A randomized trial. *Surg. Laparosc. Endosc. Percutan. Tech.,* 2014; 24:420 - 23.

[24] El-Dawlatly, A. A., Turkistani, A., Kettner, S. C. et al. (2009) Ultrasound- guided transversus abdominis plane block: Description of a new technique and comparison with conventional systemic analgesia during laparoscopic cholecystectomy. *Br. J. Anaesth.,* 102:763 - 767.

[25] Ruiz-Tovar, J., Garcia, A., Ferrigni, C. et al. Laparoscopic-guided transversus abdominis plane (TAP) block as part of multimodal analgesia in laparoscopic Roux-en-Y gastric bypass within an enhanced recovery after surgery (ERAS) program: A prospective randomized clinical trial. *Obes. Surg.,* 2018; 28:3374 - 9.

[26] Ruiz-Tovar, J., Muñoz, J. L., Gonzalez, J. et al. Postoperative pain after laparoscopic sleeve gastrectomy: Comparison of three analgesic schemes (isolated intravenous analgesia, epidural analgesia associated with intravenous analgesia and port-sites infiltration with bupivacaine associated with intravenous analgesia). *Surg. Endosc.,* 2017; 31:231 - 6.

[27] Sherwinter, D. A., Ghaznavi, A. M., Spinner, D. et al. Continuous infusion of intraperitoneal bupivacaine after laparoscopic surgery: A randomized controlled trial. *Obes. Surg.,* 2008; 18(12):1581 - 1586.

[28] Forastiere, E., Sofra, M., Giannarelli, D., Fabrizi, L., Simone, G. Effectiveness of continuous wound infusion of 0.5% ropivacaine by On-Q pain relief system for postoperative pain management after open nephrectomy. *Br. J. Anaesth.,* 2008; 101(6):841 - 847.

[29] de Raaff, C., Gorter-Stam, M., de Vries, N., Sinha, A. C., Jaap Bonjer, H., Chung, F., Coblijn, U. K., Dahan, A., van den Helder, R. S., Hilgevoord, A., Hillman, D. R., Margarson, M. P., Mattar, S. G., Mulier, J. P., Ravesloot, M., Reiber, B., van Rijswijk, A. S., Singh, P. M., Steenhuis, R., Tenhagen, M., ... van Wagensveld, B. A. Perioperative management of obstructive sleep apnea in bariatric surgery: A consensus guideline. *Surg. Obes. Relat. Dis.,* 2017; 13(7): 1095 - 1109.

[30] Epstein, L. J., Kristo, D., Strollo, P. J. Jr., Friedman, N., Malhotra, A., Patil, S. P., Ramar, K., Rogers, R., Schwab, R. J., Weaver, E. M., Weinstein, M. D., and Adult Obstructive Sleep Apnea Task Force of the American Academy of Sleep Medicine. Clinical guideline for the evaluation, management and long-term care of obstructive sleep apnea in adults. *JCSM,* 2009; 5(3): 263 - 276.

[31] Weingarten, T. N., Kendrick, M. L., Swain, J. M., Liedl, L. M., Johnson, C. P., Schroeder, D. R. et al. Effects of CPAP on gastric pouch pressure after bariatric surgery. *Obes. Surg.,* 2011; 21(12):1900 - 5.

[32] Gross, J. B., Bachenberg, K. L., Benumof, J. L., Caplan, R. A., Connis, R. T., Cote, C. J. et al. Practice guidelines for the perioperative management of patients with obstructive sleep apnea: a report by the American Society of Anesthesiologists task force on perioperative management of patients with obstructive sleep apnea. *Anesthesiology,* 2006; 104(5):1081 - 93.

In: Enhanced Recovery after Surgery ... ISBN: 978-1-53619-976-5
Editor: Jaime Ruiz-Tovar

Chapter 12

DIET IN BARIATRIC SURGERY: PROGRESSION AND LIFESTYLE MODIFICATION - A MULTIDISCIPLINARY APPROACH

Virginia Esperanza Fernández Ruiz*[1], *RD, PhD, and Maria Dolores Frutos Bernal*[2,*], *MD, PhD

[1]Bariatric Surgery Unit, Hospital Clínic Universitary "Virgen de la Arrixaca," Murcia, Spain

[2]Department of General Surgery, Bariatric and Advanced Laparoscopic Surgery Unit. University of Murcia, Hospital Clínic Universitary "Virgen de la Arrixaca," Murcia. Spain

ABSTRACT

In this chapter we have tried to design a useful tool for health professionals who start or perform their work in bariatric surgery units and do not know how to carry out the modification of unhealthy

[*] Corresponding Author's Email: mfb25s@gmail.com.

habits in people who have undergone surgical treatment for morbid obesity and associated metabolic comorbidity.

Thus, a succinct description is given of the objectives to be established for dietary and sports treatment and the safe progression from the initial post-surgical phase to adherence to the new lifestyle.

Keywords: diet, bariatric surgery, progression, lifestyle modification

INTRODUCTION

Bariatric surgery (BS) has proven to be an effective tool in the face of the therapeutic failure of conservative treatment of morbid obesity (MO), achieving a reduction of excess body weight, between 60%-70%, which is equivalent to an average weight loss of 40Kg [1, 2]; overcoming, in addition, factors inherent to human beings such as sex or age [3]. On the other hand, it has shown results beyond weight loss, with the reduction and/or resolution of comorbidities associated with obesity [Diabetes Mellitus (DM), dyslipidemia (DLP), arterial hypertension (HTN), hyperuricemia, among others]; hence, different authors call it metabolic surgery (MS) [4-8].

However, some long-term limitations have been described, in terms of psychiatric comorbidity [anxiety, depression and eating disorders (ED)] and even weight gain, nutritional deficits, sarcopenia and musculoskeletal injuries [9, 10]. This fact justifies the need for a multidisciplinary team [surgeon, endocrinologist, psychiatrist, clinical psychologist, nutrition nurse, dietitian-nutritionist, and physical activity and sports science professional (PAS] [10-13], able to instruct the patient ensuring commitment and adherence to the new lifestyle; thus, correcting the original problem and avoiding the complications described in the long term [14, 15]. Although the individual and short-term objectives of each member of the team vary at different times, the ultimate goal is the same, the patient's quality of life [15, 16].

It is essential that the multidisciplinary team knows the anatomical and functional modifications of the different surgical techniques in the gastrointestinal tract (restrictive, malabsorptive and mixed) to be able to detect possible surgical complications, make the appropriate modifications in the pharmacological treatment of comorbidities associated with obesity, to carry out a correct progression in the diet (in terms of both nutrients and textures) that allow the patient to reach the caloric-protein nutritional requirements, as well as a safe evolution of physical activity, guaranteeing the psychological well-being of the patient in the different stages of the post-surgical process [9, 17].

PHASE 0. PRE-SURGICAL

As mentioned, the patient who is to undergo BS should be approached by a multidisciplinary team and, ideally, assessment and follow-up would begin before surgery (Table 1) [9, 10, 12, 13, 17]; so that it is possible to identify whether the origin that has led to the development of obesity [18] and its comorbidity is psychological or behavioral, due to lack of knowledge in terms of healthy eating, immobility or sedentary lifestyle, sleep deprivation, biological (endocrine disruptors, hormonal disorder, genetic disorders), socioeconomic or others; since the correction/modification of the underlying problem will guarantee the success of the surgery as well as the prevention of potential complications in the short and long term [11, 14, 19, 20].

In addition, current scientific evidence has shown that patients before undergoing surgery present vitamin-mineral deficiencies and protein malnutrition and even sarcopenia; situations that compromise surgery and favor the appearance of immediate and late complications [11, 21, 22]. Similarly, it has been found that weight loss between 10-15% prior to surgery reduces potential intra- and post-surgical complications [23, 24]. These facts confirm the importance of communication with the patient [25] and the presence of a multidisciplinary team in this first stage (3 to 6 months prior to surgery). The inclusion of these patients in programs such as the I^2AO^2 [26-30], before and after surgery, could benefit both the patient and the public health system in terms of cost-effectiveness.

Table 1. Assessment and follow-up of the patient undergoing BS [11, 13, 19, 31-36]

	Before Surgery	3 months	6 months	12 months	18 months	24 months	annual
Biochemistry (pre-albumin, albumin and transferrin) blood count, Fe, Ca, P and Mg. Hormones (thyroid, insulin and parathormone)	X	X		X		X	X
Water-soluble vitamins (A,D,E,K) and fat-soluble (B1,B9,B12) trace elements (Cu, Zn, Se)	X	X	X	X		X	X
Indirect calorimetry, anthropometry and bioelectrical impedance	X	X	X	X	X	X	X
Sarcopenia screening (SARC-F), gait test and saddle test	X	X	X	X	X	X	X
Dynamometry, muscle ultrasound	X	X	X	X	X	X	X
Evaluation of aerobic capacity (maximum heart rate) and strength capacity (% maximum power)	X	X	X	X	X	X	X
Food frequency survey	X		X	X		X	X
Survey of dietary and sporting habits	X		X	X		X	X
Quality of life survey	X		X	X		X	X

Based on the healthcare reality, where it is not always possible to have a multidisciplinary team at the beginning, we propose the progression of the medical, dietetic and sports treatment, starting from a patient with bad habits and without psychological alteration.

Phase 1. Protection of Surgery and Detection of Potential Complications (Infections, Bleeding, Suture Dehiscence and Thrombotic Complications)

Duration: initial 7 days [11, 13, 19, 31-36].

Medical treatment: prophylactic anticoagulation, proton pump inhibitor, adjustment of treatment for DM (Table 2), DLP (initially withdrawn) and HTN (unchanged), among others [4, 13, 17, 31, 33, 34, 35, 37].

In this phase, the effect of BS on the pharmacokinetics of drugs that may modify their bioavailability should be assessed:

- There is a decrease in gastric disintegration.
- Large tablets may obstruct the gastrojejunal anastomosis, so they should be crushed or liquid and/or dilutable formulations should be sought.
- Modification of gastric pH by exclusion of the duodenum and first jejunal loops interfering with the bioavailability of minerals such as iron and calcium.
- In restrictive techniques, the decrease of intrinsic factor may alter the absorption of vitamin B12.
- Possible decrease in the absorption of fat-soluble drugs by reducing the activity of bile salts [13, 19, 31, 33, 34].

Sports treatment: the aim will be to promote physical activity, the patient will be asked to take short walks at home, under supervision, according to tolerance (count the minutes he/she is able to maintain a continuous walk). The patient should be accompanied and driving is not recommended [11, 13, 17, 33-35].

Table 2. Modifications of treatment for DM in the patient undergoing BS [4]

Treatment for DM Prior to BS	Therapeutic Approach after BS	BS Control
GLP-1 analog	Withdraw	Not needed
1 OAD	Withdraw	Not needed
2 OAD	Maintain: Metformina	BG
3 OAD	Maintain: Dapagliflozin, canaglifozin and empaglifozin / Metformin	BG
Basal Insulin + Bolus Insulin	Maintain 1/3 and administer of basal insulin	BG y prepandrial lunch and dinner
Target blood glucose (90-140 mg/dl)	2 days de BG>140mg/dl increase 2 UI of basal insulin	BG y prepandrial lunch and dinner
Target blood glucose (90-140 mg/dl)	1 day de BG <90mg/dl decrease 2 UI of basal insulin	BG y prepandrial lunch and dinner
OADvs BASAL INSULIN	After 6 months, due to the reduction of insulin treatment, its modification by an ADO is evaluated if necessary	BG

OAD: Oral Antidiabetic; BG: Basal Glycemia.

Table 3. Volume restriction and protein requirements according to the surgical technique applied [11, 13, 17, 19, 31-36, 38]

	Technique	Volume	Proteins Requirements
Restrictive	Adjustable gastric banding (AGB)	25-50 ml	1g/Kg corrected weight /day
	Tubular Gastrectomy (TG)	100-150ml	
Mixed	Roux-en-Y Gastric Bypass (RYGB)	50ml	1,2g/Kg corrected weight/day
Malabsortive	Biliopancreatic diversion (BPD)*	150-200ml	1,5g/Kg corrected weight/day

*Although BPD has a restrictive component, its main mechanism is malabsorptive.

Dietary treatment: the main objectives of this phase in terms of surgery protection are: to guarantee the consolidation of the anastomosis sutures (liquid texture diet) and the protection of the gastric reservoir, prevention of the dilatation of the gastric residue (limitation of the volume of liquid per ingestion). 24 hours after the end of the surgical procedure, a liquid-textured diet with volume control is established. The volume of liquid to be ingested per intake will depend on the surgical technique performed (Table 3). However, it is recommended to start with intakes of 30 ml and progress with the same amount (30 ml) according to tolerance, without forcing gastric capacity (the patient should not reach the sensation of fullness or pain) [11, 13, 19, 31-36].

It is essential to train the patient in slow and fractioned intake (6-8 intakes/day), completing hydration with water outside these intakes. It should be noted that water is the most difficult liquid to tolerate. Although there is no scientific evidence to corroborate this, clinical experience has shown that flavoring water with a few drops of lemon or orange can help the patient to achieve the hydration objective. To ensure hydration, 30 ml of liquid/kg of corrected weight/day should be ingested.

Difficulty in hydration, limited mobility and the absence of residue favor the appearance of constipation in this first phase [11, 13, 19, 31-36].

Regarding the composition of the diet, the foods or products to be included in this phase are: water, infusions, diluted and strained natural juices, skimmed liquid dairy products (in certain cases there is a better tolerance to these, if they are lactose-free), soy vegetable drink or nuts (almonds or cashews), vegetable broths and defatted chicken or turkey broths (Table 4). It is recommended to avoid coffee or other infusions with diuretic effect, until water requirements are met [11, 13, 19, 31-36].

Table 4. Example of liquid diet during the first days after surgery

9h: 50-100 ml of skimmed milk (add grams of protein module*).
11h: 50-100 ml of diluted and strained natural juice (add gr of protein module*).
13h: 50-100ml of liquid yogurt (add gr of protein module*).
15h: 50-100 ml of defatted chicken broth (add gr of protein module*).
17h: 50-100ml of diluted and strained natural juice (add gr of protein module*).
19h: 50-100ml of liquid yogurt (add gr of protein module*).
21h: 50-100ml of vegetable broth (add gr of protein module*).
23h: 50-100ml skimmed milk (add gr of protein module*).

*The protein module can be diluted in water or other liquid, according to the patient's preference.

Another fundamental objective is to avoid protein malnutrition and to favor surgical wound healing. To guarantee the consumption of the patient's daily protein requirements (1-1.5g protein/kg corrected weight/day, depending on the type of surgical technique performed, (Table 3); to ensure that the requirements are met, the prescription of a protein module is necessary. In order to prevent specific nutritional deficiencies, a multivitamin-mineral intake is required. In our clinical experience, we have noted the difficulty of the patient to introduce the protein module and the multivitamin-mineral supplement at the same time, so our team prioritizes the insertion of the protein supplementation for Phase 1, leaving the insertion of the multivitamin-mineral for Phase 2 [11, 13, 19, 31-38].

One of the objectives in this phase in terms of "nutritional education" will be to eliminate the intake of ultra-processed products. Therefore, priority will be given to the purchase of natural or fresh products rather than processed ones; to introduce the patient to the reading of nutritional labeling, an app will be provided to help him/her discern between good processed (healthy foods/products) and ultra-processed (unhealthy foods/products), fundamental in this phase the scanning by app of vegetable drinks, liquid yogurts and processed broths. Another of the first measures, will be to eliminate sugar from the diet, it will be modified by Ceylon cinnamon powder, stevia, sucralose or erythritol; 100% pure cocoa could also be used. The adaptation of the palate will be worked on by educating it, under the premise of enjoying the own and natural flavor of the food consumed [26-30, 39-41].

Table 5. General recommendations to promote gastrointestinal tolerance [11, 13, 19, 31-36]

- Each time a new food is incorporated, it is advisable to incorporate it one at a time to detect any intolerance problems. In case of intolerance, wait a few days and try again.
- Ingest water separately from the main feedings to avoid the sensation of nausea, regurgitation or vomiting; stop drinking liquids 30 minutes before the feeding and restart 1 hour after the end of the feeding.
- The intake intended for one feeding should last between 30 and 45 minutes.
- Do not drink liquids quickly.
- Do not drink a large amount of liquid in one sip.
- Do not drink liquids at extreme temperatures (cold liquids should be allowed to cool down and hot liquids should be allowed to cool down).
- Do not drink sugary drinks.
- Do not drink fizzy drinks or foods with meteorizing or flatulent capacity.
- Do not drink alcohol.
- Stop eating if you notice a significant sensation of fullness, swelling or pain.
- Avoid bending or lying down immediately after ingestion (at least 1 hour sitting down after ingestion).

To ensure gastrointestinal tolerance, dietary recommendations should be maintained and healthy behavioral habits should be acquired (Table 5).

One week after surgery (unless there is a previous incidence), the patient should be re-evaluated by the multidisciplinary team; if there is no contraindication (immediate surgical complication or gastrointestinal intolerance), he will progress to the next phase (Phase 2); in case of gastrointestinal intolerance, he will remain one more week at Phase 1 (total of 14 days, or more if necessary) [11, 13, 19, 31-36].

PHASE 2. SURGERY PROTECTION

Duration: initial 15 days [11, 13, 19, 31-36].

Medical treatment: prophylactic anticoagulation, proton pump inhibitor, adjustment of treatment for DLP, HTN Regarding the treatment of DM, if the patient is administered insulin during Phase 1 and pre-prandial blood glucose levels are in the normal range, it will be limited to WBC control. A regimen of insulin treatment will be applied according to Table 2 [4].

Sports treatment: the physical exercise indicated up to three months will be solely aerobic, and the progression of this will be individualized; during this phase, light aerobic exercise (walking) will be recommended, and the target (minutes/day) will be established based on what has been achieved in the previous phase. Although it is true that there is scientific evidence that recommends early initiation of strength exercises (from one month after the intervention), including at the abdominal level, our clinical experience makes us advise against initiating strength exercises until three months, both because of the patient's weakness and because of progressive adherence to sports practice, under the premise that we are dealing with sedentary patients who are not trained in a pre-surgical stage [11, 17, 19, 33-35].

Dietary treatment: the priority of protection of the surgical procedure is maintained, so the progression in texture is to a semi-liquid diet (cream) and the volume according to tolerance but limited between 100 and 150ml. As in the previous phase, reiterate the importance of slow and fractioned intake (5-6 intakes/day), completing hydration with water outside these intakes [11, 13, 19, 31-36].

Regarding the composition of the diet, the products or foods to be included in this phase are: potato and vegetables (cooking culinary technique) and fruits (cooking or baking culinary technique), limiting those with a high content of insoluble fiber (Table 6); the shortage of hydrochloric acid does not allow the cell walls to digest well, causing a sensation of gastric heaviness and flatulence. Yogurt, cottage cheese and clear (few) and thin ("0") noodle soup are also included, with the precaution that they should be "very cooked" and not "al dente" to favor their tolerance.

Table 6. Classification of vegetables and fruits according to dietary fiber and meteorizing capacity [46, 46]

SOLUBLE OR FERMENTABLE FIBER (high viscosity, delays gastric emptying, slows intestinal transit, increases water and sodium absorption, decreases nutrient absorption, little effect on fecal bolus)	*Vegetables:* garlic, onion, carrot, pumpkin, artichoke, beet, asparagus, tomato, chicory root. *Cereals*: oats, buckwheat, rye, millet, barley, potato, rice and pasta (cooked and cooled). *Fruits*: citrus fruits, apple (without skin), grapes, plums, strawberries, banana. Nuts: almonds, hazelnuts. *Legumes:* lentils (without skin).
INSOLUBLE OR NON-FERMENTABLE FIBER (low viscosity, accelerates gastric emptying, accelerates intestinal transit, increases fecal bolus and decreases intraluminal pressure)	*Cereals*: whole grains (rice and pasta), quinoa, wheat bran and corn. *Legumes*: peas, dried beans. *Seeds:* (sesame or flax) and nuts. *Green vegetables*: lettuce, endive, cabbage, celery, turnips, radish, broccoli. Fruits with skin (apple and pear) and plant stems.
MIXED FIBER	White bread, pasta, white rice, carrots, asparagus, beans and corn.
RESISTANT SULFUR (resists digestion and acts as soluble fiber)	*Legumes*: peas, lentils, chickpeas, white beans. *Cereals*: rice, wheat, rye, buckwheat, tapioca, oats, pasta and corn flour. *Tubers:* potato, cassava, sweet potato. *Fruits:* green banana (unripe), plantain.
WEATHERING	*Vegetables:* cabbage, cauliflower, broccoli, onion, paprika, garlic, cilantro, cucumber, corn, asparagus, artichoke and lettuce. *Fruits:* melon, watermelon, cucumber, pear, banana. *Fresh and dried legumes*: beans, lentils and chickpeas.

In addition, it could include as a non-semi-liquid food the toasted bread type biscote, NOT WHOLE (Table 7) [11, 13, 19, 31-36]. In addition, the protein module should be maintained and a multivitamin-mineral supplement should be started to meet daily requirements according to the Recommended Daily Allowance (RDA), preferably in a dilutable solution for better tolerance. In the case of malabsorptive techniques at the distal level, the dose of the multivitamin-mineral is doubled and the need for preventive supplementation with iron (45-60mg/day), calcium (1200-1500mg/day), vitamin B12 (350g/day) and vitamin D (2,000-3,000 IU/day) will be assessed; these recommendations will be assessed in restrictive techniques if the patient presents vomiting or intolerance [11, 13, 17, 19, 31-38, 41, 43, 44].

In relation to the objectives of "nutritional education" in this phase, the behaviors acquired in Phase 1 will be reinforced (label reading for elimination of ultra-processed foods and sugar withdrawal) and the insertion of vegetables and fruits at least 5 times a day will be worked on (Phase 2 objective) [26-30, 39-41].

Keys to success for gastrointestinal tolerance: stress on "chewing" or retention of the cream bolus in the mouth, together with those described in Table 5.

Unless there are previous incidences, in the third week the patient will be re-evaluated. If he/she manifests post-ingestion intolerances, he/she will remain at least seven more days in Phase 2, until total tolerance. Otherwise, the patient will go on to Phase 3 [11, 13, 19, 31-36].

Table 7. Example of semi-liquid diet (cream) after BS

9h: 100 ml of skimmed milk (add gr of protein module*) and a biscuit (not wholemeal) with cottage cheese.
12h: 100-150ml of natural juice diluted and strained (add gr of protein module*).
15h: 100ml of defatted vegetable and chicken broth with noodles and a roasted pear.
18h: 100-150ml of natural juice diluted and strained (add gr of protein module*).
21h: 100ml of vegetable and root vegetable cream (add gr of protein module*) and apple compote.
24h: 125g of non-fat yogurt (add gr of protein module*).

*The protein module can be diluted in cream or any liquid, according to the patient's preference.

PHASE 3. SURGERY PROTECTION

Duration: initial 15 days [11, 13, 19, 31-36].

Medical treatment: antithrombotic prophylaxis is maintained for 30 days after surgery. The proton pump inhibitor is maintained during the first year. In the case of dyslipidemic and anitihypertensive treatment, it will be modified based on postoperative evolution, referring the follow-up to the primary care physician. Regarding the treatment of DM, if the patient is administered insulin during Phase 2 and basal and pre-prandial blood glucose levels are in the normal range, it will be limited to the control of BG. A tapering regimen of insulin treatment will be applied according to Table 2. [4].

Sports treatment: the objective of promoting daily physical activity will be maintained. Maintain light aerobic activity (walking) 5 days a week (30 minutes/day), increasing to moderate intensity (40% of maximum heart rate) 3 times a week for a total of 90 minutes a week [11, 17, 19, 33-35].

Dietary treatment: the priority of protection of the surgical procedure is maintained, so we will progress to a semi-solid texture (puree). As for the volume, tolerance will be tested, without exceeding 150-200ml per feeding in any case. As in the previous phase, reiterate the importance of slow and fractioned intake (5-6 intakes/day), completing hydration with water outside these intakes.

Regarding the composition of the diet, the products or foods to incorporate in this phase are: skinless legumes (chickpeas, lentils, beans, peas), white meats (turkey or chicken), white fish (hake, halibut, sole, others) and eggs. All foods included in this phase must be subjected to a cooking technique that allows maintaining hydration (boiling, steaming, oven or microwave), in such a way as to avoid protein coagulation; therefore, the grilling cooking technique is discarded (Table 8). In addition, uncooked fruit is introduced (avoiding fruit with insoluble fiber) (Table 6). The supplementation with the protein module was replaced by the insertion of protein foods (meat, fish, eggs and legumes). Multivitamin-mineral supplementation is maintained [11, 13, 19, 31-36].

In this phase, the patient is often constipated, so insoluble fiber is introduced progressively: first through vegetables and then legumes with skin, leaving as a last measure the fiber from fruit.

Table 8. Example of semi-solid diet (puree) after BS

9h: 100 ml of skimmed milk, a biscuit (not whole meal) with fresh cheese and 50 ml of fruit puree.
12h: 150-200ml of fruit puree.
15h: 150ml of puree (vegetables, skinless chickpeas and fish) and 50ml of yogurt.
18h: 150-200ml of fruit puree.
21h: 150ml of puree (vegetables, potato, chicken and egg) and 50ml of yogurt.
24h: 125ml of yogurt with 75ml of fruit puree.

In relation to the objectives of "nutritional education" in this phase, the behaviors acquired in the previous phases will be reinforced (label reading to eliminate ultra-processed foods, withdrawal of sugar and insertion of vegetables and fruits in at least 5 meals/day) and the weekly balance (objective Phase 3) between legumes (4 times a week), white fish (4 times a week), white meat (3 times a week), and the rest of the meals completed with tubers and dairy products (cottage cheese) will be worked on. A biweekly dietary record will be provided [26-30, 39-41].

Keys to success for gastrointestinal tolerance: food should be cooked using a culinary technique that allows the food to remain juicy and hydrated, even if it is subsequently to be crushed. In addition, the importance of slow ingestion should be reiterated, with emphasis on chewing and retention of the food bolus in the mouth, respecting sedentary rest for 40 minutes after ingestion, together with those described in Table 5. In the fifth week post-surgery, a new evaluation will be made, monitoring possible complications. If tolerance is good, progress to Phase 4; if complications occur, Phase 3 will be maintained for seven days or until tolerance of Phase 3 [11, 13, 19, 31-36].

PHASE 4. SURGERY PROTECTION

Duration: 15 to 30 days [11, 13, 19, 31-36].

Medical treatment: the indications presented in Phase 3 are maintained. [4].

Sports treatment: the premise of daily activity with the same intensity (light and moderate) is maintained, with the proposal to progress, individually and based on tolerance, until reaching a minimum of 150 minutes/week of moderate intensity. This can be achieved by increasing the weekly frequency and/or time per session [11, 17, 19, 33-35].

Dietary treatment: maintains the priority of protection of the surgical procedure, so the progression in texture is to an easily chewed solid diet ("manual mashing with a fork") keeping the volume limitation between 150 and 200ml. This is the first phase where the patient, having spent at least five weeks, makes the step from swallowing to chewing in terms of mashing, so it is emphasized that "his mouth should be the previous masher"; as in the previous phase, stressing slow and fractioned intake (5-6 intakes/day), completing hydration with water outside these intakes. Due to the complexity required in the chewing process, new foods are not introduced in this phase, with the exception of unprocessed vegetables in the form of puree (traditional Andalusian gazpacho type).

In relation to cooking techniques, the progression should be maintained according to the hydration of the food: boiled, steamed, oven or microwave and then grilled. For example, an egg will be introduced first cooked or poached, if it is tolerated, it will be tried in steam, oven or microwave and if there are no incidences, it will be tried in scrambled eggs and later in omelet. In relation to fruit, ripe fruit should be introduced in small pieces, applying manual crushing with a fork (Table 9) [11, 13, 19, 31-36].

Table 9. Example of solid diet (manual mashing with fork) after BS

9h: 100 ml of skimmed milk (one spoonful of powdered milk*), one biscuit (not whole meal) with cottage cheese and half a banana.
12h: an apple and a half with 50g of fresh cheese.
15h: 50g of red bell pepper and 50g of cooked beans with 100g of steamed hake.
18h: 75g of chickpea hummus with 125g of carrot sticks.
21h: 100g of cauliflower au gratin with mozzarella cheese and 2 boiled eggs.
24h: 125ml of yogurt, half a banana and half an apple.

*1 tablespoon of powdered milk = 10g of protein.

The multivitamin-mineral complex should be maintained with the indications given in Phase 2 [11, 13, 19, 31-37].

If the patient's constipation persists in this phase, fruit rich in insoluble fiber should be introduced and the 35° angle posture with stool support (sitting on the toilet leaning forward, with the knees higher than the hips and the feet resting on the step to straighten the anorectal angle) should be recommended.

In relation to the objectives of "nutritional education" all those proposed in the previous phases are strengthened, focusing on slow intake and chewing [establish a minimum time of 30 minutes for each intake, chew between twenty and thirty times each mouthful, leave the cutlery on the plate between mouthfuls, smell the food in each mouthful, if possible eat in company and in a quiet environment, if it is not possible and we eat alone, avoid distractions (television and cell phone)]. The dietary record given in the previous phase should be reviewed to identify the errors made (generally there is an abuse of tubers instead of legumes and an abuse of meat products instead of fish) [26-30, 39-41].

Keys to success for gastrointestinal tolerance: chewing and oral trituration are the key to this phase. Be warned that rapid ingestion and swallowing without proper chewing can cause the pain mentioned above and described by the patient as "it is as if a ball is stuck in the center of my chest and until I vomit, I cannot breathe" and another sensation described as "an elevator, the food goes up and down from the stomach to the throat, until I vomit". Maintain measures described in Table 5. The seventh week after surgery (unless previous incidence), the patient should be reevaluated by the multidisciplinary team, if there is no contraindication (immediate surgical complication or gastrointestinal intolerance), it will progress to the next phase (Phase 5); in case of gastrointestinal intolerance, it will remain one more week at Phase 4 (it is not unusual for the patient to require 30 days for complete adaptation to this phase) [11, 13, 19, 31-36].

PHASE 5. TOLERANCE

Duration: once Phase 4 is over, the patient returns to a normalized and healthy diet [11, 13, 19, 31-36].

Medical treatment: the indications presented in Phase 3 and Phase 4 are maintained [4].

Sports treatment: the guidelines presented in Phase 4 will be maintained up to 3 months; after this time, a sports program will be established that includes aerobic activity (walking, including cycling) 3 days a week at high intensity intervals (60% of maximum heart rate), according to individual tolerance; complemented with strength exercises (performance of dynamic or static contractions against resistance). As with aerobic exercise, start slowly with a progressive increase in intensity to avoid injury. Start with 2 or 3 days per week, trying with elastic bands and in case of using weights or resistance machines, always with lower loads than those performed before the time of surgery. The exercises will include the 8 to 10 major muscle groups and will be performed in 1-3 sets of 8-12 repetitions, with 30 to 60 seconds rest between sets. The initial goal will be to reach 50-60% of the maximum power that can be performed with that muscle group [11, 17, 19, 33-35].

Dietary treatment: this phase is the return to normality and the aim is to prevent nutritional complications (protein malnutrition and nutritional deficiencies), as well as hypoglycemia or dumping syndrome. Foods that are more difficult to tolerate are progressively inserted: white but fibrous meats (rabbit), oily fish (tuna, bonito and salmon), red meat (veal, beef, pork or lamb), hard meat fish (cuttlefish and squid), raw green leafy vegetables (lettuce, spinach, tender sprouts) or tomato (initially without skin), cereals and derivatives (rice, pasta, dry bread), cereal flakes (oats, rye, corn), fruit (citrus fruits).

At this stage, the texture of the food is not modified. However, the first time that any of them is introduced, it should be done with the progression described for the culinary techniques, respecting the hydration of the food, thus favoring its tolerance. For example, rice should be tried very cooked and with broth, before moving on to a dry rice, al dente, Spanish paella type. Regarding the volume, respect the limitation between 150 and 200 ml. If it is not possible to reach the target per intake, prioritize protein foods (eggs, fish, meat and legumes) to avoid protein malnutrition (5-6 intakes/day), completing hydration with water outside these intakes.

No modifications are established with respect to the multivitamin-mineral supplementation regimen [11, 13, 19, 31-36].

If constipation persists after having taken all the measures described in the previous phases, after three months, a glass of lukewarm water on an empty stomach could be inserted to promote intestinal transit.

In relation to the objectives of "nutritional education", we insist on the points worked on in the previous phases and work on the weekly planning (Annex I), varied and balanced: white fish (3 times a week), blue fish (once a week), white meats (maximum 3 times a week), red meats (maximum once a month), legumes (3 times a week), eggs (3 times a week), cereals, pasta or rice (once a week), eggs (3 times a week): pasta or rice (once a week), tubers (potato, cassava, sweet potato) once a week, greens, vegetables and fruits (5 times a day), skimmed/skimmed dairy (0-2 times a day) [26-30, 39-41].

Keys to success for gastrointestinal tolerance: as in the previous phase, oral chewing and mashing are the key when a food cooked by the griddle cooking technique is to be ingested because it is harder and drier. Maintain the measures described in Table 5 [11, 13, 19, 31-36].

After nine weeks, the review with the Dietitian-Nutritionist and the PAS professional will depend on the difficulties of each patient and should be maintained every 15 days to ensure adherence to the dietary and sports treatment.

After three months, a complete re-evaluation by the multidisciplinary team should be carried out (Table 1) in order to detect nutritional complications (protein malnutrition, vitamin and mineral deficiencies, sarcopenia) and to analyze and progress with individualized objectives within the general guidelines set out. Up to 6 months the correction of minerals or vitamins will be done through supplements due to the difficulty of gastrointestinal tolerance, as described in Phase 2 [11, 13, 19, 31-37].

PHASE 6. RETURN TO NORMALITY

Duration: this phase begins when the patient has tolerated all the foods described in Phase 5 (at approximately 6 months) and a healthy lifestyle is established [11,13,19, 31-36].

Medical treatment: the pharmacological reduction protocol described after BS has proven to be effective and safe. At 9 months after surgery the comorbidities associated with obesity were reduced by 100% for AHT ($p < 0.001$), 99.3% for DLP and hyperuricemia ($p < 0.001$), as well as

97.9% for DM ($p < 0.001$); which means that only 1.4% of patients require OAD, with 100% elimination of insulin treatment ($p < 0.001$) [4].

Sports treatment: after 6 months, it is recommended to maintain 3 days a week of aerobic activity with moderate intensity, increasing the time to 200 minutes/week and 3 days a week of exercises 3-4 series of 8-12 repetitions with an individualized progression, setting the objective of reaching 80% of the maximum power that can be achieved with each muscle group [11, 17, 19, 33-35].

Dietary treatment: after six months, in general, the risks involved in surgery and the tolerance problems have been overcome in terms of reduced gastric capacity and low acidity of the medium which hinder the digestion of insoluble fiber (in malabsorptive and mixed techniques) or the delay in gastric emptying which aggravates the symptoms of gastroesophageal reflux (restrictive techniques), so that healthy fat can be inserted. However, it would be unrealistic not to mention that, in certain cases, up to one year is required for the tolerance of rice or pasta and red meat. At six months, the patient does not require texture adaptation and will maintain the volume limitation outlined in Phase 5 [11, 13, 19, 31-36]. During the previous phases the patient should have reached the basic goal of having eliminated sugar and achieved a structured and balanced diet with a weekly schedule (fruits and vegetables, legumes, fish, fish, egg and dairy products).

In this phase, refined cereals will be replaced by whole grains (pasta, rice, bread) or legume flour (lentil or chickpea) and tubers (potato, cassava, sweet potato) will be refrigerated for 24 hours after cooking to obtain resistant starch. Similarly, healthy fats are inserted as a source of satiety (to avoid the habit of snacking out of meals), avocado, nuts, seeds and fermented dairy products.

Regarding "nutrition education," since Phase 1, the patient has been asked to scan the products during the time of purchase to classify them as: healthy products (natural or well processed product) or unhealthy (ultra-processed); now, label reading training in terms of ingredients is initiated, for example, when faced with the purchase of a yogurt, the patient should look for that among the ingredients only "whole milk" and "lactic ferments" appear, discarding all those with a proportion higher than 5g of sugar/100g of product and which are sweetened, sweetened, flavored or include any other compound; the patient will be recommended to modify the yogurt the same by adding: Ceylon cinnamon, pure cocoa or chocolate >85%, fruit, nuts or others [26-30, 39-41].

The points mentioned above will be worked on until approximately one year after surgery (depending on each patient) for the consolidation of a healthy lifestyle (Table 10).

In addition, we start healthy cooking by inserting simple and unusual recipes (Annex 2), progressively increasing in complexity so that after two years the patient is autonomous and independent. The first recipe we insert is the manufacture of their own whole wheat bread (Table 11), due to the difficulty of finding it in supermarkets and, sometimes, its high cost.

Table 10. Consolidation of a healthy lifestyle [26-30, 39-41]

- Make a shopping list based on the weekly dietary schedule. - Avoid creating a dispensary with "unhealthy" foods for visitors; in the end they never come and we end up consuming them ourselves. - Prioritize in the purchase products that do not contain labels, this will indicate that they are "fresh". Without forgetting the good processed products (canned vegetables, legumes, frozen fruits, yogurt, cheese, canned fish, dark chocolate, etc.) and discarding the ultra-processed ones. - Eliminate sugar and refined flours. - Extra virgin olive oil for raw consumption and cooking and cold-pressed virgin coconut oil for home baking. - Homemade pastries, although homemade, should not be consumed daily (maximum once a week). - Eliminate alcohol and carbonated beverages. - Limit salt intake. - The intake of healthy sausages will be allowed, they are considered those with a minimum of 92% meat product expressed in the food label (Serrano ham, Iberian ham, turkey ham, among others). - Decrease the amount of animal protein in the diet, especially meat, milk and sausages. - Increase the intake of vegetable protein (legumes). - Increase consumption of fruits and vegetables (5 times a day). - Intake of one serving of raw and one cooked vegetable per day. - Increase the intake of probiotics.

Table 10. (Continued)

- Make a shopping list based on the weekly schedule of the diet. - Avoid creating a dispensary with "unhealthy" foods for visitors, in the end they never come and we end up consuming them ourselves. - Prioritize in the purchase products that do not contain labels, this will indicate that they are "fresh". Without forgetting the good processed products (canned vegetables, legumes, frozen fruits, yogurt, cheese, canned fish, dark chocolate, etc.) and discarding the ultra-processed ones. - Eliminate sugar and refined flours. - Extra virgin olive oil for raw consumption and cooking and cold-pressed virgin coconut oil for home baking. - Homemade pastries, although homemade, should not be consumed daily (maximum once a week). - Eliminate alcohol and carbonated beverages. - Limit salt intake. - The intake of healthy sausages will be allowed, they are considered those with a minimum of 92% meat product expressed in the food label (Serrano ham, Iberian ham, turkey ham, among others). - Decrease the amount of animal protein in the diet, especially meat, milk and sausages. - Increase the intake of vegetable protein (legumes). - Increase consumption of fruits and vegetables (5 times a day). - Intake of one serving of raw and one cooked vegetable per day. - Increase probiotic intake: kefir, yogurt, sauerkraut or fermented cabbage, kimchi, natto, kombucha, miso, cheeses, pickles, unfiltered apple cider vinegar, cocoa (>85%), tempeh. - Increase the intake of prebiotics: broccoli, seaweed, artichoke, beets, onions, pumpkin, chicory, asparagus, rye, ripe banana, wheat, flakes (oats, rice, potato, sweet potato, legumes) and pulses (beans, beans, lentils, chickpeas, peas, soybeans). - Natural coffee (preferably, buy the bean and grind it before drinking it) and infusions (green tea, ginger, fennel, anise, among others). - Maintain regular physical activity (indicated by your CAFD professional). - Avoid stress, incorporate relaxation techniques among your habits, yoga is a good alternative. - Achieve a restful sleep using 6 to 8 hours/day.

Table 11. Recipe for whole wheat spelt bread

Ingredients: 600ml of warm water, 1Kg of wholemeal spelt flour and 25g of fresh yeast.

Preparation:

1. Preheat the oven to 200°C up and down.
2. Heat 600ml of water in a glass bowl.
3. On a baking tray place parchment paper and put a little bit of flour.
4. Introduce the 25g of yeast in the water until it dissolves.
5. Introduce 1 kg of whole wheat flour and knead it.
6. Once the dough has the desired shape, place it on the baking tray and cover it with a kitchen towel for 40 minutes.
7. After the 40 minutes of rest, place in the oven at 180° for 40 minutes.
8. After this time, remove from the oven and let it cool. Once cooled, slice and freeze, if desired.

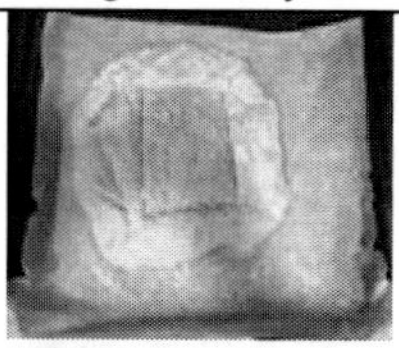

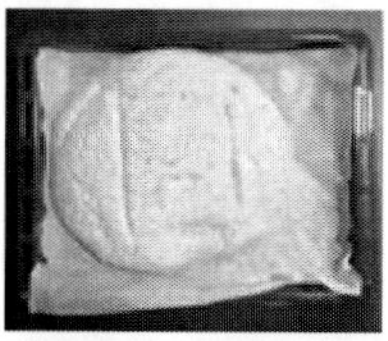

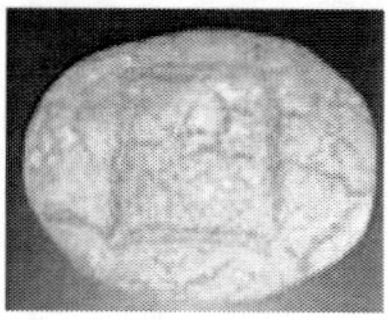

Table 12. Most common nutritional deficiencies, causes and surgical technique involved [17, 34-38, 41, 47]

Nutritional Deficiency	Cause	Surgical Technique
Iron	Frequent due to decreased intake of iron-rich foods, modification of gastric pH and exclusion of preferential absorption site (duodenum and jejunum)	MALABSORPTIVE MIXED
Calcium	Gastric resection, exclusion of the first part of the small intestine and steatorrhea	MALABSORPTIVE MIXED
Magnesium	Infrequent, caused by diarrhea	MALABSORPTIVE
Zinc, Copper, Selenium	Asymptomatic	MALABSORPTIVE
Thiamine (B1)	Insufficient intake or vomiting	MALABSORPTIVE MIXED RESTRICTIVE
Folic Acid (B9)	Insufficient intake	MALABSORPTIVE MIXED RESTRICTIVE
Vitamin B12	Gastric resection	MALABSORPTIVE MIXED RESTRICTIVE
Vitamin D	Malabsorption due to inadequate mixing with biliopancreatic secretions in distal jejunum (RYGB) or ileum (DBP)	MALABSORPTIVE MIXED
Vitamin A, E, K	Infrequent	MALABSORPTIVE

Table 13. Vitamin-mineral supplementation through diet [41, 43, 44, 48-52]

Deficiency	Place of Absorption	Food
Iron	Absorption in duodenum and first jejunal sections, requiring an acid gastric pH.	*Meat:* red meat (beef, pork, lamb and poultry); viscera (liver, heart and kidney). *Fish and shellfish*: oysters, clams, cockles, mussels, snails, beef, shrimp, crayfish, prawns, lobster, whiting, sardines and anchovies. *Legumes*: soybeans, lentils, white beans, chickpeas, broad beans and peas. Vegetables: black currants, broccoli, Brussels sprouts and peppers. *Nuts:* pistachios, almonds, cashew nuts, hazelnuts and walnuts. Dried fruits: dried peaches, raisins, plums, apricots, dates. *Egg yolk.* Whole grains: bread, rice or pasta. Chelators (oxalates, phytates and phosphates) and insoluble fiber: spinach, celery, currant, beet, chard, cocoa powder, tea or coffee, bran and walnut, pomegranate, grape, quince, persimmon, green apple, blueberry, strawberry. Substances rich in calcium. *Adjuvants (vitamin C):* green leaves (parsley, basil), peppers and citrus fruits (orange, tomato, lemon).
Calcium	Absorption in duodenum and jejunum.	*Canned fish*: herring or sardines. *Seafood and crustaceans:* whitebait, langoustines, shrimps, prawns, shrimps, mussels, squids. *Fish with bones*: anchovies and sardines. *Green leafy vegetables*: broccoli, thistle, spinach, chard, artichoke, leek, cabbage, cabbage, lettuce. *Nuts:* almond, walnut, date. Seeds: chia, flax or sesame. Legumes: lentils, white beans, chickpeas, soybeans. Dairy products. *Chelators (oxalates, phytates and phosphates) and insoluble fiber*: spinach, celery, currant, beet, chard, cocoa powder, tea or coffee, bran and walnut, pomegranate, grape, quince, persimmon, green apple, blueberry, strawberry. *Adjuvants (vitamin A, D and C, lactose and protein foods):* leafy greens (spinach, parsley, basil), peppers and citrus fruits (orange, tomato, lemon). Sun exposure to ensure vitamin D dosage (20 min/day).

Deficiency	Place of Absorption	Food
Magnesium	Absorption in duodenum and jejunum	*Fish:* swordfish and sardines in olive oil. *Green leafy vegetables:* spinach and chard. *Vegetables:* lettuce, endive and chicory. *Legumes*: chickpeas, white beans, peas and lentils. *Nuts:* walnuts, cashew nuts, almonds. Dairy products and eggs. Whole grains. Chocolate.
Zinc	Absorption in duodenum and jejunum	*Meats:* veal and offal and lamb meat. *Shellfish and crustaceans*: oyster, clam, scallop, mussel, crayfish, lobster, spider crab, red shrimp, prawn. *Dairy products:* especially cheeses: parmesan, blue cheese, manchego, cheddar, gouda. *Nuts:* pumpkin seeds and pine nuts. *Legumes:* chickpeas, lentils, white and pinto beans and peas. *Egg yolk*. Whole grains
Copper	Absorption in duodenum and jejunum	*Seafood:* oysters. Animal viscera: liver and kidneys. *Nuts:* walnut, hazelnut, almond, peanut and chestnut. *Cheese*: Emmental cheese. Chocolate or cocoa powder.
Selenium	Absorption in duodenum and jejunum	*Meats:* red meat, chicken and liver. *Fish:* canned tuna. Seafood. *Vegetables*: garlic and mushroom. *Nuts:* Brazil nuts or Amazonian chestnuts. *Eggs*. Whole grains.
Thiamine (B1)	Absorption in jejunum and ileum.	*Fish:* pompano and tuna. *Meat and offal*: pork. Legumes: black beans and soybeans. *Seeds:* sunflower. *Nuts*: pine nuts, pecans, macadamia nuts and pistachios. Whole grains.
Folic acid (B9)	Absorption in the proximal third of the small intestine	*Fruits*. Dark leafy vegetables. Legumes. Eggs. Nuts: peanuts and hazelnuts. Liver. cereals

Table 13. (Continued)

Deficiency	Place of Absorption	Food
Vitamin B12	Complex absorption, occurs in the distal ileum	*Foods of animal origin:* eggs, milk, meat and seafood.
Vitamin D	Partial absorption in duodenum, mainly in jejunum	*Cod liver oil. Fish:* bonito in oil, smoked salmon, anchovies in oil, sardines, salmon, pickled herring, mackerel, swordfish, tuna, anchovies. *Vegetables:* Fresh Shiitake mushroom and dried Shiitake mushroom. *Legumes:* Reinforced tofu. Egg yolk. Beverages: reinforced soy or rice beverage.
Vitamin A	Absorption in duodenum and jejunum	*Fish:* elver, conger eel, clams, clams and cockles. *Meat:* turkey and beef liver. *Fruits*: mango, melon, peach, papaya. *Vegetables:* carrots, spinach, lettuce, turnip greens, dandelion greens, cabbage, red peppers, pumpkin, sweet potato, tomatoes, *Legumes*: peas, *Dried fruits*: apricots. Eggs and dairy products: whole milk, cream and butter. Cod liver oil
Vitamin E	Absorption in duodenum and first jejunal sections	*Nuts*: pine nuts and peanuts, hazelnut and sunflower seeds. *Oils:* soybean oil, sunflower oil, corn oil, cod liver oil, olive oil.
Vitamin K	Absorption in duodenum and jejunum (food origin) and ileum and colon (microbiota)	*Meat:* beef and liver. *Vegetables (green leafy vegetables):* spinach, chard, watercress, parsley, cabbage, lettuce, Brussels sprouts, broccoli. *Fruits*: avocado, kiwi and green grapes. *Herbs*: parsley and coriander. Green tea.

If the constipation persists after the adoption of the described measures, after 6 months we would have the option of ingesting a spoonful of olive oil on an empty stomach or a spoonful of chia or flax in three spoonfuls of water leaving it to rest for 10 hours in the refrigerator and take it on an empty stomach.

As has been mentioned on different occasions, multivitamin-mineral supplementation should be maintained as a chronic prophylactic treatment due to the complications described at the level of vitamin and mineral deficiency (Table 12) [17, 34-38, 41, 47].

From 6 months onwards, the initial dose of the multivitamin-mineral established in Phase 2 will be maintained and an attempt will be made to reach the requirements through the diet (Table 13).

Based on our experience, we suggest that two years of follow-up by the Dietitian-Nutritionist or Nurse specialized in Nutrition is required to achieve healthy eating and learn not only what to eat and how to cook it, but also what utensils to use and how to preserve them [frying pans and casseroles (they should be made of iron, 18/10 stainless steel or titanium reinforced and free of perfluorooctanoic acid), glass containers (for preserving and cooking) or plastic containers valid for food preservation (not for heating food inside the container), avoiding aluminum, boards (wood or tempered glass), spatulas, ladles, skimmers (wood, platinum silicone, stainless steel and ceramic knives), cleaning and maintenance of kitchen towels, cloths, scouring pads or sponges, preservation of food, among other measures to work with] [53, 54].

ANNEX 1. WEEKLY DIET TABLE

A balanced menu is presented that complies with the rations described: vegetables and fruit 5 times a day, vegetables one serving raw and one cooked, legumes 3 times a week, dairy products 2 times a day, eggs 3 times a week, meat maximum 3 times a week, fish minimum 4 times a week and a blue portion (tuna spread over 3 breakfasts), homemade pastries (not daily) and nuts to increase satiety.

	Monday	**Tuesday**	**Wenesday**	**Thursday**	**Friday**	**Saturday**	**Sunday**
Breakfast	Coffee (plain) with milk (whole) Wholemeal toast: tomato, tuna (plain) and oregano	Oat Porridge (whole milk) Kiwi	Coffee (plain) with milk (whole) Wholemeal toast: tomato, tuna (plain) and oregano	Oat Porridge (whole milk) Kiwi	Coffee (plain) with milk (whole) Wholemeal toast: tomato, tuna (plain) and oregano	Coffee (natural) with milk (whole) 2 Banana tartlets (see recipe)	Coffee (plain) with milk (whole) Pancakes with 85% chocolate syrup (see recipe)
Lunch	Apple and cottage cheese	Kefir with strawberries	Apple and cottage cheese	Kefir with mango	Apple and cottage cheese	Strawberries	Apple
Lunch	Baked stuffed aubergine (onion, peppers, tomato and turkey)	Baked rooster. Salad: tomato, cabbage, endive and grated carrot.	Crafty" spaghetti carbonara (see recipe)	Stewed white beans with vegetables (carrot, onion, garlic, red pepper, leek).	Sea bass on the back Spinach, mushroom, caper and beetroot salad	Garden lentils with cheese (see recipe)	Seafood and vegetable rice (brown).
Mid-Afternoon	Kiwi and 6 pistachio nuts	Orange and 2 walnuts	Kiwi and 6 cashew nuts	Orange and 4 hazelnuts	Kiwi and 2 walnuts	Chocolate ice cream (see recipe)	Berries ice cream (see recipe)
Dinner	Tomato Scrambled eggs with asparagus and prawns	Zucchini strips with leek. Mini pizza with chicken breast, tomato, onion and mozzarella	Asparagus and artichokes. Fresh cod.	Cold carpaccio with courgette, tomato, onion and garlic. Pea omelette.	Broccoli pizza with vegetables and mozzarella (see recipe)	Tomato. Mushroom scrambled eggs.	Artichoke hummus with carrot sticks. Fresh cheese

ANNEX 2. RECIPE BOOKLET

Garden lentils with cheese (2 persons)

Ingredientes: Ingredients: 120 g lentil paste, 200 g cherry tomatoes, 100 g green pepper, 100 g onion, 200 g feta cheese, basil to taste, extra virgin olive oil, 1 tablespoon, salt, oregano and pepper.

Preparation:

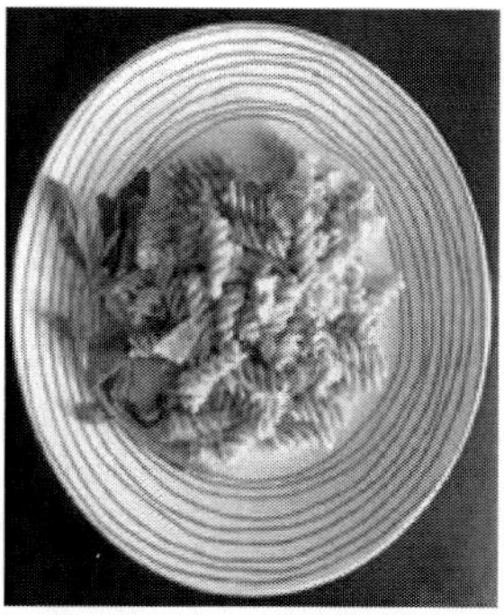

1. Preheat the oven to 200°C top and bottom
2. In a glass dish, place the tomatoes, pepper, onion, oil, oregano, salt and pepper.
3. Place the feta cheese in the centre of the tray and season with salt and pepper.
4. Bake for 30 minutes at 200°C.
5. Cook the pasta for 10 minutes and drain.
6. Once baked, mix all the ingredients in the tray to create a sauce.
7. Add the pasta and basil to the sauce, mix everything together and ready to serve!

Spaghetti carbonara "Crafty" (2 persons)

Ingredients: 250g Konjac spaghetti, 200g mushrooms, 100g onion, 4 cloves of garlic, 150g pork shoulder, extra virgin olive oil 1 tablespoon, kefir 4 tablespoons, salt, oregano and pepper.

Preparation:

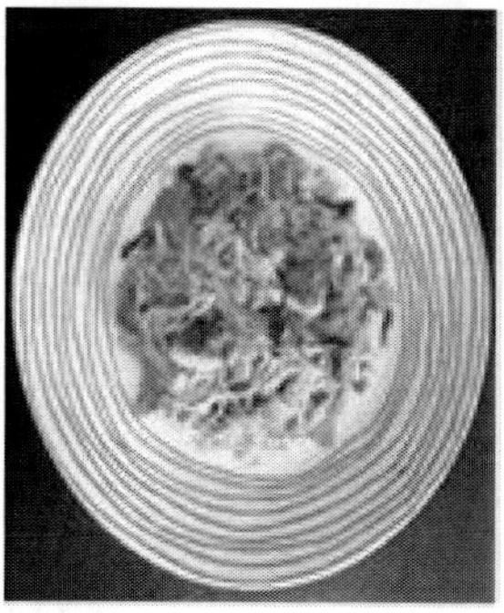

1. Peel the onion and garlic cloves.
2. Chop the onion, mushrooms, garlic and pork shoulder.
3. In a frying pan, add the oil and the onion and fry.
4. When the onion is golden brown, add the mushrooms, garlic and pork shoulder; add the oregano and season with salt and pepper.
5. Once everything is poached, add the 4 spoonfuls of kefir.
6. Boil the Konjac for 3 minutes.
7. After this time, drain and add to the frying pan with the stir-fry.
8. Poach everything for 10 minutes and it's ready to serve!

Broccoli pizza with vegetables and mozzarella (4 persons)

Ingredients: 350g broccoli, 90g oats, extra virgin olive oil one tablespoon, oregano, salt, pepper, basil, vegetable ratatouille 380gr (good processed), 6 cherry tomatoes and 6 mushrooms, 150gr mozzarella cheese and basil to taste.

Preparation:

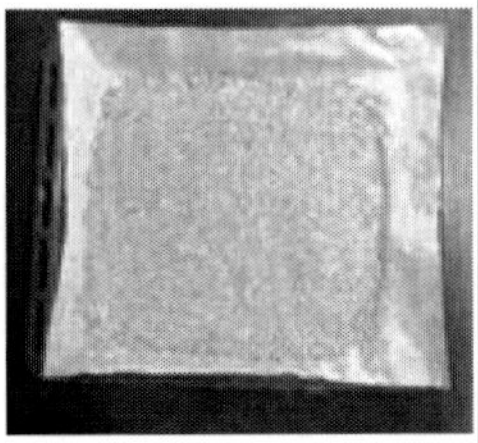

1. Preheat the oven to 200°C (top and bottom).
2. Place baking paper on a baking tray.
3. Place the broccoli in a blender and blend.
4. Add the oatmeal, oregano, salt, pepper and oil to the blender and blend.
5. Pour the mixture onto the parchment paper on the baking tray and roll out until you have a thin, even dough.
6. Bake for 20 minutes at 180°C (top and bottom).
7. Slice the cherry tomatoes and mushrooms.
8. Once this time has elapsed and the dough has browned, add the vegetable ratatouille, mozzarella cheese and a little more oregano, the cherry tomatoes and mushrooms.
9. Bake for X minutes and add the basil, ready to serve!

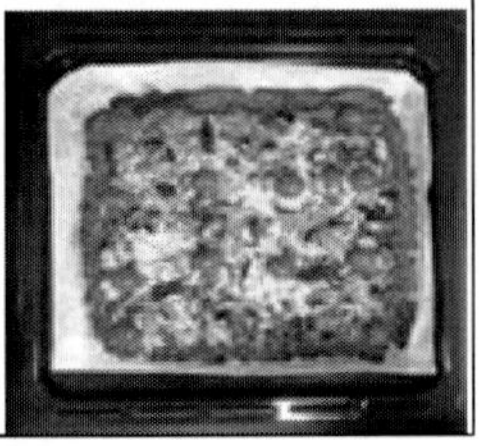

Banana and chocolate tartlet (5 units)

Ingredients: one ripe banana, one egg, 40g of oats, 8g of yeast, 4 tablespoons of kefir, 2 ounces of 85% chocolate, 5ml of olive oil and Ceylon cinnamon (to taste).

Preparation:

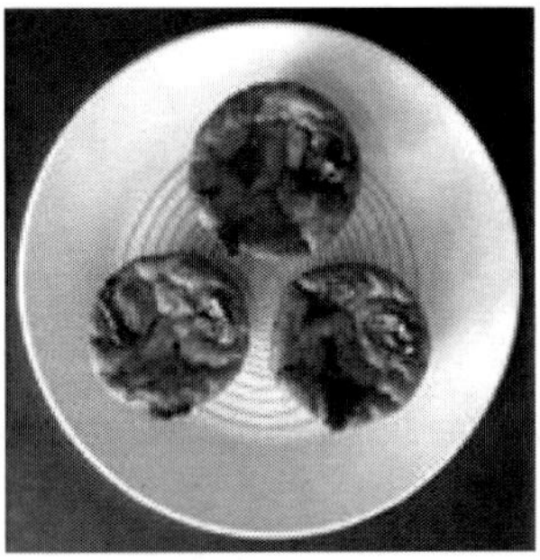

1. Preheat the oven to 200°C (top and bottom).
2. Place baking paper on a baking tray.
3. Place the moulds on top of the parchment paper and apply the oil with a brush to grease them.
4. Place the banana, egg, oats, yeast, kefir and Ceylon cinnamon in a blender and blend.
5. Pour the batter into the moulds (leaving 2cm to the surface).
6. Chop the ounces of chocolate and place in the batter.
7. Bake for 20 minutes at 180°C (top and bottom).
8. Leave to cool, unmould and ready to serve!

*The oats can be replaced by wholemeal flour and the banana by baked apple.

Banana and chocolate pancakes (2 units)

Ingredients: one ripe banana, one egg, 20g oats, 4g yeast, 2 tablespoons kefir, 2 ounces 85% chocolate, 5ml olive oil and Ceylon cinnamon (to taste).

Preparation:

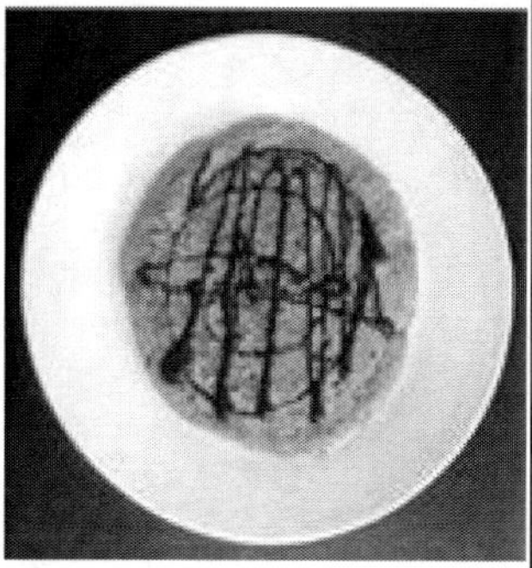

1. In a blender add: banana, egg, oats, yeast, kefir and Ceylon cinnamon; blend.
2. Heat a frying pan over medium heat.
3. When hot, pour in oil and rub with a napkin.
4. Pour in half of the dough and when holes appear, turn it over.
5. Do this process on both sides (approximately 2 minutes per side).
6. Heat the 2 ounces of chocolate in the microwave for 2 minutes.
7. Serve the pancake on a plate and with a spoon add the chocolate on top to taste.

Chocolate ice cream

Ingredients: two bananas, a spoonful of 100% cocoa, 3 tablespoons of kefir, 3 cashew nuts and Ceylon cinnamon to taste.

Preparation:

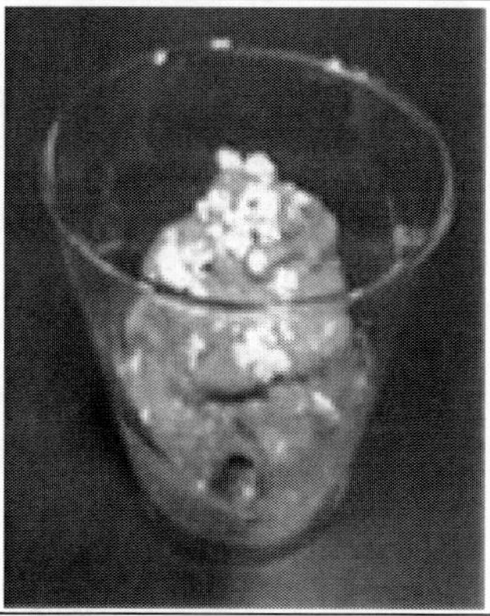

1. Leave the fruit out of the freezer for 15 minutes to decrystallise.
2. Crush 3 pistons and set aside.
3. Place the banana, kefir, cocoa and cinnamon in a blender and blend until creamy.
4. Pour the ice cream into a glass.
5. Add the pistachios.
6. Ready to taste!

Berries ice cream

Ingredients: one banana, 3 strawberries, 3 raspberries, 3 blackberries, 3 tablespoons of kefir, 3 pistachios and Ceylon cinnamon to taste.

Preparation:

1. Leave the fruit out of the freezer for 15 minutes to decrystallise.
2. Crush 3 cashew nuts and set aside.
3. Place the banana, strawberries, raspberries, blackberries, blackberries, kefir and cinnamon in a blender and blend until creamy.
4. Pour the ice cream into a glass.
5. Add the cashew nuts.
6. Ready to taste!

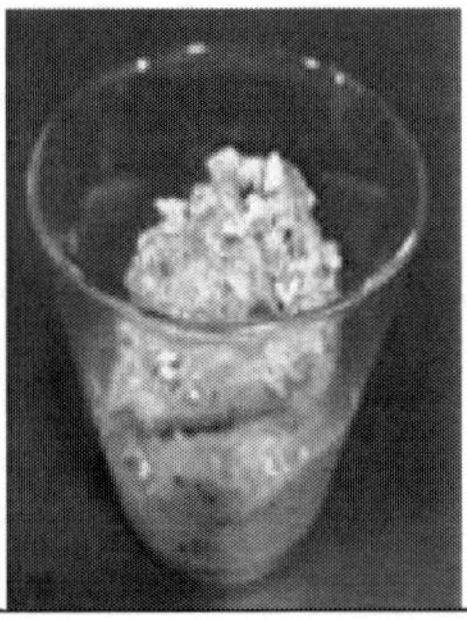

REFERENCES

[1] Nguyen, N. T., & Varela, J. E. (2017). Bariatric surgery for obesity and metabolic disorders: state of the art. *Nature reviews Gastroenterology & hepatology*, *14*(3), 160.

[2] Arterburn, D. E., Telem, D. A., Kushner, R. F., & Courcoulas, A. P. (2020). Benefits and risks of bariatric surgery in adults: a review. *Jama*, *324*(9), 879-887.

[3] Fernandez-Ruiz, V. E., Armero-Barranco, D., Xandri-Graupera, J. M., Paniagua-Urbano, J. A., Sole-Agusti, M., & Mulero, J. (2016). Bariatric and cardiovascular efficacy of long-limb Roux-en-Y gastric bypass: Overcoming the limitations inherent in individuals. *Bariatric Surgical Practice and Patient Care*, *11*(2), 49-55.

[4] Fernández-Ruiz, V. E., Armero-Barranco, D., Xandri-Graupera, J. M., Paniagua-Urbano, J. A., Solé-Agustí, M., & Mulero, J. (2017). Roux-en-Y Gastric Bypass: Effective against Metabolic and Psychiatric Comorbidity? *Biological research for nursing*, *19*(2), 162-169.

[5] Le Roux, C. W., & Heneghan, H. M. (2018). Bariatric Surgery for Obesity. *The Medical Clinics of North America*, *102*(1), 165-182.

[6] Jakobsen, G. S., Småstuen, M. C., Sandbu, R., Nordstrand, N., Hofsø, D., Lindberg, M., & Hjelmesæth, J. (2018). Association of

bariatric surgery vs medical obesity treatment with long-term medical complications and obesity-related comorbidities. *Jama*, *319*(3), 291-301.

[7] Ruiz-Tovar, J., Carbajo, M. A., Jimenez, J. M., Castro, M. J., Gonzalez, G., Ortiz-de-Solorzano, J., & Zubiaga, L. (2019). Long-term follow-up after sleeve gastrectomy versus Roux-en-Y gastric bypass versus one-anastomosis gastric bypass: a prospective randomized comparative study of weight loss and remission of comorbidities. *Surgical endoscopy*, *33*(2), 401-410.

[8] Oliveira, S. C., Neves, J. S., Souteiro, P., Pedro, J., Magalhães, D., Guerreiro, V., & Carvalho, D. (2020). Impact of bariatric surgery on long-term cardiovascular risk: comparative effectiveness of different surgical procedures. *Obesity surgery*, *30*(2), 673-680.

[9] Ho, K., Hawa, R., Wnuk, S., Okrainec, A., Jackson, T., & Sockalingam, S. (2018). The psychosocial effects of perioperative complications after bariatric surgery. *Psychosomatics*, *59*(5), 452-463.

[10] Li, Z. J., & Yu, J. C. (2018). Multidisciplinary Team and Nutrition Management for Bariatric Surgery. *Zhongguo yi xue ke xue yuan xue bao. Acta Academiae Medicinae Sinicae*, *40*(5), 577-580.

[11] Heber, D., Greenway, F. L., Kaplan, L. M., Livingston, E., Salvador, J., & Still, C. (2010). Endocrine and nutritional management of the post-bariatric surgery patient: an Endocrine Society Clinical Practice Guideline. *The Journal of Clinical Endocrinology & Metabolism*, *95*(11), 4823-4843.

[12] Bullen, N. L., Parmar, J., Gilbert, J., Clarke, M., Cota, A., & Finlay, I. G. (2019). How Effective Is the Multidisciplinary Team Approach in Bariatric Surgery?. *Obesity surgery*, *29*(10), 3232-3238.

[13] Mechanick, J. I., Apovian, C., Brethauer, S., Garvey, W. T., Joffe, A. M., Kim, J., & Still, C. D. (2019). Clinical practice guidelines for the perioperative nutrition, metabolic, and nonsurgical support of patients undergoing bariatric procedures–2019 update: cosponsored by American Association of Clinical Endocrinologists/American College of Endocrinology, The Obesity Society, American Society for Metabolic & Bariatric Surgery, Obesity Medicine Association, and American Society of

Anesthesiologists. *Surgery for Obesity and Related Diseases*, *16*(2), 175-247.

[14] Tabesh, M. R., Maleklou, F., Ejtehadi, F., & Alizadeh, Z. (2019). Nutrition, physical activity, and prescription of supplements in pre- and post-bariatric surgery patients: a practical guideline. *Obesity surgery*, *29*(10), 3385-3400.

[15] Marshall, S., Mackay, H., Matthews, C., Maimone, I. R., & Isenring, E. (2020). Does intensive multidisciplinary intervention for adults who elect bariatric surgery improve post-operative weight loss, co-morbidities, and quality of life? A systematic review and meta-analysis. *Obesity Reviews*, *21*(7), e13012.

[16] Paul, M. A., Opyrchał, J., Knakiewicz, M., Jaremków, P., Duda-Barcik, Ł., Ibrahim, A. M., & Lin, S. J. (2020). The long-term effect of body contouring procedures on the quality of life in morbidly obese patients after bariatric surgery. *Plos one*, *15*(2), e0229138.

[17] Fried, M., Hainer, V., Basdevant, A., Buchwald, H., Deitel, M., Finer, N., & Widhalm, K. (2007). Interdisciplinary European guidelines for surgery for severe (morbid) obesity. *Obesity Surgery*, *17*(2), 260-270.

[18] Qasim, A., Turcotte, M., De Souza, R. J., Samaan, M. C., Champredon, D., Dushoff, J., & Meyre, D. (2018). On the origin of obesity: identifying the biological, environmental and cultural drivers of genetic risk among human populations. *Obesity reviews*, *19*(2), 121-149.

[19] Rubio, M. A., Martínez, C., Vidal, O., Larrad, A., Salas-Salvadó, J., Pujol, J., & Moreno, B. (2004). Documento de consenso sobre cirugía bariátrica. *Revista Española Obesidad*, *4*, 223-249.

[20] Hasan, N. A., Freije, A., Abualsel, A., Al-Saati, H., & Perna, S. (2020). Effect of Bariatric Surgery on Weight Loss, Nutritional Deficiencies, Postoperative Complications and Adherence to Dietary and Lifestyle Recommendations: A retrospective cohort study from Bahrain. *Sultan Qaboos University Medical Journal*, *20*(3), e344.

[21] Al-Mutawa, A., Anderson, A. K., Alsabah, S., & Al-Mutawa, M. (2018). Nutritional status of bariatric surgery candidates. *Nutrients*, *10*(1), 67.

[22] Ben-Porat, T., Weiss, R., Sherf-Dagan, S., Nabulsi, N., Maayani, A., Khalaileh, A., & Elazary, R. (2020). Nutritional deficiencies in patients with severe obesity before bariatric surgery: what should be the focus during the preoperative assessment?. *Journal of the Academy of Nutrition and Dietetics*, *120*(5), 874-884.

[23] Lecube, A., Monereo, S., Rubio, M. Á., Martinez-de-Icaya, P., Marti, A., Salvador, J., & Casanueva, F. F. (2017). Prevention, diagnosis, and treatment of obesity. 2016 position statement of the Spanish Society for the Study of Obesity. *Endocrinologia, diabetes y nutricion*, *64*, 15-22.

[24] Romeijn, M. M., Kolen, A. M., Holthuijsen, D. D. B., Janssen, L., Schep, G., Leclercq W. K. G., van Dielen, F. M. H. (2021) Effectiveness of a Low-Calorie Diet for Liver Volume Reduction Prior to Bariatric Surgery: a Systematic Review. *Obesity Surgery*, *31*(1), 350-356.

[25] Ruiz de Angulo, D., Munitiz, V., Ortiz, M. Á., Martínez de Haro, L. F., Frutos, M. D., Hernández, A., Parrilla, P. (2015). Communication between the obese patient and bariatric surgeon. *Cirugía Española*, *93*(8), 492-5.

[26] Fernández-Ruiz, V. E., Armero-Barranco, D., Paniagua-Urbano, J. A., Sole-Agusti, M., Ruiz-Sánchez, A., & Gómez-Marín, J. (2018). Short-medium-long-term efficacy of interdisciplinary intervention against overweight and obesity: Randomized controlled clinical trial. *International journal of nursing practice*, *24*(6), e12690.

[27] Fernández-Ruiz, V. E., Paniagua-Urbano, J. A., Solé-Agustí, M., Ruiz-Sánchez, A., Gómez-Marín, J., & Armero-Barranco, D. (2018). Effectiveness of the I2AO2 interdisciplinary programme led by nurses on metabolic syndrome and cardiovascular risk: a randomized, controlled trial. *Journal of International Medical Research*, *46*(6), 2202-2218.

[28] Fernández-Ruiz, V. E., Paniagua-Urbano, J. A., Solé-Agustí, M., Ruiz-Sánchez, A., Gómez-Marín, J., & Armero-Barranco, D. (2018). Impact of the I2AO2 interdisciplinary program led by nursing on psychological comorbidity and quality of life: Randomized controlled clinical trial. *Archives of psychiatric nursing*, *32*(2), 268-277.

[29] Fernández-Ruiz, V. E., Ramos-Morcillo, A. J., Solé-Agustí, M., Paniagua-Urbano, J. A., & Armero-Barranco, D. (2020). Effectiveness of an interdisciplinary program performed on obese people regarding nutritional habits and metabolic comorbidity: A randomized controlled clinical trial. *International journal of environmental research and public health*, *17*(1), 336.

[30] Fernández-Ruiz, V. E., Solé-Agustí, M., Armero-Barranco, D., & Cauli, O. (2021). Weight Loss and Improvement of Metabolic Alterations in Overweight and Obese Children through the I2AO2 Family Program: A Randomized Controlled Clinical Trial. *Biological Research for Nursing.*

[31] Stein, J., Stier, C., Raab, H., & Weiner, R. (2014). The nutritional and pharmacological consequences of obesity surgery. *Alimentary pharmacology & therapeutics*, *40*(6), 582-609.

[32] Leahy, C. R., & Luning, A. (2015). Review of nutritional guidelines for patients undergoing bariatric surgery. *AORN journal*, *102*(2), 153-160.

[33] Thorell, A., MacCormick, A. D., Awad, S., Reynolds, N., Roulin, D., Demartines, N., & Lobo, D. N. (2016). Guidelines for perioperative care in bariatric surgery: enhanced recovery after surgery (ERAS) society recommendations. *World journal of surgery*, *40*(9), 2065-2083.

[34] Busetto, L., Dicker, D., Azran, C., Batterham, R. L., Farpour-Lambert, N., Fried, M., & Yumuk, V. (2017). Practical recommendations of the obesity management task force of the European Association for the Study of obesity for the post-bariatric surgery medical management. *Obesity facts*, *10*(6), 597-632.

[35] Sherf Dagan, S., Goldenshluger, A., Globus, I., Schweiger, C., Kessler, Y., Kowen Sandbank, G., & Sinai, T. (2017). Nutritional recommendations for adult bariatric surgery patients: clinical practice. *Advances in nutrition*, *8*(2), 382-394.

[36] Bettini, S., Belligoli, A., Fabris, R., & Busetto, L. (2020). Diet approach before and after bariatric surgery. *Reviews in Endocrine and Metabolic Disorders*, *21*(3), 297-306.

[37] Di Lorenzo, N., Antoniou, S. A., Batterham, R. L., Busetto, L., Godoroja, D., Iossa, A., & Silecchia, G. (2020). Clinical practice guidelines of the European Association for Endoscopic Surgery

(EAES) on bariatric surgery: update 2020 endorsed by IFSO-EC, EASO and ESPCOP. *Surgical endoscopy*, *34*(6), 2332-2358.

[38] Parrott, J., Frank, L., Rabena, R., Craggs-Dino, L., Isom, K. A., & Greiman, L. (2017). American Society for Metabolic and Bariatric Surgery integrated health nutritional guidelines for the surgical weight loss patient 2016 update: micronutrients. *Surgery for Obesity and Related Diseases*, *13*(5), 727-741.

[39] Grupo Colaborativo de la Sociedad Española de Nutrición Comunitaria (SENC). Guías alimentarias para la población española; la nueva pirámide de la alimentación saludable. Nutr Hosp 2016;33(Supl 8):1-48.

[40] Ruiz, E., & Varela-Moreiras, G. (2017). Adecuación de la ingesta de azúcares totales y añadidos en la dieta española a las recomendaciones: estudio ANIBES. *Nutrición Hospitalaria*, *34*, 45-52.

[41] Amaya García, M., Vilchez López, F. J., Campos Martín, C., Sánchez Vera, P., & Pereira Cunill, J. L. (2012). Micronutrientes en cirugía bariátrica. *Nutrición Hospitalaria*, *27*(2), 349-361.

[42] Redondo-Cuevas, L., Castellano, G., Torrens, F., & Raikos, V. (2018). Revealing the relationship between vegetable oil composition and oxidative stability: A multifactorial approach. *Journal of Food Composition and Analysis*, *66*, 221-229.

[43] Abellan, I., Luján, J., Frutos, M. D., Abrisqueta, J., Hernández, Q., López, V., & Parrilla, P. (2014). The influence of the percentage of the common limb in weight loss and nutritional alterations after laparoscopic gastric bypass. *Surgery for Obesity and Related Diseases*, *10*(5), 829-833.

[44] Durán, B., de Angulo, D. R., & Parrilla, P. (2015). Beriberi: an uncommon complication of sleeve gastrectomy. *Surgery for Obesity and Related Diseases*, *11*(6), e53-e55.

[45] Bermejo-López, L. M. (2015). Fiber-type indication among different pathologies. *Nutricion hospitalaria*, *31*(6), 2372-2383.

[46] Dong, Y., Chen, L., Gutin, B., & Zhu, H. (2019). Total, insoluble, and soluble dietary fiber intake and insulin resistance and blood pressure in adolescents. *European journal of clinical nutrition*, *73*(8), 1172-1178.

[47] Antoniewicz, A., Kalinowski, P., Kotulecka, K. J., Koconń, P., Paluszkiewicz, R., Remiszewski, P., & Zieniewicz, K. (2019). Nutritional deficiencies in patients after Roux-en-Y gastric bypass and sleeve gastrectomy during 12-month follow-up. *Obesity surgery*, *29*(10), 3277-3284.
[48] Trumbo, P., Yates, A. A., Schlicker, S., & Poos, M. (2001). Dietary reference intakes: vitamin A, vitamin K, arsenic, boron, chromium, copper, iodine, iron, manganese, molybdenum, nickel, silicon, vanadium, and zinc. *Journal of the American Dietetic Association*, *101*(3), 294-301.
[49] Singh, P. (2018). Treatment of vitamin D deficiency and comorbidities: A review. *The Journal of the Association of Physicians of India*, *66*(1), 75-82.
[50] Mangan, A., Le Roux, C. W., Miller, N. G., & Docherty, N. G. (2019). Iron and vitamin D/calcium deficiency after gastric bypass: mechanisms involved and strategies to improve oral supplement disposition. *Current drug metabolism*, *20*(3), 244-252.
[51] Base de datos Española de Composición de Alimentos (BEDCA). https://www.bedca.net/bdpub/index_en.php. (Accessed february 1st, 2021).
[52] Domellöf, M., Thorsdottir, I., & Thorstensen, K. (2013). Health effects of different dietary iron intakes: a systematic literature review for the 5th Nordic Nutrition Recommendations. Food & nutrition research, 57(1), 21667.
[53] Choi, J. C., Park, S. J., Goh, H., Lee, J. Y., Eom, M. O., & Kim, M. (2014). A study on migration of heavy metals from kitchen utensils including glassware, ceramics, enamel, earthenware and plastics. *Journal of Food Hygiene and Safety*, *29*(4), 334-339.
[54] Kim, H., Park, S. Y., Jo, Y. E., Park, Y., Park, S. J., & Kim, M. (2018). Monitoring of heavy metals migrated from polylactide (pla) food contact materials in Korea. *Journal of Food Hygiene and Safety*, *33*(2), 102-109.

In: Enhanced Recovery after Surgery ... ISBN: 978-1-53619-976-5
Editor: Jaime Ruiz-Tovar

Chapter 13

DISCHARGE CRITERIA AND FOLLOW-UP

Covadonga Martín Garrido*
Nursing Department, Hospital del Tajo, Madrid, Spain

ABSTRACT

This chapter details the care of the surgical wound. Immediate postoperative management is also addressed. Finally, the discharge criteria are described along with their indications and the postoperative approach based on the ERAS protocol is specified.

Keywords: surgical wound, postoperative management, discharge criteria

INTRODUCTION

Due to the increasing rate of bariatric surgery, this chapter has been written to detail the care of surgical wounds, as well as discharge care.

* Corresponding Author's Email: covadonga1995_mg@hotmail.com.

The Surgical Wound. Surgical Wound Control

Despite the advances applied in surgical techniques, antibiotics and sterile methods, there is a high number of surgical procedures that lead to a relevant complication: Surgical site infection (SSI) [1].

SSI is considered to duplicate the time spent in hospital as well as its economic cost. To consider a surgical wound as infected, the following conditions must be met: it occurs within 30 days postoperatively, involves the skin and soft tissues, and presents at least one sign / symptom of infection (purulent drainage, isolation of the causative microorganism, pain, inflammation, erythema…) [1].

The diagnosis of SSI can be determined by a medical or nurse staff. The pillars of treatment are to establish adequate antibiotic treatment, surgical drainage (if applicable) and ensure the hemodynamic and metabolic support of the patient [1].

Different types of risk factors are distinguished:

- Dependent on the patient (immune status, usual treatment, toxic habits, nutritional status...).
- Dependent on the surgical act (surgical technique, duration of surgery, location of the surgical wound, use of antibiotic prophylaxis, asepsis and antisepsis of the operating room, personnel and instrumental material...).
- General factors (postoperative care, length of hospital stay, operation of drains...) [1].

Therefore, surgical wounds are a potentially lethal problem that represents a significant increase in morbidity, cost, and hospital stay; their prevention must be carried out actively and continuously by all the personnel involved in the pre, intra and postoperative period [1].

Surgical Wound Healing

The healing process is a dynamic and complex process, so it is important to assess the needs of each stage of said healing. Currently, we have a wide variety of materials and dressings with different functions (protect the wound from possible infection and / or trauma, provide compression if necessary due to bleeding or inflammation, allow the administration of medications, absorb exudate...) [5].

Healing represents the physiological process of tissue repair until a complete closure of the wound is achieved. This applies to any surgical wound. The following factors are determiniant in healing process [5]:

- Physiological humid environment (healing in a humid environment is faster than if it is done in a dry environment). It involves less pain, thermal insulation, autolytic debridement, faster healing speed and better quality of the scar, since the humid environment provides a wound as natural as possible for tissue repair to develop without alterations [5].
- Dressings: they should maintain the physiological moist environment. They are an insulating and protective barrier that allows gas exchange and adequate blood circulation. They must be adaptable, flexible and easy to manipulate, with an adhesive that does not injure or involve trauma or pain when changing to perform the cure. The decision of the dressing to use depends on the evolutionary stage of the wound, also based on the advantages and disadvantages offered by each of them as well as the objective to be achieved [5].

At the time of healing, we carry out an exhaustive assessment of the wound, taking into account whether it is an open or closed wound [5].

Closed Surgical Wound Care

Various items can be used to close a surgical incision: stitches or sutures, staples, or adhesives (skin glue) [6].

For the care of the surgical wound, a bandage may be applied, whose functions are to protect the wound from microbes, reduce the risk of infection, cover the wound so that the sutures or staples are not in contact with clothing, protect the healthy area and absorb any fluid that exudates from the wound [6].

It is very important to perform proper hand hygiene prior to handling the surgical wound [6].

The warning signs of a surgical wound are [6]:

- Redness or pain of the wound.
- Swelling or bleeding.
- Increase in the size or depth of the wound.
- Variation in the content drained by the wound (thicker, change in pain or density).
- Fever [6].

Open Surgical Wound Care

In case of being an open wound, the cares to follow are [7]:

- Use a saline solution or soapy water to wash the wound.
- Use topical disinfectant.
- Eliminate suppuration or any rest of dried blood or other biological content that may have accumulated on the skin.
- Do not use alcohol, iodine solutions or soaps with antibacterial chemicals as they can damage the wound tissue and delay its healing.
- Do not apply any lotion, cream or herbal remedies on or around the wound without prior medical authorization [7].

Immediate Postoperative and Discharge Criteria

First postoperative day:

- Evaluation of constants, diuresis and quantification of the drainage (if it was placed).
- Anamnesis and physical examination of the patient.
- Analytical control, if applicable [3].

If the clinical evolution is favorable, continue with the established clinical pathway. In the event of any clinical or analytical alteration, an individual evaluation will be carried out [3].

Medical indications [3]:

- Beginning of standing and ambulation.
- Use of the respiratory incentive.
- Checking the integrity of the sutures with methylene blue dye or contrast X-ray films is controversial.
- Examination of the surgical wound.
- Beginning of tolerance with oral fluids.
- Gastrointestinal thromboembolic prophylaxis.
- Medical prescription:
  - Oral or intravenous analgesia regimen (according to patient pain and oral tolerance).
  - Antiemetic regimen.
  - Insulin regimen (according to metabolic needs of the patient) [3].

Second and third postoperative days:

As on the first postoperative day, an evaluation of constants, diuresis and drainage is carried out; Anamnesis accompanied by physical examination of the patient and analytical control. If there is any alteration from normal evolution, the patient must be carefully observed [3].

Medical indications [3]:

- Active mobilization.
- Use of respiratory incentive.
- Evaluate drainage removal.
- Liquid diet, and stop of intravenous fluid therapy.
- The thromboembolic prophylaxis regimen is continued.
- Oral analgesia regimen.
- Insulin regimen according to the metabolic needs of the patient.
- The patient's usual medical treatment is restarted (except antiplatelet drugs and anticoagulation).

- Explain indications at discharge and type of diet to maintain in the immediate postoperative period. If the evolution is favorable, hospital discharge can be considered from the second post-surgical day [3].

Indications at Discharge [3]

- Liquid diet and follow the indications of the endocrinology and nutrition service.
- Use of respiratory incentivator.
- Omeprazole orally every 24h and Low molecular weight heparin subcutaneously every 24h (for 4-6 weeks).
- Progressive physical activity.
- Attend to the Emergency department in case of fever > 38°C, persistent vomiting, abdominal pain or worsening of the general condition.
- Revision in the outpatient clinics (approximately one week after discharge from hospital), in surgery, endocrinology and nutrition ones (review with nursing the first month, and medical consultation three months after discharge with complete blood analysis) [3].

Postoperative Approach Based on ERAS Protocol

The recommendations based on the ERAS protocol focused on the bariatric postoperative period are [4]:

- Early catheter removal: early removal of the epidural catheter as well as the bladder catheter is recommended (delayed removal of the bladder catheter is associated with an increase in urinary tract infections, lengthening the duration of hospital admission) [4].

- Multimodal analgesia and epidural anesthesia: multimodal postoperative analgesia consists of the combination of epidural anesthesia or port-site infiltration with local anesthetics, associated with intravenous anesthesia. Epidural analgesia, when applied; is maintained for the first 48 hours and then the catheter is removed. The use of opioids is associated with delayed return of normal bowel function, so they are usually left as rescue analgesic treatment. If the surgery has been performed with a laparoscopic approach, the patient usually presents less postoperative pain, so analgesia needs are reduced and the patient is discharged from the hospital earlier [4].
- Avoid the use of nasogastric tube: it is recommended to avoid its use, and in case it is necessary for gastric decompression during surgery, it can be used temporarily but will be removed at the end of the surgical procedure. There is scientific evidence supporting that the routine use of nasogastric catheterization delays the recovery of intestinal function, increases the risk of pulmonary complications and prolongs hospital stay, without avoiding vomiting, abdominal distension or anastomosis dehiscence. In addition, it causes discomfort to the patient and may delay early mobility [4].
- Early restarting of the oral diet: the ERAS protocol proposes starting the diet four hours after surgery, since it has been proven that early ingestion is safe and reduces postoperative complications, as well as hospital stay. In addition, tolerance to the diet is a good indicator of recovery of normal bowel function [4].
- Early mobilization: it has been proven that even short periods of immobilization in the postoperative period can cause morbidity. Such immobility triggers various events (increased insulin resistance, decreased muscle strength, worsened respiratory function and increased risk of thromboembolism, etc.). It is recommended that on the first postoperative day the patient remains seated as long as he can and active mobiliozation must be encouraged [4].

Therefore, the ERAS protocol establishes 3 fundamental criteria for hospital discharge: tolerance to diet, determination of effective oral analgesia and correct mobilization [4].

Postoperative Follow-Up After Hospital Discharge

Continued postoperative care is vital for the long-term success of surgery. Such care involves the participation of the entire multidisciplinary team, and its objectives are to assess the variation in weight, assess possible comorbidities associated with surgery, monitor the actual or potential appearance of surgical complications or nutritional deficits, and provide the patient with support to implant changes in the lifestyle [2].

Regarding metabolic and nutritional management, close monitoring is recommended for possible protein depletion, imbalances in skeletal homeostasis, fat malabsorption, nutritional anemia, or alterations in vitamin and mineral levels. As a general rule, vitamin and mineral supplementation is recommended in the postoperative period, even more strictly in malabsorptive procedures [2].

After being discharged from the hospital, the patient will be followed up on a regular basis. Usually these revisions are the first month after surgery, the third, the sixth, the ninth and the twelfth. After these check-ups, the patient is usually scheduled for a check-up every 6 or 12 months until the clinical evolution is favorable and advisable [8].

The follow-up of patients corresponds mainly to the endocrinology and nutrition service. The first review, which is scheduled in the first month after surgery, is carried out by the nursing staff of this medical service. The nursing staff will evaluate the correct progression of the diet as well as the intake of multivitamins, and will immediately notify the medical staff of any problem or incident detected. The second check-up will take place 3 months after the intervention and a complete blood analysis will be carried out beforehand, including vitamin determinations in order to address any vitamin deficiency [8].

In each of the aforementioned reviews, different interventions will be performed [3]:

- Assessment of the clinical situation:
    - General condition.
    - Surgical wound status.
    - Food tolerance.
    - Digestive symptoms.
    - Psychological situation (to be accompanied by psychiatric evaluation according to clinical evolution).
- Evolution of secondary pathologies and those associated with obesity, as well as cardiovascular risk factors.
- General examination, together with anthropometric parameters.
- Complementary examinations (blood analysis).
- Dietary survey to assess established eating habits and will be reinforced with nutritional counseling.
- Physical exercise program (it is recommended to incorporate it as a progressive habit, so as to improve the patient's functional capacity and at the same time avoid excessive loss of muscle mass) [3].

In a complementary manner, the following will be carried out [3]:

- Annual densiometry.
- Pneumology evaluation and polysomnographic study (according to clinical evolution).
- Referral to plastic surgery (to assess abdominoplasty in patients who present abdominal skin flap and are in a weight maintenance phase).

Finally, the stable patients will be scheduled annually with complete analytical tests. Communication between hospital outpatient care and primary care is crucial to favor joint management of patients [3].

METHODS

For the writing of this chapter, a bibliographic search of articles related to surgical wound care and bariatric surgery protocols was carried out in order to reach a consensus on the best postoperative and discharge care.

REFERENCES

[1] Santalla A., López-Criado M. S., Ruiz M. D., et al. Infección de la herida quirúrgica. Prevención y tratamiento. *Clin. Invest. Gin. Obst.* 2007;34(5):189-96.

[2] Maluenda F. Cirugía bariátrica. *Rev. Méd. Clín. Las. Condes.* 2012;23(2):180-188.

[3] Priego P. Protocolo de cirugía bariátrica/metabólica del Hospital Universitario Ramón y Cajal. http://www.pablopriego.com/wp-content/uploads/2016/01/Protocolo-de-cirug%C3%ADa-bari%C3%A1trica-del-Hospital-Ram%C3%B3n-y-Cajal.pdf (Accessed 08/03/2021).

[4] Carrillo Esper I., Espinoza de los Monteros E., Pérez Calatayud A. Una nueva propuesta de la medicina perioperatoria. El protocolo ERAS. *Revista Mexicana de Anestesiología.* 2013;36(1):296-301.

[5] Flores Montes I. Manejo avanzado de heridas. *Rev. Mex. Enferm. Cardiol.* 2006;14(1):24-28.

[6] https://medlineplus.gov/spanish/ency/patientinstructions/000738.htm (Accessed 08/03/2021).

[7] https://medlineplus.gov/spanish/ency/patientinstructions/000040.htm (Accessed 08/03/2021).

[8] Protocolo de Cirugía Bariátrica. Scledyn. Sociedad Castellano-Leonesa de Endocrinología, *diabetes y nutrición.* 2013; 1(1): 1-18.

In: Enhanced Recovery after Surgery ... ISBN: 978-1-53619-976-5
Editor: Jaime Ruiz-Tovar

Chapter 14

POSTOPERATIVE RECOMMENDATIONS OF PHYSICAL ACTIVITY

Artur Marc Hernández[1,*], PhD, Eva Hernández-García[2], PhD and Jaime Ruiz-Tovar[3], MD, PhD

[1]Faculty of Humanities and Social Sciences, University Isabel I, Burgos, Spain
[2]University College London, London, UK
[3]Department of Surgery, University Rey Juan Carlos, Móstoles, Spain

ABSTRACT

Currently, it is widely accepted that bariatric surgery generates great benefits for patients who undergo it. This surgical intervention greatly improves the patients' health status and has proved to be cost-effective.

However, this type of surgery has several disadvantages since, after surgery, there are large reductions in fat-free mass, as well as reductions in bone mineral density, while some patients do not achieve an optimal weight loss. Likewise, in the medium and long-

* Corresponding Author's Email: arturmarc.hernández@gmail.com.

term after bariatric surgery, weight regain is a common problem in bariatric patients, which, in turn, can lead to a relapse in the different comorbidities related with obesity.

Although the disadvantages that have been mentioned are relatively common, there are strategies that can be used with the aim of reducing or avoiding them, where physical activity and exercise are useful tools for these goals.

Nowadays, several studies have emerged to clarify the effects of exercise in patients undergoing bariatric surgery, and have tried to provide adequate guidelines for exercise to be performed in this population. Therefore, this chapter will mainly focus on the post-surgery disadvantages, which can be prevented through exercise and physical activity. Thus, these drawbacks will be carefully described, in order to analyze the effects that exercise can have on bariatric patients. In turn, based on studies available in scientific literature, a series of guidelines and exercise considerations to be performed in these patients will be provided.

Keywords: bariatric surgery, cardiovascular risk factors, exercise, physical activity, weight regain

1. Introduction

Patients awaiting bariatric surgery have different obesity-related comorbidities that greatly aggravate their health status, affecting both their quality of life and their life expectancy. On the one hand, obesity is associated with depression [1], while, on the other hand, obese patients have lower scores in variables related to quality of life, especially in variables related to physical components [2]. For instance, it has been reported that obesity increases by 76% the probability of obtaining poor evaluations of the general health of patients, while it can increase by 97% the probability of presenting deficient values in physical function [3].

In turn, patients with morbid obesity have their life expectancy seriously compromised. Studies have shown that subjects suffering from morbid obesity have a decrease in life expectancy of 7.7 years in women and 9.1 years in men [4]. However, these data get worse the higher the individuals' body mass index (BMI). It has been reported that, while in patients with a BMI of between 40-44.9 kg·m^{-2}, the risk of mortality increases by 2.52 times, in patients with a BMI of between 55-55.9 kg·m-

^{2}, this risk of mortality increases up to 6.42 times [5]. This shows the great importance of BMI in these patients, and the need for them to undergo surgical intervention, since in patients with a BMI of between 55-55.9 $kg \cdot m^{-2}$, life expectancy is reduced in 13.7 years compared to an individual with a normal weight [5].

Therefore, it is necessary that patients with morbid obesity reduce their body weight, and bariatric surgery is an excellent method to achieve this goal. At this point, it is required to define the concept of excess weight loss (EWL), used in bariatric surgery to determine if a surgery can be considered successful. It has been established that, for a surgery to be successful, the patient undergoing bariatric surgery must achieve ≥ 50% of the EWL [6]. To calculate the percentage of excess weight, the following formula is used:% EWL = (Initial weight - Current weight)/(Excess body weight) × 100, where excess body weight refers to the difference between the patient's current weight and the weight they should have with a BMI equal to 25 $kg \cdot m^{-2}$ if patients manage to achieve 50% or more of the excess weight lost (Excess body weight = actual weight - (25 × height^{2})) [7].

In this regard, it has been shown that bariatric surgery can generate reductions of approximately 30 kg after 3 months of it [8], reaching up to 40 kg at 6 months. These weight reductions last over time, and it has been observed that these weight losses continue until 1-2 years after surgery. Recently, a meta-analysis found that, even 12 months after surgery, patients undergoing sleeve gastrectomy present an EWL of between 69.7-83%, while in patients undergoing gastric bypass, the EWL is 60.5-86.4% [9]. These data show the great efficacy of bariatric surgery to achieve significant weight loss in individuals with morbid obesity.

In addition to being effective in weight loss, this surgical intervention has a great impact in reducing the obesity-related comorbidities, especially in the short-term. A 5-unit decrease in BMI after bariatric surgery has been reported to involve a reduction of 33%, 27%, and 20% in the risk of diabetes, hypertension, and hyperlipidaemia, respectively [10]. This contributes to remission of obesity-related comorbidities after surgery. In the short-term, bariatric surgery generates complete remissions of type 2 diabetes mellitus, hypertension, and dyslipidaemia in 91.5%, 84.3%, and 78.3% of patients, respectively [11]. In this regard, an interesting meta-analysis showed that obstructive sleep apnea was resolved in approximately 85% of patients after surgery [12]. Equally, a resolution of diabetes, hyperlipidaemia and hypertension was in 76.8%, 70% and 61.7% of patients undergoing bariatric surgery [12], also improving hepatic steatosis in 90% of patients [13]. In turn, it should be noted that these cardiometabolic improvements affect the risk of cardiovascular disease, which decreases after the operation in 82% of patients [13]. Although, bariatric surgery causes great improvements in the in physical and physiological parameters, patients undergoing this surgery also present great improvements in the psychological variables, and a decrease in depression levels after surgery has been reported, accompanied of increases in the self-esteem [14, 15].

All these improvements result in several benefits for patients. On the one hand, it is observed that approximately 95% of patients undergoing bariatric surgery surgery have improvements in their quality of life [13]. On the other hand, this surgical procedure leads to a significant increase in life expectancy. Studies have found that patients undergoing bariatric surgery reduce their 5-year mortality relative risk by 89% [16]. In this respect, other studies have shown a gain of between 2.6 and 3.4 years in life expectancy after bariatric surgery [17, 18]. Furthermore, these effects on life expectancy increase if patients undergoing bariatric surgery have some obesity-related comorbidity, and it has been reported that in women with morbid obesity and type II diabetes mellitus, life expectancy after surgery increases by 6.7 years [19].

Therefore, bariatric surgery is a method that can greatly improve the health of patients with morbid obesity, since it generates large reductions in weight and obesity-related comorbidities, leading to increases in both quality of life and life expectancy.

2. Bariatric Surgery Disadvantages

As previously reported, bariatric surgery is a procedure that provides great advantages, and it should be used in individuals with morbid obesity who are not able to reduce their body weight by other methods. However, this surgery also has several disadvantages.

First, it should be noted that after this surgical intervention, especially if it has been of the malabsorptive procedures (gastric bypass, biliopancreatic diversion or one anastomosis gastric bypass anastomosis), great deficiencies of determined micronutrients can occur. On the one hand, after gastric bypass, iron and calcium deficiencies occur in approximately 50% and 10% of patients, respectively [20, 21]. Furthermore, between 37-50% and 20-51% of patients undergoing gastric bypass have shown to have vitamin B12 and vitamin D deficiencies after surgery [20, 21]. Equally, other studies have determined that after 24 months of one gastric bypass anastomosis, 37.5%, 23% and 10.5% of patients need supplements of vitamin D, iron and vitamin B12 [11]. However, this chapter will focus on the disadvantages of surgery, which can be improved or avoided through exercise and physical activity.

These drawbacks produced by bariatric surgery will be shown divided into 2 parts, depending the amount of time that has elapsed since surgery: a) short-term disadvantages after surgery; b) medium and long-term disadvantages after surgery.

2.1. Short-Term Disadvantages

Fat Free Mass Loss

One of the biggest short-term disadvantages produced by bariatric surgery is the loss of fat free mass (FFM). It has been widely reported that, when there are large weight reductions, especially if these are in a short period of time, in addition to reducing fat mass levels, FFM levels are also reduced, which means around 25% of weight lost [22]. In bariatric patients there is this same trend, producing large reductions in FFM after surgery. These losses of FFM occur mainly during the first year after surgery, and reductions of between 6.95 and 12.7 kg a year after surgery have been shown, although most studies agree that this loss of FFM is approximately 10 kg at 12 months after bariatric surgery [23–32].

These reductions in FFM can lead to different disadvantages. On the one hand, they may predispose the patient to relapse in the different obesity-related comorbidities, since FFM is closely associated to cardiovascular risk factors. FFM is composed mainly by skeletal muscle, which means 40% of the total weight of an individual [33]. In turn, skeletal muscle is currently considered a powerful endocrine organ [34, 35], since it is responsible for storing around 80% of the body's glycogen, being able to store approximately 500 g of this nutrient [36]. On the other hand, skeletal muscle is responsible offor removing around 75% of post-prandial glucose [37].

In the same way, FFM has a decisive role in weight control, since it is directly associated with the basal metabolic rate, being responsible for 95% of it [33]. Therefore, the reductions in the FFM after surgery will lead to large decreases in the basal metabolic rate. Significant reductions have been observed one month after surgery, with the FFM being the component that presents a greater association with this reduction (r = .640) [26]. Unfortunately, the basal metabolic rate progressively decreases until approximately 6-12 months after surgery, at which point it seems to reach its maximum reduction [26, 38]. This lower basal metabolic rate predisposes the body to a gain in fat mass, and different studies in bariatric patients have shown how a basal metabolic rate is associated with weight regain after bariatric surgery [39–41]. In turn, this weight gain will also influence the comorbidities associated with obesity, increasing the probability of relapse. Therefore, it is of great importance to prevent the reduction of FFM after surgery, since it has been observed that for each kilogram of FFM, the basal metabolic increases by 10.78 kcal [41].

Another of the disadvantages caused by FFM reductions is a decrease in the functional capacity of patients. FFM is associated with strength levels [42], so that reductions in these can occur after surgery [25]. In fact, several studies have shown reductions in strength levels after bariatric surgery, both in the short-term [43, 44] and medium and long-term [25], showing associations between FFM and strength levels [25]. This can negatively affect the functional capacity of patients. Moreover, some studies have determined that 36 months after surgery, only 53.3% of patients had normal strength levels for their age [25].

Finally, an excessive loss of FFM can lead to sarcopenic obesity, which has been defined as an imbalance between the amount of fat mass and muscle mass, in which the muscle mass cannot support all the weight generated by the fat mass [45]. This sarcopenic obesity can generate different disadvantages, since it has been associated with low functional capacity [45], higher levels of systolic and diastolic blood pressure, higher insulin resistance, and an increased risk of developing type II diabetes mellitus [46–48].

Bone Mineral Density Reduction

Currently, there is already enough scientific evidence to affirm that after bariatric surgery there is a reduction in bone mineral density. Some studies have reported reductions of approximately 10% in bone content at 6 months after bariatric surgery, increasing to 12.9% at 12 months [49]. Other studies have observed reductions of between 8% and 11% of hip bone mineral density and of 8.8% of spine bone mineral density at 12 months after surgery [50, 51]. Furthermore, these reductions persist over time, and it has been shown that significant reductions in bone mineral density of the femur or spine continue to occur between 2 and 5 years after the surgical procedure [52].

These data show significant reductions in bone mineral density after surgery, which in turn, can generate different disadvantages. On the one hand, the risk of suffering from osteopenia or osteoporosis after surgery is increased [52], and it has been shown that after surgery, 1.7% and 6.8% of patients developed osteoporosis in the femoral neck and lumbar spine [53]. These reductions in bone mineral density increase the risk of suffering any fracture, showing that one year after surgery, the risk of fracture increases significantly from 1.5% to 2.1% [54]. In turn, other studies have concluded that the relative risk of suffering any type of fracture increases by 2.3 times after surgery [55].

Recently, different meta-analyses have also been performed on this topic, obtaining interesting conclusions. On the one hand, it has been concluded that the risk of fracture after bariatric surgery increases 1.41 times [56]. In addition, in this same meta-analysis it is concluded that malabsorptive techniques generate greater increases in the risk of fracture after surgery. In this regard, it has been reported that biliopancreatic diversion and gastric bypass have a relative risk of fracture of 2.44 and 1.33 compared to subjects who have not undergone surgery [56].

Suboptimal Weight Loss

Although bariatric surgery has been shown to be an effective technique in weight reduction, some patients are unable to achieve successful weight loss or *optimal* resolution of comorbidities after surgery. Some authors have referred to these patients as “bariatric surgery resistant” [57]. In this regard, several investigations have been carried out, showing that between 11% and 18.3% of patients have a suboptimal weight loss one year after surgery [58, 59], while in other studies this figure increases up to 22.3% [60]. Similarly, it has been determined that approximately 25% of patients undergoing gastric bypass do not achieve adequate weight loss or have weight regain [6]. It is important to highlight that this suboptimal weight loss may influence the remission of obesity-related comorbidities. For example, it has been reported that one year after surgery, 27% and 49% of patients who had a successful weight loss had diabetes and hypertension, however, these figures increase to 53% and 62%, respectively, in patients with suboptimal weight loss [58].

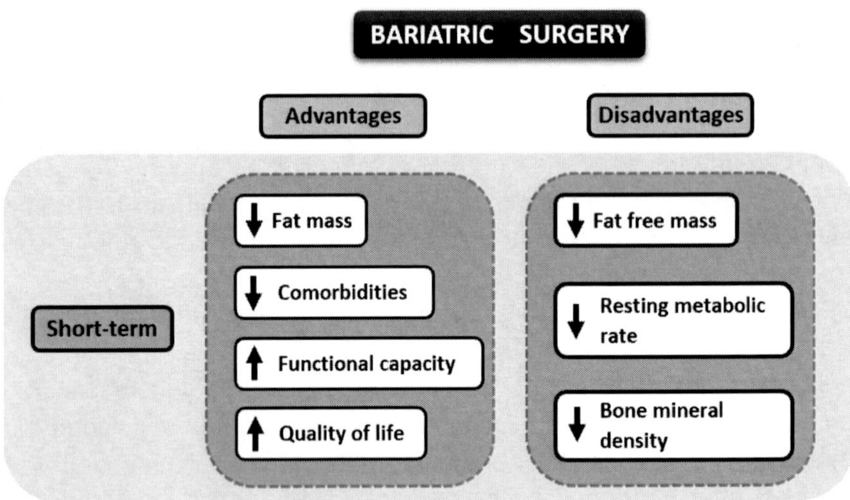

Figure 1. Main short-term advantages and disadvantages of bariatric surgery.

2.2. Medium and Long-Term Disadvantages

Weight Regain

As previously described, large reductions in total weight occur after surgery, resulting in successful surgery in a large proportion of patients. A recent meta-analysis has shown that patients achieve approximately 70% of the EWL one year after surgery [61]. Therefore, it can be stated that this surgery is effective in short-term weight loss. Most studies show that after the surgical procedure, there is a rapid loss of weight, being more pronounced in the first months after surgery (0-6 months). After this time, weight losses continue for up to 1-2 years after surgery, but at this time, these weight reductions are slower. [62].

However, the results of several studies show a weight regain process. It has been reported that, one year after a sleeve gastrectomy, patients had reached 84.8% of the EWL, while this was reduced up to 71.5% and 57.3% at 3 and 5 years after surgery, respectively [63]. This same trend occurs after gastric bypass, in which patients reach 88% of the EWL one year after surgery, and this decreases to 63% at 5 years after surgery [64]. Nevertheless, these results worsen over time and some studies have reported that the postoperative period is positively associated with weight regain [65, 66]. Equally, other studies have reported that in patients who showed weight regain, the time that had elapsed since surgery was higher compared to patients who had no weight regain [41]. In this regard, it has been shown that weight regain begins to gain great importance from 5 years after surgery [67], when many subjects with an EWL less than 50% begin to be observed. Some studies have concluded that 6 years after a sleeve gastrectomy, 64% of patients had an EWL of less than 50% [68]. Other studies have reported that these results worsen over time, and it has been obtained that 5 years after surgery, 18% of the patients did not achieve adequate weight loss, while this value increased to 35% after surgery at 10 years after surgery [69]. In turn, different studies show that the mean percentage of EWL is reduced to approximately 50% at 10 years after gastric bypass [70, 71], with 41% of patients with weight regain [71]. These decreases continue over time, and for instance, a mean of 48.9% of the EWL was obtained at 20 years of laparoscopic gastric banding [72].

Therefore, after surgery, there is a high percentage of weight regain, which occurs in 19.2%-58.5% of patients [65, 73–75]. However, this is not the only disadvantage, since these weight gains are mainly produced by increases in fat mass [25]. After bariatric surgery, there are large reductions in fat mass, which persist for up to 1–2 years [76–78]. Nevertheless from this time on, a process of fat mass regain begins in bariatric patients. [79–82]. For example, a study obtained that at 12 months after bariatric surgery, patients reached their lowest point of fat mass (27.7 kg) and FFM (56.1 kg). However, these patients showed a significant increase in fat mass (up to 33.1 kg), without an increase in FFM [25], results that have been obtained in other studies [24, 83]. In turn, this trend persists over time [82]. Other study shown that, at one year after surgery, patients had 58.6 kg of FFM and 35.5 kg of fat mass, while at 9 years, the FFM decreased to 53.9 kg, and fat mass levels increased up to 44.1 kg [81].

All this can lead to several disadvantages. On the one hand, weight regain, especially if they are mainly due to increases in fat mass, can contribute to the appearance of different comorbidities. On the other hand, it can lead to sarcopenic obesity. It should be noted that sarcopenic obesity in bariatric patients can occur in different ways. The first one is that there is a great decrease in FFM, which in bariatric patients occurs in the short-term after surgery. The second is the result of a weight regain exclusively generated by fat mass gains, which usually occurs in the medium-long term after surgery.

Finally, it should be noted that this weight regain can lead to other inconveniences. On the one hand, weight regain is one of the main reasons for revisional surgery [84], representing 7.4% of all bariatric interventions [85]. In reference to this, some studies have reported that revision surgery may be needed in up to 10.4-36% of patients [73, 75, 84, 86]. In turn, it has been shown that 63% of revisional surgery are due to the weight of the patients, either because they have not reached an optimal weight, or because a weight regain has occurred [85]. However, researches have concluded that 21% of revisional surgeries are due exclusively to weight regain [73]. Similarly, these weight increases affect the quality of life of the patients, and decreases in the quality of life have been observed in the long-term after bariatric surgery [87]._[64, 71, 88–90]

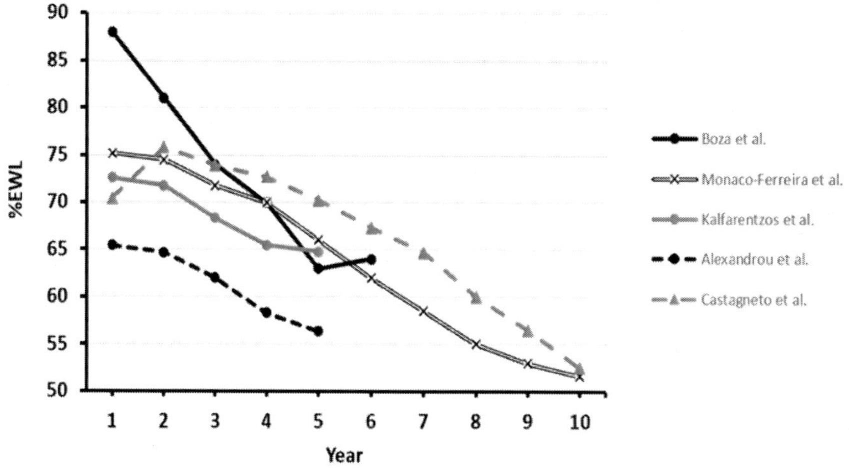

Figure 2. Percentage excess weight loss after bariatric surgery [64, 71, 88–90]. EWL, excess weight loss.

Cardiovascular Risk Factors

After bariatric surgery there is a great improvement in cardiometabolic parameters [23], with a high percentage of remissions of obesity-related comorbidities. Although, in many cases, these improvements are maintained over time, when analysing the bibliography two aspects can be extracted that must be considered. On the one hand, there are patients who do not achieve a remission in the comorbidities they suffer, while on the other hand, in the medium-long term there is a relapse in the comorbidities in numerous patients. Some studies have reported significant increases in total cholesterol, LDL cholesterol, triglycerides, and blood glucose levels between the first and third year of a sleeve gastrectomy [25]. Other studies have shown a remission of hypertension one year after a gastric bypass in 68.1% of patients, while at 3 years, a relapse hypertension was obtained in 21.9% of these patients [91].

Similarly, it has been reported that approximately 50% and 40% of patients have a total remission of type II diabetes mellitus and cholesterolemia one year after surgery, unfortunatelythese values at 5 years after surgery were reduced to 20% and 26.1% of patients, respectively [92]. Furthermore, these relapses varies depending on the different surgeries, observing relapses of type II diabetes mellitus in 17% of patients undergoing gastric bypass and in 38% of patients undergoing vertical gastrectomy 6 years after surgery [93]. In turn, this level of relapse in the different comorbidities increases over time, showing a relapse in type II diabetes mellitus after 1, 3 and 5 years in 7.9%, 22.1% and 35.1% of patients [94]. These trends persist over the years, and it has been reported that from the second to the tenth year after surgery, the number of patients with diabetes increased from 1% to 7%, while the number of patients with hypertension raised from 24% to 41% [95].

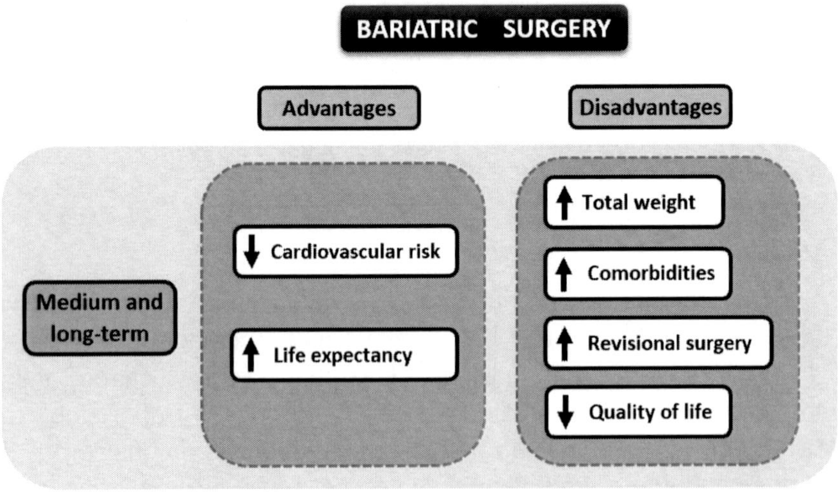

Figure 3. Medium and long-term advantages and disadvantages after bariatric surgery.

In this regard, it appears that weight regain is of great importance. On the one hand, it has been reported that at 3 years after surgery, male patients with a high EWL have glucose levels of 84 mg/dl, total cholesterol levels of 149 mg/dl or systolic blood pressure of 111 mmHg, compared to glucose values of 102 mg/dl, 171 mg/dl of total cholesterol or 123 mmHg in the systolic blood pressure in patients with a low EWL [83]. Another study showed that at 3 years after surgery, patients who had obtained a remission of hypertension had an EWL of approximately 80% compared to an EWL of approximately 70% in patients who did not present a remission in the hypertension [91]. In fact, weight regain correlates with comorbidities in the long-term after surgery [95], and different studies have found positive correlations between weight regain and relapses in diabetes mellitus type II [93, 96].

3. Pysical Activity and Exercise in Bariatric Patients

3.1. Benefits of Physical Activity and Exercise

As previously shown, bariatric surgery can generate a series of drawbakcs on which it is necessary to intervene. This chapter has focused on the disadvantages that can be prevented or reduced through physical activity. In the short-term, these disadvantages are mainly the loss of FFM, the reduction in bone mineral density, and occasionally, suboptimal weight loss of individuals undergoing bariatric surgery. In the medium-long term, there are other types of disadvantages, the most relevant being weight regain or relapse in different comorbidities.

Exercise has proven to be a method that can greatly contribute to preventing all these drawbacks. On the one hand, when there is a weight loss process, performing exercise can prevent or reduce the loss of FFM [22]. This can be achieved through resistance training. Several studies have shown that adding resistance training to a weight loss programme can avoid the loss of FFM [97]. In addition, it has been shown that if resistance training is performed appropriately in obese and untrained subjects, an increase in FFM can even occur in parallel with the loss of fat mass. As example, in the study by Sanal et al., resistance training was added to a weight loss programme, performed at an initial intensity of 50% of one repetition maximum (1RM), and progressed to 75-80% of 1RM. The results of this study showed in these subjects a loss of fat mass of approximately 5 kg and an increase in FFM of 3 kg [98]. However, it should be noted that for these effects to occur, two factors must be considered. On the one hand, it is necessary that resistance training is carried out at high intensities, and that progress is made until training is achieved at 70-80% of 1RM [98–100]. On the other hand, it is necessary to add protein supplementation. In this regard, some studies have indicated that a minimum of 1.5 g per kg of body mass is required to prevent losses in FFM [100], while other studies conclude that to generate gains in fat-free mass, they must be ingested between 1.7-1.8 grams per kg of total weight [101].

Likewise, resistance training has also been shown to be an effective method to prevent loss of bone mineral density [102]. In this regard, although some studies have recommended using intensities lower than 60% of 1RM for safety reasons [103], it has been reported that moderate and high intensities, between 70-80% of 1RM, seem to have better effects on bone health [102, 104].

Another benefit that exercise can generate in the short-term is to contribute to a greater loss of fat mass. For this, endurance training has been shown to be a highly effective method, and different studies have reported that adding an endurance training programme to a weight loss process, greater losses of fat mass are generated [105]. This would not be the case in all bariatric patients, since bariatric surgery itself presents large losses of fat mass. However, there is a percentage of bariatric patients, in whom the expected improvements are not obtained either in weight loss or in the improvement of cardiovascular risk factors [57]. In this regard, it should be noted that training volume can be a determinant factor, and it has been shown that performing between 150-250 minutes per week of exercise at moderate intensity can generate modest weight losses, however, weight losses increase when more than 250 minutes of physical activity are performed per week [106]. Therefore, the performance of endurance training after bariatric surgery, in addition to causing greater losses of fat mass, could contribute to the improvement of health in "bariatric surgery resistant".

In turn, in the medium and long-term after surgery, there is a weight regain in a large proportion of patients, which can determine to some extent the relapse in different comorbidities. At this point, the exercise can have a role of great relevance. On the one hand, it has been shown that, after a significant weight loss, it is common for a weight regain to occur and that it increases over time [107], being inversely associated with the performance of physical activity [108]. In addition, it has been reported that 150-250 minutes of exercise per week can prevent weight gain [106]. However, the prevention guidelines for weight regain after weight loss in bariatric patients are still undetermined. First, it is recommended to maintain the FFM in order to avoid or prevent large reductions in the basal metabolic rate after weight loss. In turn, it should be noted that this maintenance of the FFM will contribute to the prevention of relapse comorbidities, since the skeletal muscle presents several endocrine functions that could improve cardiovascular risk factors. Second, some studies have reported that 200-300 minutes of physical activity should be performed at a moderate intensity per week to avoid weight gain [106].

3.2. Levels of Physical Activity in Patients Undergoing Bariatric Surgery

Despite all the benefits that physical activity can generate after surgery, patients undergoing bariatric surgery have low levels of physical activity.

First, it should be noted that there is some controversy regarding short-term changes in physical activity levels after surgery. Some studies have not observed significant increases in physical activity levels after surgery [109, 110], while other studies have reported certain increases. For example, it has been observed an increase from 7140 daily steps performed before surgery to 8430 daily steps at 8 months after surgery [111]. Equally, other studies found a similar change, obtaining an increase from 7563 steps per day prior to surgery to 8788 steps per day after one year after surgery [112]. Despite this controversy in the results, and regardless of whether there are changes or not in the levels of physical activity after surgery, it is observed that these levels of physical activity are still insufficient. According to the classification provided by Freedson et al. (1998), a subject is considered to be active if 10,000 or more steps per day are performed [113], while other authors define a subject as physically inactive if 150 minutes of moderate-vigorous physical activity a week are not reached [114].

However, in the studies that have been cited, patients have a range of between 8000 and 9000 steps per day, so it can be observed that they are not physically active subjects [111, 112]. In turn, other researches have reported that one year after surgery, 56% of the subjects performed less than 150 minutes of physical activity per week [111], while other studies have obtained that at 6 months after surgery, only 5% of patients performed more than 150 minutes of physical activity per week [110]. Likewise, Wefers et al. (2016) reported significant changes in physical activity levels after surgery, observing how the performance of moderate-vigorous physical activity increased from 72 to 89.1 minutes per week, but this is still insufficient, and this study also reported that only 12% of patients performed more than 150 minutes of physical activity per week [115]. In addition, these patients spend a large part of their time in sedentary behaviours, and it has been shown that at 14 months after surgery, bariatric patients spent 72% of their waking hours in sedentary behaviours [116].

Unfortunately, these low levels of physical activity are maintained over time. In patients evaluated between 18-24 months after surgery, it was found that only 17.9% of them were considered physically active subjects [117], while other studies have found that only 33% of patients undergoing gastric bypass meet the recommendations for weekly physical activity (≥150 minutes moderate-vigorous physical activity) at 4 years after surgery [118]. In the long-term (9 years after surgery), the mean number of daily steps per patient is 6375, with only 11.27% of patients performing more than 10,000 daily steps [119]. However, the main issue is not only that the subjects are not physically active, but that many of them have a completely sedentary behaviour. It should be remembered that an individual is considered to be sedentary if he performs less than 5,000 steps a day [113]. In this regard, it has been obtained that approximately 2 years after surgery, 19.6% of patients performed less than 5000 steps per day [117], while this figure increases to 36.62% after approximately 9 years of surgery [119].

Therefore, bariatric patients have low levels of physical activity, both in the short, medium and long-term after surgery. This behaviour should be avoided since physical activity can bring several benefits in these patients. On the one hand, physical activity can lead to greater weight loss ater surgery. As shown in the study carried out by Wefers et al. (2016), patients with higher levels of physical activity showed a weight reduction of 27.2 kg at 9 months after surgery compared to reductions of 21.5 kg and 17.2 kg in patients with medium and low physical activity levels, respectively [115]. In addition, this same study reported significant and negative associations between levels of physical activity and changes in fat mass of patients [115]. As evidence of the importance of physical activity, a study showed that at one year after surgery, patients who had achieved more than 50% reduction in EWL performed an average of 150 and 120 minutes of moderate and intense physical activity per week. In contrast, patients with an EWL below than 50%, the levels of moderate and vigorous physical activity were 68 and 40 minutes per week, respectively [120].

Likewise, it has been reported that subjects with optimal weight loss after surgery have an average of 61.5 minutes of moderate physical activity per day, while in patients with a suboptimal weight loss, the average of moderate physical activity was 35 minutes per day, showing an average of 4775 steps per day [60]. In the same way, compliance with the guidelines for recommending physical activity seems to be of great importance. On the one hand, it has been concluded that both at 6 and 12 months after surgery, patients who performed more than 150 minutes of weekly physical activity had greater weight loss than those who did not reach these levels of physical activity (6 months: 56% EWL versus 50.5% EWL; 12 months: 67.4% EWL versus 61.7% EWL) [121]. On the other hand, other studies have shown that at 3 years after surgery, patients who acieve these recommendations had an EWL of 54.1%, while in patients who only performed between 0-59 minutes of physical activity, the EWL was 33% [122]. Similarly, it has been shown that at approximately 3 years after surgery, patients who performed less than 90 minutes per week of exercise had an EWL of 57% compared to an EWL of 63% in patients who performed more than 200 minutes of weekly exercise [123]. Supporting these arguments, other studies have concluded that changes in energy intake and physical activity explain 93% of the individual variations in weight loss 6 years after surgery, indicating inverse associations between levels of physical activity and changes of weight [108].

These levels of physical activity also have a great influence on weight regain. In studies that have analysed patients with weight regain at 2 years after surgery, 73.5% of the patients who showed weight regain were physically inactive [66]. Likewise, it has been concluded that, 6 years after surgery, the subjects who managed to maintain the lost weight had physical activity levels of 12.2 kcal/kg/day compared to an energy consumption of 8 kcal/kg/d in patients with weight regain [108]. In the long term (8 years after surgery), 80.8 of the patients with weight regain are more than 3 hours a day sitting, while inactive subjects have a 2 times greater risk of suffering weight regain than active subjects [124]. In another interesting study, it was reported that at 8-9 years after surgery, patients with weight regain performed an average of 41 minutes of moderate physical activity and 4919 daily steps, compared to 81 minutes and 5686 daily steps of the subjects who did not present weight regain [60].

In turn, physical activity levels after bariatric surgery can also influence cardiometabolic parameters. One year after surgery, resolutions of diabetes, obstructive sleep apnea and hypertension were shown in 20%, 11.8%, and 21.9% of patients, while these values increased to 36.4%, 28.6%, and 31.6% in patients who performed more than 150 minutes of exercise per week [122]. On the other hand, it has been reported that after surgery, the improvement in insulin sensitivity by skeletal muscle is only observed in patients who increased their levels of physical activity, while the performance of physical activity was associated with visceral fat loss [125]. Likewise, changes in physical activity levels are associated with changes in insulin sensitivity and HDL cholesterol levels, being greater in patients who report higher levels of physical activity [125]. Finally, sedentary lifestyle is also a determining factor in cardiovascular risk factors, showing that sedentary patients present higher levels of total cholesterol and LDL cholesterol (220 mg/dl and 133 mg/dl) than active subjects (182.8 mg/dl and 103.2 mg/dl) at one year after surgery [126].

3.3. Exercise Programmes in Bariatric Patients

Once the observational studies on the subject and the additional benefits that physical activity can bring to bariatric patients have already been reviewed, the exercise programmes performed in this population should be analysed. Although there are few studies that have carried out an experimental intervention, in recent years some studies have emerged that show the effects of applying different exercise programmes after surgery, both in the short and medium long-term.

3.3.1. Short-Term Exercise Programmes after Bariatric Surgery

Effects on Body Composition

Exercising after surgery has been shown to be useful tool for improving different variables. On the one hand, various studies have reported that exercising, especially endurance training, can generate additional losses of fat mass. In one study, a 3-month endurance training programme was implemented with 40-minute sessions at an intensity between 50-70% of the maximal heat rate (HR_{max}) 3 days a week, it was found that at 4 months after surgery, the group that performed the exercise programme had greater losses in fat mass and lower reductions in FFM compared to the control group, although these differences were not significant [127]. Likewise, other studies have shown that at 12 weeks after surgery, patients who performed between 150-200 minutes of physical activity per week (walking) had greater losses of fat mass, observing among these patients a loss of more than 5.4 kg of fat mass, compared to physical inactive patients [128]._Similar results have been obtained at 6 months after surgery, reporting that patients who performed a minimum of 120 minutes of stationary walking or cycling showed greater reductions in fat mass [129]. In turn, resistance training by itself also seems to generate additional losses of fat mass, and it has been demonstrated that at 6 months after surgery, patients who performed this type of training had an additional loss of fat mass of 2.3 kg [130].

Although, these additional losses of fat mass are not sometimes significant among experimental group (patients on an exercise programme) to a control group, physical activity can have a great relevance in the prevention of FFM loss. In an interesting study, the effects on body composition after bariatric surgery were compared according to the type of exercise performed, and the following groups were compared: 1) endurance training; 2) endurance more resistance training; 3) control group (group that did not participate in any exercise program). The results showed how the group that did not exercise lost 2.4 kg more of FFM than the endurance training group, while, when compared with the group that performed endurance more resistance training, this difference increased to 3.7 kg [128]. In the same way, other researches in which resistance training was applied 3 times a week at an intensity of between 50-75% of the 1RM, it was shown that the experimental group had lower reductions in the FFM at 6 months after surgery [130].

Although there have been no studies in which the frequency of training necessary to reduce FFM is studied, an investigation showed how with only 2 days per week of resistance training, the loss of FFM can be reduced. In this regard, it has been obtained that the patients who performed resistance training after bariatric surgery had 2.17 kg of FFM, while in the group that did not exercise this reduction was 4.64 kg [131]. On the other hand, in another study in which combined training (endurance and resistance training) was used, although differences between the groups were not significant, it was observed that at 4 months after surgery, the exercising group lost 2.2 kg less than FFM than the control group [132].

Effects on the Bone Health

To our knowledge, there are few experimental studies that analyse this variable in the short-term; however, it seems that exercising after surgery can reduce the loss of bone mineral density. The results of the study conducted by Campanha-Versiani et al. concluded that through the resistance training carried out 2 days a week at high intensity, smaller reductions in bone mineral density are produced at one year after surgery[131]. For example, in this study was reported that patients who participated in resistance training had reductions in bone mineral density in lumbar spine and in right hip of 0.02 g/cm^3 and 0.04 g/cm^3 respectively, while in subjects who did not perform resistance training these reductions increased to 0.09 g/cm^3 for both variables, being these differences between experimental and control group significant [131].

Effects on Quality of Life

Most of the studies that have been analysed show greater improvements in functional capacity in subjects who have carried out an exercise programme after surgery. On the one hand, improvements have been shown in the 6-minute walk test and in maximal oxygen consumption only in groups that have exercised after surgery[132–135]. However, different factors must be taken into consideration, since endurance training does not prevent against the loss of strength that occurs after surgery. In this regard, it has been shown that adding resistance training to an exercise programme prevents reductions in strength levels after the surgical procedure[128]. For example, it has been reported that after surgery, handgrip strength and lower limb maximum repetition decreased significantly, however, in patients who performed resistance training at an intensity of 50-70% of the 1RM, the handgrip strength was maintained, and the lower limb strength increased by 17.6 kg[130]. Other studies in which were also used high intensities in resistance training (70-80% 1RM), shown benefits in strength levels only in groups that performed tis type of training[136].

Effects on Cardiovascular Risk Factors

Currently, there are few studies in the literature that have analysed the effects of a short-term supervised exercise programme on cardiovascular risk factors in bariatric patients. In this regard, a study determined that performing 120 minutes of aerobic training at an intensity between 60-70% of HR_{max} can generate additional benefits in glucose effectiveness and insulin sensitivity [137]. In turn, other studies have found that area under the postprandial blood glucose curve is higher in patients consuming ≥2,000 kcal/week performing endurance training at an intensity between 60-70% of VO_{2max} [138]. Finally, it has been showed that the subjects who performed an aerobic training programme lasting 3 months, 3 days a week, 40 minutes at an intensity between 50-70% of the peak heart rate, showed greater reductions in diastolic blood pressure 4 months after surgery [127].

3.3.2. Medium and Long-Term Exercise Programmes after Bariatric Surgery

Unfortunately, there is little research addressing the effects of exercise in bariatric patients at medium and long-term after surgery, although the studies that have been carried out on the subject have provided information of great interest. On the one hand, Marchesi et al. (2015), enrolled patients between 1 and 3 years after surgery, and applied an aerobic training programme to the experimental group, in which training intensity progressed from 55-65% of the HR_{max} to 70-90% of HR_{max}. The results of this study showed that the control group kept their weight stable at the end of the study, however, the experimental group decreased their fat mass and waist circumference, while showing a tendency to increase their FFM [139].

In another study, in which patients who underwent surgery between 12 and 24 months after the study were enrolled, a combined training intervention of 12 weeks duration was carried out, with 3 weekly sessions of 60 minutes each session. Endurance training was performed at an intensity between 64-77% of HR_{max}, while for resistance training, two exercises were performed per session, with 12 repetitions at 60% of 1RM. The results of this study showed that the experimental group lost 2 kg of fat mass, with no decreases in FFM, while in the control group an increase of approximately 1 kg of fat mass was obtained [140]. In addition, the experimental group had decreases in both systolic (-7.4 mmHg) and diastolic (-5.3 mmHg) blood pressure, while in control group, these variables increased in 3.7 and 3.3 mmHg, respectively [140].

In another investigation, an exercise program was applied after bariatric surgery that combined endurance training (at least 3 days a week, 45 minutes per session) and resistance training (at least 2 days a week, 30 minutes per session) and the results were observed 24 months after surgery. These results showed how the experimental group had a 3.5% decrease in lean mass, while this reduction was 12.4% in the control group [141]. In this same study, resistance training also had effects on bone mineral density, reporting that the group that carried out exercise programme had reductions of 4.9% on BMD total hip and 3.2% on BMD femoral neck, compared to a reduction of 9.9% and 6.7% in these same variables in patients who did not participate in the exercise programme after surgery [141].

Finally, Marc-Hernández et al. carried out an exercise programme in patients who presented weight regain at 3 years after surgery. The exercise programme consisted of combined training, progressing to high intensities both endurance (60-95% VO_{2peak}) and resistance training (50-75% 1RM). The results of this study showed significant reductions in fat mass, an increase of 1.3 kg in FFM in the experimental group, along with other anthropometric improvements (reduction in waist circumference, visceral fat, etc.). In contrast, patient in the control group showed a significant increase in total weight and fat mass in the same period. In turn, the experimental group had significant reductions in blood glucose and total cholesterol, and a tendency to reduce blood pressure, in addition to improving their cardiorespiratory capacity and their quality of life. In addition, it should be noted that these improvements disappeared 2 months after completing the exercise program [142].

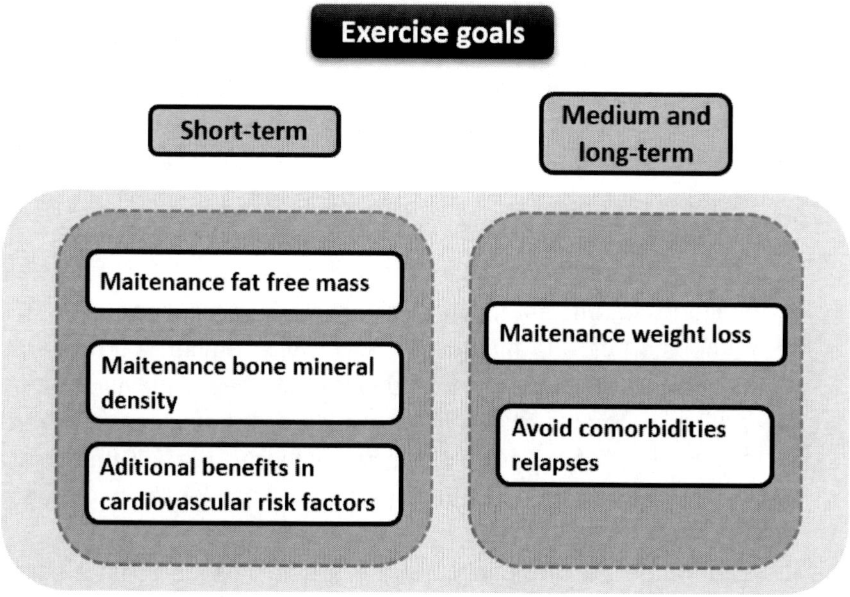

Figure 4. Main exercise goals after bariatric surgery.

3.4. Guidelines and Recommendations for Exercise after Bariatric Surgery

As has been widely described, exercise can generate great benefits in patients undergoing bariatric surgery and can prevent the disadvantages associated with it. On the one hand, it has been shown that, in the medium term, exercise can generate greater losses of fat mass, reduce the reduction in FFM and bone mineral density and improve the functional capacity of patients. On the other hand, in the medium and long-term, exercise programmes can prevent weight regain and relapse in the different obesity-related comorbidities, as well as maintaining an adequate quality of life in patients. Some guidelines and considerations for the performance of exercise in this type of patients will be provided, retrieved from the latest updates on exercise and the existing bibliography on the subject.

Short-Term Exercise Guidelines and Recommendations

- Special attention should be paid to resistance training.
- Resistance training is essential to reduce losses of FFM, bone mineral density, basal metabolic rate and strength levels. It should be started early, one month after surgery. It must be done, at least, 3 days a week, working the large muscle groups. This type of training should be started at moderate intensities (~ 50% 1RM) and progressed to high intensities (70-80% 1RM).
- Training volume is an important factor for fat mass loss. The completion of 120 minutes per week of exercise at a moderate intensity can influence the loss of fat mass, however, most studies recommend a minimum of 150 minutes per week for greater loss of fat mass to occur. If more than 250 minutes a week are performed, it can increase fat mass losses to a greater extent.
- Endurance training can generate greater losses of fat mass. It can be started before resistance training, at the 2nd week after surgery. Start at moderate intensity and progress. Studies have shown ranges between 40-80% of HR_{max}.
- Ingest a minimum of 1.5 grams per kg of body mass, trying to reach 1.8-1.9 grams per kg of body mass.

Medium and Long-Term Exercise Guidelines and Recommendations

- It is important to combine both types of training: resistance and endurance training.
- The main objectives of resistance training are to maintain the FFM, the basal metabolic rate and the bone mineral density, in addition to helping to avoid relapse in the different comorbidities. It is recommended 3 days a week of resistance training, although 2 days a week have been shown to have positive effects on FFM and bone health. Performing 4 sets per large muscle group, progressing from 20 to 10 repetitions and from 60% to 75% of

1RM has been shown to be highly effective. One component that seems to be essential is that intensities of between 70-80% of 1RM are achieved.

- The main objectives of endurance training are to avoid weight regain and relapse in different comorbidities. It should be started at moderate intensities, and progress to higher intensities (55-90% HR_{max}; 60-90% VO_{2max})
- The volume of exercise is a fundamental aspect to prevent weight regain, recommending the performance of between 200-300 minutes per week of physical activity to maintain the lost weight.
- Ingest a minimum of 1.5 grams per kg of body mass, trying to reach 1.8-1.9 grams per kg of body mass.

References

[1] Milaneschi Y, Simmons WK, van Rossum EFC, et al. Depression and obesity: evidence of shared biological mechanisms. *Mol Psychiatry*. 2019; 24: 18–33.

[2] Huang IC, Frangakis C, Wu AW. The relationship of excess body weight and health-related quality of life: Evidence from a population study in Taiwan. *Int J Obes*. 2006; 30: 1250–1259.

[3] García-Mendizábal MJ, Carrasco JM, Pérez-Gmez B, et al. Role of educational level in the relationship between Body Mass Index (BMI) and health-related quality of life (HRQL) among rural Spanish women. *BMC Public Health*. 2009; 9: 1–10.

[4] Bhaskaran K, dos-Santos-Silva I, Leon DA, et al. Association of BMI with overall and cause-specific mortality: a population-based cohort study of 3·6 million adults in the UK. *Lancet Diabetes Endocrinol*. 2018; 6: 944–953.

[5] Kitahara CM, Flint AJ, Berrington de Gonzalez A, et al. Association between Class III Obesity (BMI of 40-59 kg/m2) and Mortality: A Pooled Analysis of 20 Prospective Studies. *PLoS Med*.; 11. Epub ahead of print 2014. DOI: 10.1371/journal.pmed.1001673.

[6] Uittenbogaart M, Leclercq WK, Luijten AA, et al. Laparoscopic Adjustable Gastric Banding After Failed Roux-En-Y Gastric Bypass. *Obes Surg*. 2016; 1–6.

[7] Kruseman M, Leimgruber A, Zumbach F, et al. Dietary, weight, and psychological changes among patients with obesity, 8 years after gastric bypass. *J Am Diet Assoc*. 2010; 110: 527–34.

[8] Benaiges D, Flores-Le-Roux JA, Pedro-Botet J, et al. Impact of restrictive (Sleeve Gastrectomy) vs hybrid bariatric surgery (roux-en-y gastric bypass) on lipid profile. *Obes Surg*. 2012; 22: 1268–1275.

[9] Osland E, Nutr B, Mphil D, et al. Weight Loss Outcomes in Laparoscopic Vertical Sleeve Gastrectomy (LVSG) Versus Laparoscopic Roux-en-Y Gastric Bypass (LRYGB) Procedures : A Meta-Analysis and Systematic Review of Randomized Controlled Trials. *Surg Laparosc Endosc Percutan Tech*. 2017; 27: 8–18.

[10] Ricci C, Gaeta M, Rausa E, et al. Early impact of bariatric surgery on type II diabetes, hypertension, and hyperlipidemia: a systematic review, meta-analysis and meta-regression on 6,587 patients. *Obes Surg*. 2014; 24: 522–8.

[11] Tovar JR, Angel M, Jose C, et al. Long-term follow-up after sleeve gastrectomy versus Roux-en-Y gastric bypass versus one-anastomosis gastric bypass : a prospective randomized comparative study of weight loss and remission of comorbidities. *Surg Endosc*. 2018; 33: 401–410.

[12] Buchwald H, Avidor Y, Braunwald E, et al. Bariatric Surgery: A Systematic Review and Meta-analysis. *Jama*. 2004; 292: 1724–1737.

[13] Fouse T, Brethauer S. Resolution of Comorbidities and Impact on Longevity Following Bariatric and Metabolic Surgery. *Surg Clin North Am*. 2016; 96: 717–732.

[14] Omotosho P, Mor A, Shantavasinkul PC, et al. Gastric bypass significantly improves quality of life in morbidly obese patients with type 2 diabetes. *Surg Endosc*. 2016; 30: 2857–64.

[15] Burgmer R, Petersen I, Burgmer M, et al. Psychological Outcome Two Years after Restrictive Bariatric Surgery. *Obes Surg*. 2007; 17: 785–791.

[16] Christou N V., Sampalis JS, Liberman M, et al. Surgery decreases long-term mortality, morbidity, and health care use in morbidly obese patients. *Ann Surg.* 2004; 240: 416–424.
[17] Carlsson LMS, Sjöholm K, Jacobson P, et al. Life Expectancy after Bariatric Surgery in the Swedish Obese Subjects Study. *N Engl J Med.* 2020; 383: 1535–1543.
[18] Pope DG, Finlayson SRG, Kemp JA, et al. Life expectancy benefits of gastric bypass surgery. *Surg Innov.* 2006; 13: 265–273.
[19] Schauer DP, Arterburn DE, Livingston EH, et al. Impact of bariatric surgery on life expectancy in severely obese patients with diabetes: A Decision analysis. *Ann Surg.* 2016; 261: 914–919.
[20] Abdeen G, le Roux CW. Mechanism Underlying the Weight Loss and Complications of Roux-en-Y Gastric Bypass. Review. *Obes Surg.* 2016; 26: 410–421.
[21] Weng TC, Chang CH, Dong YH, et al. Anaemia and related nutrient deficiencies after Roux-en-Y gastric bypass surgery: A systematic review and meta-analysis. *BMJ Open.* 2015; 5: 1–11.
[22] Dixon JB, Lambert EA, Grima M, et al. Fat-free mass loss generated with weight loss in overweight and obese adults: What may we expect? *Diabetes, Obes Metab.* 2015; 17: 91–93.
[23] Sans A, Bailly L, Anty R, et al. Baseline Anthropometric and Metabolic Parameters Correlate with Weight Loss in Women 1-Year After Laparoscopic Roux-En-Y Gastric Bypass. *Obes Surg.* 2017; 27: 2940–2949.
[24] Nuijten MAH, Monpellier VM, Eijsvogels TMH, et al. Rate and Determinants of Excessive Fat-Free Mass Loss After Bariatric Surgery. *Obes Surg.* 2020; 30: 3119–3126.
[25] Sherf-Dagan S, Zelber-Sagi S, Buch A, et al. Prospective Longitudinal Trends in Body Composition and Clinical Outcomes 3 Years Following Sleeve Gastrectomy. *Obes Surg.* 2019; 29: 3833–3841.
[26] Carey DG, Pliego GJ, Raymond RL. Body composition and metabolic changes following bariatric surgery: effects on fat mass, lean mass and basal metabolic rate: six months to one-year follow-up. *Obes Surg.* 2006; 16: 1602–1608.
[27] Otto M, Elrefai M, Krammer J, et al. Sleeve Gastrectomy and Roux-en-Y Gastric Bypass Lead to Comparable Changes in Body

Composition after Adjustment for Initial Body Mass Index. *Obes Surg.* 2015; 26: 479–485.

[28] Calleja-Fernández A, Pintor-de-la-Maza B, Diez-Rodríguez R, et al. Relationship Between Diet and Body Composition After Biliopancreatic Diversion. *Obes Surg.* 2015; 25: 2093–2099.

[29] Olbers T, Björkman S, Lindroos A, et al. Body composition, dietary intake, and energy expenditure after laparoscopic Roux-en-Y gastric bypass and laparoscopic vertical banded gastroplasty: A randomized clinical trial. *Ann Surg.* 2006; 244: 715–722.

[30] Ciangura C, Bouillot J-L, Lloret-Linares C, et al. Dynamics of change in total and regional body composition after gastric bypass in obese patients. *Obes (Silver Spring).* 2010; 18: 760–5.

[31] Carrasco F, Ruz M, Rojas P, et al. Changes in bone mineral density, body composition and adiponectin levels in morbidly obese patients after bariatric surgery. *Obes Surg.* 2009; 19: 41–46.

[32] Andreu A, Moizé V, Rodríguez L, et al. Protein intake, body composition, and protein status following bariatric surgery. *Obes Surg.* 2010; 20: 1509–1515.

[33] Dulloo AG, Jacquet J, Solinas G, et al. Body composition phenotypes in pathways to obesity and the metabolic syndrome. *Int J Obes.* 2010; 34: S4–S17.

[34] Pedersen BK, Febbraio MA. Muscles, exercise and obesity: Skeletal muscle as a secretory organ. *Nat Rev Endocrinol.* 2012; 8: 457–465.

[35] Kim TN, Choi KM. The implications of sarcopenia and sarcopenic obesity on cardiometabolic disease. *J Cell Biochem.* 2015; 116: 1171–1178.

[36] Jensen J, Rustad PI, Kolnes AJ, et al. The role of skeletal muscle glycogen breakdown for regulation of insulin sensitivity by exercise. *Front Physiol.* 2011; 2: 1–11.

[37] Houmard JA, Pories WJ, Dohm GL. Severe obesity: evidence for a deranged metabolic program in skeletal muscle? *Exerc Sport Sci Rev.* 2013; 40: 204–210.

[38] Wolfe B, Schoeller D, McCrady-Spitzer S, et al. Resting metabolic rate, total daily energy expenditure, and metabolic adaptation 6-

months and 24-months after bariatric surgery. *Obes (Silver Spring).* 2018; 26: 862–868.

[39] da Silva FBL, Gomes DL, e Carvalho KMB. Poor diet quality and postoperative time are independent risk factors for weight regain after Roux-en-Y gastric bypass. *Nutrition.* 2016; 32: 1–4.

[40] Odom J, Zalesin KC, Washington TL, et al. Behavioral Predictors of Weight Regain after Bariatric Surgery. *Obes Surg.* 2010; 20: 349–356.

[41] Faria SL, Kelly E, Faria OP. Energy Expenditure and Weight Regain in Patients Submitted to Roux-en-Y Gastric Bypass. *Obes Surg.* 2009; 19: 856–859.

[42] Alba DL, Wu L, Cawthon PM, et al. Changes in Lean Mass, Absolute and Relative Muscle Strength, and Physical Performance After Gastric Bypass Surgery. *J Clin Endocrinol Metab.* 2019; 104: 711–720.

[43] Hue O, Berrigan F, Simoneau M, et al. Muscle force and force control after weight loss in obese and morbidly obese men. *Obes Surg.* 2008; 18: 1112–1118.

[44] Handrigan G, Hue O, Simoneau M, et al. Weight loss and muscular strength affect static balance control. *Int J Obes (Lond).* 2010; 34: 936–942.

[45] Cauley JA. An Overview of Sarcopenic Obesity. *J Clin Densitom.* 2015; 18: 499–505.

[46] Curvello-silva K, Barreto-medeiros JM. Association between sarcopenic obesity and cardiovascular risk : where are we ? *Nutr Hosp.* 2016; 33: 1245–1255.

[47] Srikanthan P, Hevener AL, Karlamangla AS. Sarcopenia exacerbates obesity-associated insulin resistance and dysglycemia: Findings from the national health and nutrition examination survey III. *PLoS One.*; 5. Epub ahead of print 2010. DOI: 10.1371/journal.pone.0010805.

[48] Parr EB, Coffey VG, Hawley JA. 'Sarcobesity': A metabolic conundrum. *Maturitas.* 2013; 74: 109–113.

[49] Marc-hernández A, Ruiz-tovar J, Jimenez JM, et al. Short-Term Changes on Body Composition and Bone Mass After One-Anastomosis Gastric Bypass : a Prospective Observational Study. *Obes Surg.* 2020; 30: 3514–3521.

[50] Stein EM, Silverberg SJ. Bone Loss After Bariatric Surgery: Causes, Consequences and Management. *Lancet Diabetes Endocrinol.* 2014; 2: 165–174.

[51] Obinwanne KM, DM, Riess KP, et al. Effects of laparoscopic Roux-en-Y gastric bypass on bone mineral density and markers of bone turnover. *Surg Obes Relat Dis.* 2014; 10: 1056–1062.

[52] Raoof M, Näslund I, Rask E, et al. Effect of Gastric Bypass on Bone Mineral Density, Parathyroid Hormone and Vitamin D: 5 Years Follow-up. *Obes Surg.* 2016; 26: 1141–1145.

[53] Vilarrasa N, José PS, García I, et al. Evaluation of bone mineral density loss in morbidly obese women after gastric bypass: 3-year follow-up. *Obes Surg.* 2011; 21: 465–472.

[54] Adamczyk P, Buzga M, Holeczy P, et al. Body Size, Bone Mineral Density, and Body Composition in Obese Women After Laparoscopic Sleeve Gastrectomy: A 1-Year Longitudinal Study. *Horm Metab Res.* 2015; 47: 873–879.

[55] Nakamura K, Haglind E, Clowes J, et al. Fracture risk following bariatric surgery : a population-based study. *Osteoporos Int.* 2014; 25: 151–158.

[56] Zhang Q, Dong J, Zhou D, et al. Comparative risk of fracture for bariatric procedures in patients with obesity: A systematic review and Bayesian network meta-analysis: Bariatric procedures and fracture risk. *Int J Surg.* 2020; 75: 13–23.

[57] Gilbertson NM, Paisley AS, Kranz S, et al. Bariatric Surgery Resistance: Using Preoperative Lifestyle Medicine and/or Pharmacology for Metabolic Responsiveness. *Obes Surg.* 2017; 27: 3281–3291.

[58] Melton GB, Steele KE, Schweitzer MA, et al. Suboptimal weight loss after gastric bypass surgery: Correlation of demographics, comorbidities, and insurance status with outcomes. *J Gastrointest Surg.* 2008; 12: 250–255.

[59] Lutfi R, Torquati A, Sekhar N, et al. Predictors of success after laparoscopic gastric bypass: A multivariate analysis of socioeconomic factors. *Surg Endosc Other Interv Tech.* 2006; 20: 864–867.

[60] Amundsen T, Strømmen M, Martins C. Suboptimal Weight Loss and Weight Regain after Gastric Bypass Surgery—Postoperative

Status of Energy Intake, Eating Behavior, Physical Activity, and Psychometrics. *Obes Surg.* 2017; 27: 1316–1323.

[61] Kang JH, Le QA. Effectiveness of bariatric surgical procedures: A systematic review and network meta-analysis of randomized controlled trials. *Medicine (Baltimore).* 2017; 96: e8632.

[62] Park CH, Nam SJ, Choi HS, et al. Comparative Efficacy of Bariatric Surgery in the Treatment of Morbid Obesity and Diabetes Mellitus: a Systematic Review and Network Meta-Analysis. *Obes Surg.* 2019; 29: 2180–2190.

[63] Braghetto I, Csendes A, Lanzarini E, et al. Is laparoscopic sleeve gastrectomy an acceptable primary bariatric procedure in obese patients? Early and 5-year postoperative results. *Surg Laparosc Endosc Percutan Tech.* 2012; 22: 479–86.

[64] Boza C, Daroch D, Barros D, et al. Long-term outcomes of laparoscopic sleeve gastrectomy as a primary bariatric procedure. *Surg Obes Relat Dis.* 2014; 10: 1129–1134.

[65] Freire RH, Borges MC, Alvarez-Leite JI, et al. Food quality, physical activity, and nutritional follow-up as determinant of weight regain after Roux-en-Y gastric bypass. *Nutrition.* 2012; 28: 53–8.

[66] Gomes DL, de Almeida Oliveira D, Dutra ES, et al. Resting Energy Expenditure and Body Composition of Women with Weight Regain 24 Months After Bariatric Surgery. *Obes Surg.* 2015; 26: 1443–7.

[67] Magro DO, Geloneze B, Delfini R, et al. Long-term weight regain after gastric bypass: A 5-year prospective study. *Obes Surg.* 2008; 18: 648–651.

[68] Himpens J, Dobbeleir J, Peeters G. Long-term results of laparoscopic sleeve gastrectomy for obesity. *Ann Surg.* 2010; 252: 319–324.

[69] Christou N V., Look D, Maclean LD. Weight gain after short- and long-limb gastric bypass in patients followed for longer than 10 years. *Ann Surg.* 2006; 244: 734–740.

[70] O'Brien PE, Mcphail T, Chaston TB, et al. Systematic Review of Medium Term Weight loss after Bariatric Surgery. *Obes Surg.* 2006; 16: 1032–1040.

[71] Monaco-Ferreira DV, Leandro-Merhi VA. Weight Regain 10 Years After Roux-en-Y Gastric Bypass. *Obes Surg.* 2017; 27: 1137–1144.

[72] O'Brien PE, Hindle A, Brennan L, et al. Long-Term Outcomes After Bariatric Surgery: a Systematic Review and Meta-analysis of Weight Loss at 10 or More Years for All Bariatric Procedures and a Single-Centre Review of 20-Year Outcomes After Adjustable Gastric Banding. *Obes Surg.* 2019; 29: 3–14.

[73] Felsenreich DM, Langer FB, Kefurt R, et al. Weight loss, weight regain, and conversions to Roux-en-Y gastric bypass: 10-year results of laparoscopic sleeve gastrectomy. *Surg Obes Relat Dis.* 2016; 12: 1655–1662.

[74] Tamboli RA, Breitman I, Marks-Shulman PA, et al. Early weight regain after gastric bypass does not affect insulin sensitivity but is associated with elevated ghrelin. *Obesity.* 2014; 22: 1617–1622.

[75] Bohdjalian A, Langer FB, Shakeri-Leiden Mühler S, et al. Sleeve gastrectomy as sole and definitive bariatric procedure: 5-Year results for weight loss and ghrelin. *Obes Surg.* 2010; 20: 535–540.

[76] Biagioni MFG, Mendes AL, Nogueira CR, et al. Bariatric Roux-En-Y Gastric Bypass Surgery: Adipocyte Proteins Involved in Increased Bone Remodeling in Humans. *Obes Surg.* 2017; 25: 2376–2385.

[77] Guida B, Belfiore A, Angrisani L, et al. Laparoscopic gastric banding and body composition in morbid obesity. *Nutr Metab Cardiovasc Dis.* 2005; 15: 198–203.

[78] Trakhtenbroit MA, Leichman JG, Algahim MF, et al. Body Weight, Insulin Resistance, and Serum Adipokine Levels 2 Years after 2 Types of Bariatric Surgery. *Am J Med.* 2009; 122: 435–442.

[79] Lubrano C, Cornoldi A, Pili M, et al. Reduction of risk factors for cardiovascular diseases in morbid-obese patients following biliary-intestinal bypass: 3 years' follow-up. *Int J Obes Relat Metab Disord.* 2004; 28: 1600–6.

[80] De Luis DA, Pacheco D, Izaola O, et al. Clinical results and nutritional consequences of biliopancreatic diversion: Three years of follow-up. *Ann Nutr Metab.* 2009; 53: 234–239.

[81] Cole AJ, Kuchnia AJ, Beckman LM, et al. Long-Term Body Composition Changes in Women Following Roux-en-Y Gastric Bypass Surgery. *J Parenter Enter Nutr.* 2016; 1–9.

[82] Laguna S, Andrada P, Silva C, et al. Body weight- independent variations in HDL-cholesterol following gastric bypass. *An Sist Sanit Navar.* 2016; 39: 23–33.

[83] Gómez-Ambrosi J, Andrada P, Valentí V, et al. Dissociation of body mass index, excess weight loss and body fat percentage trajectories after 3 years of gastric bypass: Relationship with metabolic outcomes. *Int J Obes.* 2017; 41: 1379–1387.

[84] Guan B, Chong TH, Peng J, et al. Mid-long-term revisional surgery after SG a Systematic review and meta analysis. *Obes Surg.* 2019; 29: 1965–1975.

[85] Angrisani L, Santonicola A, Iovino P, et al. IFSO Worldwide Survey 2016: Primary, Endoluminal, and Revisional Procedures. *Obes Surg.* 2018; 28: 3783–3794.

[86] Sarela AI, Dexter SPL, O'Kane M, et al. Long-term follow-up after laparoscopic sleeve gastrectomy: 8-9-year results. *Surg Obes Relat Dis.* 2012; 8: 679–684.

[87] Herpertz S, Müller A, Burgmer R, et al. Health-related quality of life and psychological functioning 9 years after restrictive surgical treatment for obesity. *Surg Obes Relat Dis.* 2015; 11: 1361–1370.

[88] Kalfarentzos F, Skroubis G, Kehagias I, et al. A prospective comparison of vertical banded gastroplasty and Roux-en-Y gastric bypass in a non-superobese population. *Obes Surg.* 2006; 16: 151–158.

[89] Alexandrou A, Athanasiou A, Michalinos A, et al. Laparoscopic sleeve gastrectomy for morbid obesity: 5-year results. *Am J Surg.* 2015; 209: 230–234.

[90] Castagneto Gissey L, Casella Mariolo JR, Genco A, et al. 10-year follow-up after laparoscopic sleeve gastrectomy: Outcomes in a monocentric series. *Surg Obes Relat Dis.* 2018; 14: 1480–1487.

[91] Benaiges D, Sagué M, Roux JAF, et al. Predictors of Hypertension Remission and Recurrence After Bariatric Surgery. *Am J Hypertens.* 2016; 29: 653–659.

[92] Golomb I, Ben David M, Glass A, et al. Long-term Metabolic Effects of Laparoscopic Sleeve Gastrectomy. *JAMA Surg.* 2015; 150: 1051–1057.

[93] Brethauer SA, Aminian A, Romero-Talamás H, et al. Can diabetes be surgically cured? Long-term metabolic effects of bariatric

surgery in obese patients with type 2 diabetes mellitus. *Ann Surg.* 2013; 258: 628–36; discussion 636-7.

[94] Arterburn DE, Bogart A, Sherwood NE, et al. A multisite study of long-term remission and relapse of type 2 diabetes mellitus following gastric bypass. *Obes Surg.* 2013; 23: 93–102.

[95] Neto RML, Herbella FAM, Tauil RM, et al. Comorbidities remission after roux-en-y gastric bypass for morbid obesity is sustained in a long-term follow-up and correlates with weight regain. *Obes Surg.* 2012; 22: 1580–1585.

[96] Jimenez A, Casamitjana R, Flores L, et al. Long-Term Effects of Sleeve Gastrectomy and Roux-en-Y Gastric Bypass Surgery on Type 2 Diabetes Mellitus in Morbidly Obese Subjects. *AnnSurg.* 2012; 256: 1023–1029.

[97] Schwingshackl L, Dias S, Strasser B, et al. Impact of different training modalities on anthropometric and metabolic characteristics in overweight/obese subjects: A systematic review and network meta-analysis. *PLoS One.* 2013; 8: e82853.

[98] Sanal E, Ardic F, Kirac S. Effects of aerobic or combined aerobic resistance exercise on body composition in overweight and obese adults: Gender differences. A randomized intervention study. *Eur J Phys Rehabil Med.* 2013; 49: 1–11.

[99] Said M, Lamya N, Olfa N, et al. Effects of high-impact aerobics vs. low-impact aerobics and strength training in overweight and obese women. *J Sports Med Phys Fitness.* 2017; 57: 278–288.

[100] Clark JE. Diet, exercise or diet with exercise: Comparing the effectiveness of treatment options for weight-loss and changes in fitness for adults (18-65 years old) who are overfat, or obese; systematic review and meta-analysis. *J Diabetes Metab Disord.* 2015; 14: 31.

[101] Urdampilleta A, Vicente-Salar N, Martínez-Sanz J. Necesidades proteicas de los deportistas y pautas diétetico-nutricionales para la ganancia de masa muscular. *Rev Española Nutr Humana y Dietética ….* 2012; 16: 25–35.

[102] Watson SL, Weeks BK, Weis LJ, et al. Heavy resistance training is safe and improves bone, function, and stature in postmenopausal women with low to very low bone mass: novel early findings from the LIFTMOR trial. *Osteoporos Int.* 2015; 26: 2889–2894.

[103] Kohrt WM, Bloomfield SA, Little KD, et al. Physical activity and bone health. *Med Sci Sports Exerc.* 2004; 36: 1985–1996.

[104] Hong AR, Kim SW. Effects of resistance exercise on bone health. *Endocrinol Metab.* 2018; 33: 435–444.

[105] Volek JS, Vanheest JL, Forsythe CE. Diet and exercise for weight loss: a review of current issues. *Sport Med.* 2005; 35: 1–9.

[106] Jakicic JM, Clark K, Coleman E, et al. American College of Sports Medicine position stand. Appropriate intervention strategies for weight loss and prevention of weight regain for adults. *Med Sci Sports Exerc.* 2001; 33: 2145–56.

[107] Wang X, Lyles MF, You T, et al. Weight Regain is Related to Decreases in Physical Activity During Weight Loss. *Med Sci Sport Exerc.* 2009; 40: 1781–1788.

[108] Kerns JC, Guo J, Fothergill E, et al. Increased Physical Activity Associated with Less Weight Regain Six Years After "The Biggest Loser" Competition. *Obesity.* 2017; 25: 1838–1843.

[109] Berglind D, Willmer M, Eriksson U, et al. Longitudinal Assessment of Physical Activity in Women Undergoing Roux-en-Y Gastric Bypass. *Obes Surg.* 2015; 25: 119–125.

[110] Bond DS, Jakicic JM, Unick JL, et al. Pre- to postoperative physical activity changes in bariatric surgery patients: self report vs. objective measures. *Obesity (Silver Spring).* 2010; 18: 2395–7.

[111] Bartsch M, Langenberg S, Gruner-Labitzke K, et al. Physical Activity, Decision-Making Abilities, and Eating Disturbances in Pre- and Postbariatric Surgery Patients. *Obes Surg.* 2016; 26: 2913–2922.

[112] King W, Hsu J, Belle S, et al. Pre- to Post-operative Changes in Physical Activity: Report from the Longitudinal Assessment of Bariatric Surgery-2. *Surg Obes Relat Dis.* 2012; 8: 522–532.

[113] Freedson PS, Melanson E, Sirard J. Calibration of the Computer Science and Applications, Inc. accelerometer. *Medicine and Science in Sports and Exercise* 1998; 30: 777–781.

[114] Tremblay MS, Aubert S, Barnes JD, et al. Sedentary Behavior Research Network (SBRN) - Terminology Consensus Project process and outcome. *Int J Behav Nutr Phys Act.* 2017; 14: 1–17.

[115] Wefers JF, SM, Woodlief TL, et al. Relationship among physical activity, sedentary behaviors, and cardiometabolic risk factors

during gastric bypass surgery – induced weight loss. *Surg Obes Relat Dis.* 2016; 13: 10–19.

[116] Chapman N, Hill K, Taylor S, et al. Patterns of physical activity and sedentary behavior after bariatric surgery: An observational study. *Surg Obes Relat Dis.* 2014; 10: 524–530.

[117] Bergh I, Kvalem IL, Mala T, et al. Predictors of Physical Activity After Gastric Bypass—a Prospective Study. *Obes Surg.* 2017; 27: 2050–2057.

[118] Sellberg F, Willmer M, Tynelius P, et al. Four years' follow-up changes of physical activity and sedentary time in women undergoing roux-en-Y gastric bypass surgery and appurtenant children. *BMC Surg.* 2017; 17: 1–7.

[119] Reid RER, Carver TE, Andersen KM, et al. Physical Activity and Sedentary Behavior in Bariatric Patients Long-Term Post-Surgery. *Obes Surg.* 2015; 25: 1073–1077.

[120] Mundi MS, Lorentz PA, Swain J, et al. Moderate physical activity as predictor of weight loss after bariatric surgery. *Obes Surg.* 2013; 23: 1645–1649.

[121] Evans RK, Bond DS, Wolfe LG, et al. Participation in 150 min/wk of moderate or higher intensity physical activity yields greater weight loss after gastric bypass surgery. *Surg Obes Relat Dis.* 2007; 3: 526–530.

[122] Shada AL, Hallowell PT, Schirmer BD, et al. Aerobic exercise is associated with improved weight loss after laparoscopic adjustable gastric banding. *Obes Surg.* 2013; 23: 608–12.

[123] Munie S, Carlin A, Keteyian S, et al. The Relationship Between Reported Exercise and Medium Term Weight Loss Following Laparoscopic Bariatric Surgery. *Surg Obes Relat Dis.* 2017; 13: S11–S12.

[124] Ryder JR, Gross AC, Fox CK, et al. Factors associated with long-term weight-loss maintenance following bariatric surgery in adolescents with severe obesity. *Int J Obes.* 2018; 42: 102–107.

[125] Savolainen AM, Karmi A, Immonen H, et al. Physical Activity Associates with Muscle Insulin Sensitivity Postbariatric Surgery. *Med Sci Sports Exerc.* 2019; 51: 278–287.

[126] Ruiz-Tovar J, Zubiaga L, Llavero C, et al. Serum cholesterol by morbidly obese patients after laparoscopic sleeve gastrectomy and additional physical activity. *Obes Surg.* 2014; 24: 385–9.
[127] Castello V, Simões RP, Bassi D, et al. Impact of aerobic exercise training on heart rate variability and functional capacity in obese women after gastric bypass surgery. *Obes Surg.* 2011; 21: 1739–49.
[128] Hassannejad A, Khalaj A, Mansournia MA, et al. The Effect of Aerobic or Aerobic-Strength Exercise on Body Composition and Functional Capacity in Patients with BMI ≥ 35 after Bariatric Surgery : a Randomized Control. *Obes Surg.* 2017; 27: 2792–2801.
[129] Carnero EA, Dubis GS, Hames KC, et al. Randomized Trial Reveals that Physical Activity and Energy Expenditure are Associated with Weight and Body Composition after RYGB. *Obes (Silver Spring).* 2017; 25: 1206–1216.
[130] Oppert JM, Bellicha A, Roda C, et al. Resistance Training and Protein Supplementation Increase Strength After Bariatric Surgery: A Randomized Controlled Trial. *Obesity.* 2018; 26: 1709–1720.
[131] Campanha-versiani L, Aparecida D, Pereira G, et al. The Effect of a Muscle Weight-Bearing and Aerobic Exercise Program on the Body Composition, Muscular Strength, Biochemical Markers, and Bone Mass of Obese Patients Who Have Undergone Gastric Bypass Surgery. *Obes Surg.* 2017; 27: 2129–2137.
[132] Stegen S, Derave W, Calders P, et al. Physical fitness in morbidly obese patients: effect of gastric bypass surgery and exercise training. *Obes Surg.* 2011; 21: 61–70.
[133] Coleman KJ, Caparosa SL, Nichols JF, et al. Understanding the Capacity for Exercise in Post-Bariatric Patients. *Obes Surg.* Epub ahead of print 2016. DOI: 10.1007/s11695-016-2240-y.
[134] Oliveira J, Freitas A, Almeida A. Postoperative effect of physical therapy related to functional capacity and respiratory muscle strength in patients submitted to bariatric surgery. *Arq Bras Cir Dig.* 2016; 29: 43–47.
[135] Onofre T, Carlos R, Oliver N, et al. Effects of a Physical Activity Program on Cardiorespiratory Fitness and Pulmonary Function in

Obese Women after Bariatric Surgery : a Pilot Study. *Obes Surg.* 2017; 27: 2026–2033.

[136] Daniels P, Burns RD, Brusseau TA, et al. Effect of a randomised 12-week resistance training programme on muscular strength, cross- sectional area and muscle quality in women having undergone Roux-en-Y gastric bypass. *J Sports Sci.* 2017; 1–7.

[137] Coen PM, Tanner CJ, Helbling NL, et al. Clinical trial demonstrates exercise following bariatric surgery improves insulin sensitivity. *J Clin Invest.* 2015; 125: 248–257.

[138] Shah M, Snell PG, Rao S, et al. High-volume exercise program in obese bariatric surgery patients: a randomized, controlled trial. *Obesity (Silver Spring).* 2011; 19: 1826–34.

[139] Marchesi F, De Sario G, Reggiani V, et al. Road Running After Gastric Bypass for Morbid Obesity: Rationale and Results of a New Protocol. *Obes Surg.* 2015; 25: 1162–1170.

[140] Herring LY, Stevinson C, Carter P, et al. The effects of supervised exercise training 12 – 24 months after bariatric surgery on physical function and body composition: a randomised controlled trial. *Int J Obes.* 2017; 41: 909–916.

[141] Muschitz C, Kocijan R, Haschka J, et al. The Impact of Vitamin D, Calcium, Protein Supplementation, and Physical Exercise on Bone Metabolism after Bariatric Surgery: The BABS Study. *J Bone Miner Res.* 2016; 31: 672–682.

[142] Marc-Hernández A, Ruiz-Tovar J, Aracil A, et al. Effects of a High-Intensity Exercise Program on Weight Regain and Cardio-metabolic Profile after 3 Years of Bariatric Surgery: A Randomized Trial. *Sci Rep.*; 10. Epub ahead of print 2020. DOI: 10.1038/s41598-020-60044-z.

In: Enhanced Recovery after Surgery ... ISBN: 978-1-53619-976-5
Editor: Jaime Ruiz-Tovar

Chapter 15

IMPLEMENTATION OF ERAS PROTOCOLS IN BARIATRIC SURGERY

Jaime Ruiz-Tovar*[1,*]*, MD, PhD
and Artur Marc Hernandez*[2]*, PhD
[1]Department of Surgery, Rey Juan Carlos University, University Rey Juan Carlos, Móstoles, Spain
[2]Faculty of Humanities and Social Sciences, University Isabel I, Burgos, Spain

ABSTRACT

Enhanced recovery after surgery (ERAS) programs are a multidisciplinary approach in the perioperative care of patients undergoing major surgery to improve their postoperative recovery. ERAS protocols are being implemented worldwide in bariatric surgery, confirming their safety and advantages on postoperative recovery. As in all surgical techniques, the implementation of ERAS protocols is sometimes a difficult issue, due to lack of acceptance by the patient, absence of enough knowledge of the protocols by the involved specialists, or even the difficulties in obtaining necessary devices to conduct certain measures included in the protocol.

---

* Corresponding Author's Email: jruiztovar@gmail.com.

In this chapter we will discuss the most relevant items included in ERAS protocols on bariatric surgery, the difficulties in their implementation and the results obtained.

Keywords: ERAS, implementation, bariatric surgery

INTRODUCTION

Recent improvements in the perioperative care of bariatric patients, optimization of the operative techniques, improvements in equipment, and the standardization of bariatric surgery programs have all resulted in decreased morbidity and mortality from bariatric surgery. Laparoscopic bariatric procedures are being performed with increasing frequency, the most common operations being laparoscopic Roux-en-Y gastric bypass (RYGB), laparoscopic sleeve gastrectomy (LSG) and laparoscopic One-anastomosis gastric bypass (OAGB) [1].

Given the increasing prevalence of obesity and its related diseases, and the resultant increased economic burden associated with their management, the current challenge is to increase the cost-effectiveness and efficiency of bariatric surgery, while maintaining the current low associated morbidity in this complicated patient group [1, 2].

Operation time, staff, and hospital stay are costly and scarce, and cannot be issued indefinitely. Ideally, better logistics and use of resources could increase both production and quality of care [3].

The concept of enhanced recovery after surgery (ERAS), was developed by Kehlet in 1997. ERAS program is a well-documented logistic program in colorectal surgery, demonstrating that an "evidence-based" approach of perioperative care leads to faster recovery and a shorter hospital stay, with improved patient well-being.

Although the contents of different fast track programs vary, common factors include the use of minimal invasive surgical techniques, the introduction short-acting anesthetic agents, optimal pain and antiemetic control, and aggressive postoperative rehabilitation, including early oral nutrition and ambulation. The rationale is to reduce the body's perioperative stress response and to induce early restoration of vital organ function, leading to a quicker recovery of the patient [4-6]. The essence of these programs is the multimodal approach, and many authors have demonstrated safety and feasibility in fast track bariatric surgery [7, 8].

ERAS Protocol in Bariatric Surgery

The basis of ERAS protocols, and bariatric surgery protocols are not an exception, is a multidisciplinary approach of patients using a specialized team, including surgical, anesthetic, dietician, and nursing teams. Encouraging patient self-reliance is essential in this concept. Preoperative information and preparation for surgery and hospital admission induce more adaptability for postoperative instructions and create realistic expectations about hospital stay, analgesia, mobilization, and discharge.

Working with the help of protocols improves the reproducibility of the operative procedure and leads to less room for failure or mistakes and increased speed [1, 7, 9].

Actually, most of the reported evidence on ERAS protocols is based on individual programs developed at single institutions [3, 5-10]. In Spain, the Spanish Enhanced Recovery Group (GERM-ERAS Spain) developed in 2014 the first national ERAS protocol in bariatric surgery. Since then, it has been updated every 2 years [11].

An ERAS protocol implies a perioperative care. Thus, the intervention must be applied in the preoperative, intraoperative and postoperative stages. The components of the Spanish ERAS protocol in bariatric surgery is summarized in Table 1.

Discharge criteria include absence of surgical complications, no fever, pain controlled with oral analgesia, full deambulation and obviously the patient acceptance.

At discharge, it is recommended to maintain the thromboprophylaxis for 28 days after surgery and the nutritional recommendations include a liquid hypocaloric hyperproteic diet, with intake in divided doses.

Table 1. Spanish ERAS protocol in bariatric surgery

Preoperative	• Provision of verbal and written information to patients regarding the ERAS. Collection of signed consent. • Preoperative evaluation. Nutritional, cardiologic, anemia, and comorbidity optimization, if required. • Laboratory data: glycemic, lipid, hepatic, and iron profiles. Basal arterial gasometry endocrinologic assessment. • Polisomnographic study to control and/or diagnosis of SAHS. Start CPAP at least 4-6 wk before surgery. • Hypocaloric diet (800 kcal/d) and nutritional supplementation 2-4 wk before surgery. 10% weight loss before intervention is advised
Day before surgery	• Low-residue diet • Dietary supplements • Thromboprophylaxis • Fasting 6 h solid. 2 h clear liquid • Avoid anxiolytic drugs
Intraoperative	• Placement of compression stockings or intermittent pneumatic compression according thromboembolic risk. • Peripheral catheter placement. Antibiotic prophylaxis 1 h before surgical incision. • Intraoperative administration of antireflux prophylaxis (metoclopramide+ranitidine 30 min before anesthetic • induction) • Usual measures for orotracheal intubation in patients with difficult airway. Rapid sequence orothacheal intubation. • Alveolar recruitment maneuvers after orothacheal intubation. • Maintenance: oxygen/air with FiO2 60%-80% • Hemodynamic optimization: goal-directed fluids administration (Cardio Q, Flo Track, Vigileo) • Analgesia: remifentanil perfusion. • Deep neuromuscular block • Active heating with thermal fluid heater and thermal blanket • No nasogastric tube • Prophylaxis of postoperative nausea and vomits following Apfel scale • Multimodal postoperative analgesia: port-sites infiltration with local anesthetics (bupivacaine 0.5%, maximum 20 mL). Immediate postoperative period • Maintenance of FiO2 50% for 2 h after surgery. • Incentive spirometry • In case of atelectasis or hypoxemia, start noninvasive mechanic ventilation (inspiratory positive airway pressure 12, expiratory positive airway pressure). CPAP in all the patients using it previously. • Avoid morphic drugs • Oral fluids 6 h after surgery • Sit patient in seat 8 h after surgery • Thromboprophylaxis
Postoperative day 1	• Liquid diet • Active mobilization • Intravenous analgesia • Analytic evaluation of C-reactive protein and/or procalcitonin
Postoeprative day 2	• Start oral analgesia • Analytic evaluation of C-reactive protein

Telephone monitoring for 48 hours to confirm the patient´s well being is recommended and the first outpatient visit must be scheduled 15 days after discharge.

RESULTS OF THE IMPLEMENTATION OF ERAS PROTOCOL IN BARIATRIC SURGERY

Bamgbade et al. [12] carried out an observational study examining the perioperative outcome data of 406 consecutive bariatric patients over a 4-year period. Their intraoperative complication rate was 0.5%. Postoperative complications occurred in 3.4% of patients with 60% within 24 h. Mean length of hospital decreased from 2 to 1 day. They concluded that establishing a fast-track bariatric service requires a learning curve of 100 cases, and a good indicator is length of hospital stay, which decreases as the service matures. Most patients can be safely discharged by 24 h.

Geubbels et al. [10] conducted a retrospective study investigating fast track care, evaluating the implementation of fast track care in unselected bariatric patients in a high volume teaching hospital in the Netherlands. They identify fast track as the banning of tubes/catheters, anesthetic management and early ambulation. They observed that the median length decreased after implementation of fast track, whereas overall complication rate remained stable after implementation of fast track care, readmission rate did not differ, but more grades I-IVa complications occurred outside the hospital. However, they concluded that this did not lead to adverse outcomes.

Conversely, other groups have also reported hospital stays <24 hours and some authors even defend that bariatric surgery can become a day-case surgery [13]. The literature shows that most of the complications occur in the first 24 hours after surgery and that complications causing readmissions could not have been avoided by longer hospitalization [1].

Dogan et al. [14] conducted prospective matched cohort study to objectify the effect of the fast-track surgery (FTS) programme in patients undergoing primary Laparoscopic Roux-en-Y Gastric Bypass (LRYGB) surgery compared to conventional perioperative care (CPC). This study compared the perioperative outcome data of two groups of 75 consecutive morbid obese patients who underwent a primary LRYGB. The two groups were matched for age and sex. Mean hospital stay was reduced from 65 to 43 hours. Major complications occurred in 3 versus 4% in the FTS and CPC, respectively. They concluded that the introduction of a fast-track programme after primary LRYGB improves short-term recovery and may reduces direct hospital-related resources.

Results of the Implementation of the Spanish ERAS Protocol in Bariatric Surgery

Following the previously presented protocol approved and endorsed by the ERAS Spain group, we conducted a first pilot multicenter study [15] to evaluate the results and implementation of the protocol. We included 125 consecutive patients undergoing bariatric surgery at 3 Spanish hospitals between January and June 2015, following the Spanish National ERAS protocol in bariatric surgery. Compliance with the protocol, morbidity, mortality, hospital stay, and readmission were evaluated. Bariatric techniques performed included 68 Roux-en-Y gastric bypass (54.4%) and 57 laparoscopic sleeve gastrectomy (45.6%) cases. All surgeries were laparoscopically performed with conversion in only 1 case (0.8%). Median postoperative pain evaluated by visual analogic scale 24 hours after surgery was 2 (range, 0 to 5). Postoperative nausea or vomiting appeared in 7 patients (5.6%). Complications appeared in 6 patients (4.8%). The reoperation rate was 4%. The mortality rate was 0.8%. The median hospital stay was 2 days (range, 2 to 10 d) and readmission rate was 2.4%. The compliance of all the items of the protocol was achieved in 78.4% of the patients. Our results regarding the bariatric techniques performed and morbidity and mortality rates are similar to those reported by other groups after fast track protocols and similar to the actual evidence available in the literature for bariatric surgery [5, 10]. The main item that distinguishes our results from those reported by other groups is the hospital stay. As previously mentioned several groups report hospital stays <24 hours and some authors even defend that bariatric surgery can become a day-case surgery [13]. Our results show that the median hospital stay was 2 days, but no patients were discharged within the first 24 hours after surgery. We still fear the appearance of complications far from a sanitary institution that might end in a fatal outcome for the patient. The systematic review performed by Elliott et al. [1] concluded that there was no sufficient evidence to promote such an early discharge based on fast track protocols.

After having observed the safety of the implementation of the ERAS protocol, we aimed to assess the benefits obtained when compared with a standard care protocol [16]. Therefore a multi-centric prospective study was performed, including 233 consecutive patients undergoing bariatric surgery during 2015 and following ERAS protocol. It was compared with a historical cohort of 286 patients, who underwent bariatric surgery at the same institutions between 2013 and 2014 and following standard care. Compliance with the protocol, morbidity, mortality, hospital stay and readmission were evaluated.

Bariatric techniques performed were Roux-en-Y gastric bypass and sleeve gastrectomy. There were no significant differences in complications, mortality and readmission. Postoperative pain and hospital stay were significantly lower in the ERAS group. The total compliance to protocol was 80%. The most difficult ítems of the protocol to be implemented were the preoperative diet (89.6%), goal-directed fluids (80%), opioid-free analgesia (96.7%), early oral intake 6 hours after surgery (88%) and early mobilization 6 hours after surgery (89.6%). We could conclude that the Spanish National ERAS protocol is a safe issue, obtaining similar results to standard care in terms of complications, reoperations, mortality and readmissions. It is associated with less postoperative pain and earlier hospital discharge.

Significant differences between the ERAS group and the historic cohort in this study were lower postoperative pain and reduction of analytical acute phase reactants (white blood cell count and CRP). These data reflected that following the ERAS protocol, the body's perioperative stress response related to the surgical act is diminished, as long as the items included in the protocol overall tend to an immunomodulation, reducing the immune stress response and finally leading to less tissue damage and lower postoperative pain [17].

A shorter hospital stay could be probably achieved without following an ERAS protocol, 'forcing' an early discharge, but, in our opinion, a lower postoperative pain implies a patient's perception of better quality of life and improves the satisfaction with the procedure. With a better postoperative pain control, the patients accept an early discharge without a sensation of being 'forced' to it. In our opinion, the shorter length of stay in the ERAS patients is directly derived from the better control of the postoperative pain. One of the main goals of ERAS protocols is the reduction of the impact of the surgical damage, thus improving the postoperative recovery. The most important clinical feature of surgical damage is often the postoperative pain. In an effort to reduce the incidence and severity of postsurgical pain, ERAS protocols include multimodal therapy. Multimodal analgesia involves the use of two or more drugs with different mechanisms of action in an effort to maximize analgesic efficacy while reducing the risk and severity of adverse events. Moreover, these protocols defend the use of opioid-free analgesia, as opioids contribute to increasing nausea and vomiting, postoperative ileus and delay in deambulation [17]. As shown in our results, the multimodal analgesia performed in the ERAS group contributes to a significant reduction in postoperative pain.

When protocols such as the present are implemented, the goal should be a full compliance with all measures outlined. However, full compliance is often very difficult to achieve. In the present study, the total compliance was, in our opinion, high (80%). Anyway, the compliance varied in its different components. The items of the protocol with lower compliance were early oral fluid administration and goal-directed fluid therapy. The reason for this different compliance rate as compared with the protocol could be the taste of oral fluid, rejection by patients fearing complications and unavailability or lack of training with the devices. Previous studies performed by the Spanish ERAS group referring to the implementation of the protocol for colorectal surgery showed that the weaknesses were the same as in the present study. Probably the implementation could improve involving and training all professionals who assist the patients and identifying these patients with signboards on bedside [18-20]. As mentioned previously, the implementation of goal-directed fluids was the measure with the worst implementation rate (80%), probably due to the economic burden associated with the use of the necessary devices, but also because some anaesthesiologists are not used to manage these devices. The objective of the intraoperative fluid administration is to maintain an adequate circulatory volume, avoiding a volume overload and trying to obtain a perioperative balance of 0. The administration of fluids based on the patients' weight tends to be higher than necessary and this is especially relevant in morbidly obese patients undergoing bariatric surgery, because the increase of fluid requirements is not directly correlated with the weight of the patient. In several studies analyzing this method, goal-directed fluid administration has been associated with a reduction in postoperative complications, mortality and hospital stay. Excessive volumen administration determines a fluid extravasation to the bowel wall, to the lungs and to the lower limbs, leading to postoperative ileus, pulmonary edema and atelectasis, and lower limbs edemas, affecting deambulation, respectively. Many other complications may derive from these issues [21-23].

Recently, we published a prospective randomized clinical trial of patients undergoing Roux-en-Y gastric bypass. To our knowledge, this was the first prospective randomized clinical trial comparing the implementation of an ERAS program versus the application of a standard care protocol. Patients were randomized into the following 2 groups: those patients after an ERAS program and those patients after a standard care protocol. Postoperative pain, nausea or vomiting, morbidity, mortality, hospital stay, and analytic acute phase reactants 24 hours after surgery were evaluated. One hundred eighty patients were included in the study, 90 in each group. Postoperative pain (16 versus 37 mm; $P < .001$), nausea or vomiting (8.9% versus 2.2%; $P = .0498$), and hospital stay (1.7 versus 2.8 d; $P < .001$) were significantly lower in the ERAS group. There were no significant differences in complications, mortality, and readmission rates. White blood cell count, serum fibrinogen, and C reactive protein levels were significantly lower in the ERAS group 24 hours after surgery. We concluded that the implementation of an ERAS protocol was associated with lower postoperative pain, reduced incidence of postoperative nausea or vomiting, lower levels of acute phase reactants, and earlier hospital discharge. Complications, reinterventions, mortality, and readmission rates were similar to that obtained after a standard care protocol [24].

REFERENCES

[1] Elliott JA, Patel VM, Kirresh A, et al. Fast-track laparoscopic bariatric surgery: a systematic review. *Updates Surg.* 2013;65:85–94.

[2] Ashrafian H. Bariatric surgery: can we afford to do it or deny doing it? *Frontline Gastroenterol.* 2011;2:82–89.

[3] Dogan K, Kraaij L, Aarts EO, et al. Fast-track bariatric surgery improves perioperative care and logistics compared to conventional care. *Obes Surg.* 2015;25:28–35.

[4] Wilmore DW, Kehlet H. Management of patients in fast track surgery. *BJM.* 2001;322:473–476.

[5] Teeuwen PH, Bleichrodt RP, Strik C, et al. Enhanced recovery after surgery (ERAS) versus conventional postoperative care in colorectal surgery. *J Gastrointest Surg.* 2010;14:88–95.

[6] Spanjersberg WR, Reurings J, Keus F, et al. Fast track surgery versus conventional recovery strategies for colorectal surgery. *Cochrane Database Syst Rev.* 2011;2:CD007635.

[7] Jacobsen HJ, Bergland A, Raeder J, et al. High-volume bariatric surgery in a single center: safety, quality, cost-efficacy and teaching aspects in 2000 consecutive patients. *Obes Surg.* 2012;22:158–166.

[8] Lemanu DP, Srinivasa S, Singh PP. Optimizing perioperative care in bariatric surgery patients. *Obes Surg.* 2012;22:979–990.

[9] Bergland A, Gislason H, Raeder J. Fast-track surgery for bariatric laparoscopic gastric bypass with focus on anesthesia and perioperative care. Experience with 500 cases. *Acta Anaesthesiol Scand.* 2008;52:1394–1399.

[10] Geubbels N, Bruin SC, Acherman YIZ, et al. Fast track care for gastric bypass patients decreases length of stay without increasing complications in an unselected patient cohort. *Obes Surg.* 2014;24:390–396.

[11] https://www.grupogerm.es/protocolos-zaragoza-2016/ (Accessed on 02/06/2021).

[12] Bamgbade OA, Adeogun BO, Abbas K. Fast-track laparoscopic gastric bypass surgery: outcomes and lessons from a bariatric

surgery service in the United Kingdom. *Obes Surg* 2012; 22:398-402.

[13] Raeder J. Bariatric procedures as day/short stay surgery: it is possible and reasonable? *Curr Opin Anaesthesiol.* 2007;20: 508–512.

[14] Dogan K, Kraaij L, Aarts EO, et al. Fast-track bariatric surgery improves perioperative care and logistics compared to conventional care. *Obes Surg.* 2015;25:28–35.

[15] Ruiz-Tovar J, Royo P, Muñoz JL, et al. Implementation of the Spanish National Enhanced Recovery Program (ERAS) in Bariatric Surgery: A Pilot Study. *Surg Laparosc Endosc Percutan Tech.* 2016;26:439-443.

[16] Ruiz-Tovar J, Muñoz JL, Royo P, et al. Implementation of the Spanish ERAS program in bariatric surgery. *Minim Invasive Ther Allied Technol* 2018;27:365-372.

[17] Practice guidelines for acute pain management in the perioperative setting: an updated report by the American Society of Anesthesiologists Task Force on Acute Pain Management. *Anesthesiology.* 2012;116:248–273.

[18] Ramiırez JM, Blasco JA, Roig JV, et al. Enhanced recovery in colorectal surgery: a multicentre study. *BMC Surg.* 2011;11:19.

[19] Arroyo A, Ramirez JM, Callejo D, et al. Influence of size and complexity of the hospitals in an enhanced recovery programme for colorectal resection. *Int J Colorectal Dis.* 2012;27:1637–1644.

[20] Esteban F, Cerdan FJ, Garcia-Alonso M, et al. A multicentre comparison of a fast track or conventional postoperative protocol following laparoscopic or open elective surgery for colorectal cancer surgery. *Colorectal Dis.* 2014;16:134–140.

[21] Jain AK, Dutta A. Stroke volume variation as a guide to fluid administration in morbidly obese patients undergoing laparoscopic bariatric surgery. *Obes Surg.* 2010;20:709–715.

[22] Poso T, Kesek D, Aroch R, et al. Morbid obesity and optimization of preoperative fluid therapy. *Obes Surg.* 2013;23:1799–1805.

[23] Arulkumaran N, Corredor C, Hamilton MA, et al. Cardiac complications associated with goal-directed therapy in high-risk surgical patients: a meta-analysis. *Br J Anaesth.* 2014;112:466–659.

[24] Ruiz-Tovar J, Garcia A, Ferrigni C, et al. Impact of implementation of an enhanced recovery after surgery (ERAS) program in laparoscopic Roux-en-Y gastric bypass: a prospective randomized clinical trial. *Surg Obes Relat Dis* 2019;15:228– 235.

In: Enhanced Recovery after Surgery … ISBN: 978-1-53619-976-5
Editor: Jaime Ruiz-Tovar

Chapter 16

ECONOMIC ASPECTS OF ERAS PROTOCOLS IMPLEMENTATION

Alfonso Higueras*, MD
Department of Health Sciences, Universidad Alfonso X,
Madrid, Spain

ABSTRACT

The exponential growth of world health spending due to the continuous increase in patients' health needs is an important variable when evaluating the alternatives and procedures implemented by professionals in the surgical area. The introduction of new methods and techniques in routine bariatric surgical practice is urgent to ensure its sustainability in the current scenario of a scarcity of health resources.

Enhanced recovery after surgery (ERAS) protocols have shown significant benefits in safety and efficacy. Besides, these protocols can be a tool to economically optimise the current surgical model by guaranteeing an overall cost-saving for the hospital and improving the social stakeholders.

The main barriers to implementing these protocols are the lack of acceptance and understanding by patients, the lack of specialists'

* Corresponding Author's Email: Alfonso.higueras.lara@gmail.com.

know-how, and the logistical effort and previous investment necessary for their implementation.

This chapter will focus on state of the art and discuss the most relevant economic issues related to ERAS protocols, the advantages and difficulties in their implementation from a socioeconomic perspective, to better inform managers and health professionals who are considering adopting this approach in their hospitals.

Keywords: ERAS, Health economics, ERAS Implementation cost, cost savings, ERAS hospital charges

Introduction

In recent years, the number and cost of surgeries increased dramatically [1], leading to the entry into a paradigm based on the optimisation of processes and techniques. Sustainability is fundamental for the system and the surgical teams if they want to continue innovating growing [2].

We will witness a constant and rapid growth of the world population in the coming years: the United Nations estimates that in 2030 we will be about 8,500 million people [3]. Before the current COVID-19 epidemic, the global healthcare expenditure was expected to grow at an annual rate of 5.4%. It will assume around $ 10 trillion in 2022 [4]. Population ageing dramatically increases the incidence of neoplastic diseases [3], one of the most common causes of surgical interventions [5].

The constant increase in patients' health needs [6], the prevalence of chronic diseases, and their management cost are critical variables when evaluating the alternatives and procedures to be implemented by professionals in the surgical area. Thus, there is an urgent need to introduce new methods and techniques that guarantee the sustainability of routine surgical practices in this current scenario, characterised by the scarcity of healthcare resources [7].

Multiple institutions and health systems are choosing to systematically introduce enhanced recovery after surgery (ERAS) protocols after numerous studies demonstrated their cost-effective benefits for patients. Since 2010, after the publication of a study by

Sammour et al., [8], we have clear evidence to defend the hypothesis that the burden and the initial cost of setting up an ERAS program are more than offset by the savings made.

The challenge of implementing the ERAS protocol represents a major change from the current traditional practice. A successful implementation implies the participation and commitment of all stakeholders in primary, secondary and social care. High-complexity teams, coordinated through high-level management, are necessary for a change to be sustainable [9]. The work team is usually multidisciplinary, made up of surgeons, anaesthetists, specialised nurses and managers. Their function is to understand the current service, identify and implement the improvements to be made, generate changes, measure their impact and provide feedback to the clinical team [10].

Besides, the education and training of the professionals in charge are essential to successfully introducing the ERAS protocol in the long term since it will impact the clinical results and the team's motivation. All members of this multidisciplinary team must understand that their role is vital to the project's success [11].

To guarantee and facilitate the audit of the implementation of the protocols, Mahesh et al., in 2018 began to use the agile methodology, employing the Define, Measure, Analyse, Improve and Control (DMAIC) cycle of the Multi-Specialty Hospital in Bangalore [10]. The continuous monitoring and collection of reference data, which allows visualising the clinical and service evaluation results, is essential. Understanding the progress of implementation and its impact on the service is key to incorporating these protocols into routine clinical practice effectively [11]. Also, an important recommendation of the ERAS society guidelines is that ERAS programs provide an audit of clinical outcomes and make this information available to providers [12].

This article aims to explore the economic impact of the ERAS protocol in different surgical areas [13], analysing the cost savings at the perioperative level. It should be noted that the main indicators used by most of the articles in the literature are the length of hospital stay, the days of admission to intensive care, the number of complications, and the pain control. All of them are expensive and rare. Therefore, a logistical improvement could increase the volume and quality of the clinic [13]. We will only discuss on one indicator, the general cost-saving.

Area 1: Colorectal Surgery

The concept of enhanced recovery after surgery (ERAS) was firstly described by Although Kehlet in 1997, but it will not be until much later that the first significant evidence and economic analysis of the cost reduction benefits of this type of intervention appeared [14]. Starting from 2010, when Sammour et al., showed a saving per patient of $ 4,429 in their study [15], the surgical areas' managers began to have clear evidence to defend the ERAS program's creation. The estimated cost of the complications of this type of surgery was later described by Birkmeyer J. D. et al., in 2012 with an estimated cost of $ 10,000 in very conservative scenarios [16].

In 2014, Lee et al., first and Lemanu et al., later presented two systematic reviews that generated interesting evidence that, despite their limitations, defined ERAS protocol as cost-effective interventions in colorectal surgery, reporting cost savings, although with a lot of variability [17, 18]. In the same year, Feng F. et al., stated that ERAS protocols applied to laparoscopy would reduce hospital costs due to improved recovery and shorter hospital stay [19].

In 2015, Lee et al., described cost savings in colorectal surgery after implementing an ERAS program in a more structured way. This article registers a weighted direct saving close to $ 3,000 per patient [20]. That same year Keenan J. E. et al., showed that there are additive synergies between different peri-surgical care programs [21]. On the other hand, Thiele R. H. et al., create another study on the importance of standardising ERAS protocols [22].

In 2016 Nelson et al., published a multicenter study in Alberta [23], showing a net cost savings of $ 1768 (range $ 920 and $ 2619) per patient, describing how the implementation of the ERAS colorectal guide is beneficial for the improvement of the clinical results due to the scarce resources of the health system. Every $ 1 invested in ERAS would generate $ 3.8 (range $ 2.4 and $ 5.1) in terms of ROI. The following year Lau C. S. et al., presented a meta-analysis where they estimated the savings in using these protocols in colorectal surgery and where doubts were raised with the increase in readmissions at 30 days [24]. More recently, Peter A. Najjar et al., from the Massachusetts hospital presented an article addressing the savings produced by incorporating these protocols to the colectomy and showing a saving close to 9% ($ 2215 and $ 824) per patient [25].

Area 2: Hepatobiliary Surgery

In 2015 Joliat et al., published an article estimating a cost savings of about $ 7,000 per patient undergoing pancreaticoduodenectomy in Switzerland. Most of these savings came from the reduction of intensive care costs (€ 9,139 compared to € 13,793) [26]. Three years later, Jing et al., showed how the implementation of the ERAS protocol in China resulted in a cost-saving of $ 1,367.51 per patient undergoing hepatectomy, mainly due to the reduction of medication requirements [27].

Area 3: Urological Surgery

This area has not been deeply investigated from an economic point of view, but the results are similar to those presented in other surgical areas. A study published in 2016 showed how the implementation of ERAS protocol for radical cystectomy significantly reduced the overall cost per patient by $ 4,488 [28].

Area 4: Gynecological Surgery

Similarly to previous studies that demonstrated the profitability of the ERAS protocol in other general areas [9], in 2013, Kalogera E. et al., showed profitability of $ 7,600 per patient in gynaecological surgeries [5], while Relph et al., focused on its implementation in benign vaginal surgery and reached a saving of 15.2% (or $ 164.86) per patient [29]. A year later, Yoong W. et al., presented a saving of 9.25% per patient in vaginal hysterectomy [30].

Finally, in 2019 Pache et al., exhaustively analysed the costs of implementing an ERAS program in the gynaecological area and found out that the main costs were specialised personnel, administration times, consumables and investment in specific auditable software. In this article, the average overcharge per patient was estimated to be approximately $ 687. However, subsequent savings were estimated at $ 4,381 per patient, and the study follow-up was at three years [31].

Area 5: Cardiovascular Surgery

In 2012, Tatsuishi et al., published an article on the advantages of implementing ERAS and shortening the days of stay after an abdominal aortic aneurysm intervention in Japan, which resulted in an 8% reduction compared to the control group [32]. Recently, in 2021, Petersen et al., presented the effect of the implementation of the ERAS protocol in minimally invasive cardiac surgery, reaching an economic benefit of $ 1909 per patient [33].

Discussion on the Impact of the Implementation of ERAS Protocols

Although ERAS programs potentially provide better healthcare, reduce complications, and enhance the value of the patient care experience [34], the economic advantage may be compelling to increase their implementation by the hospital managers. In recent years, we have witnessed a growth in the development of this current of thought, and different workgroups specialised in ERAS consider that improving its acceptance from the hospital managers is necessary to ensure its success and durability of the program [35].

ERAS programs require an initial investment of resources: capital, leadership, and time, ranging from front-line providers and auxiliary services to personnel to the level of hospital executives [36]. The existing financing models, often conservative and monodisciplinary, complicate their implementation [37]; thus, hospital managers' support and resources are needed to implement these projects beyond pilot studies [38]. The value provided by patients in the so-called user experience is an interesting variable to measure in this communication to health managers and one of the most critical indicators in implementing this project [39].

Finally, we must understand the ERAS program's implementation as a net amalgamation of marginal gains, executed in isolation can produce incremental and quantifiable results in the results [40]. The previous data demonstrate how a greater compliance to the ERAS process measures leads to better results [41]. That is why having agile work methodologies that allow feedback and measurement of the results in real-time is a tool of high interest to be validated.

Table 1. Summary of cost-saving ERAS

Author	Year	Country	Speciality	Saving per Patient
Sammour et al.	2010	NZ	Colorectal	$ 4,429
Torbe et al.	2012	UK	Gynaecology	$ 240
Tatsuishi et al.	2012	Japan	Vascular	8%
Kalogera et al.	2013	USA	Gynaecology	$ 7,600
Relph et al.	2014	UK	Colorectal	$ 200
Yoong et al.	2014	UK	Colorectal	$ 129
Lemanu et al.	2014	NZ	Colorectal	$ 170-7,249
Feng et al.	2014	China	Colorectal	$ 708
Lee et al.	2015	Canada	Colorectal	$ 2,985
Joliat et al.	2015	Switzerland	Hepatobiliary	$ 8,317
Nelson et al.	2016	Canada	Colorectal	$ 1,768
Nabhani et al.	2016	USA	Urology	$ 4,488
Jing et al.	2018	China	Hepatobiliary	$ 1,367
Pache et al.	2019	Switzerland	Gynaecology	$ 4,381
Petersen et al.	2021	USA	Cardiovascular	$ 1,909
Peter A. Najjar et al.	2021	USA	Colorectal	$ 2,215-824

A limitation of this kind of studies is the high variability of currencies used in the existing literature, the economic adjustment due to inflation and the different models of reimbursement of the procedures. Thus, in this economic evaluation, we decided to change all currencies to dollars, at their exchange rate at the time of each study (Table 1). Because of that, we ask the scientific community to date the interventions in a percentage way, following the standards of economic analysis established for this type of study, always favouring a check-list compared to the control intervention to carry out reliable analyses in future studies [42].

Given the high savings in practically all the surgical areas studied, it should be remembered that due to methodological similarity, and even with little direct economic evidence, it is advisable to implement these ERAS protocols in other surgical areas such as bariatric surgery, where it is already present available from a variety of studies in which it has been shown to be clinically useful [41]. this implementation can be economically very productive

CONCLUSION

The existing literature clearly shows that ERAS programs are an interesting tool for optimising the economic resources of surgical areas. The cost savings make the implementation of these protocols a highly recommended practice in the usual work process for surgical teams, despite the lack of know-how of the professionals, the initial costs of the ERAS protocol, the added medication and the costs of personal.

We need new studies to understand the lack of acceptance and understanding of these protocols by patients, to improve their empowerment and implementation.

The economic analysis reveals that the implementation of ERAS protocols is a highly variable health intervention. This being a multifactorial, temporal and multidisciplinary variability, which requires specialised personnel and medication. The need arises for new studies to measure and compare the added benefit of the implementation of this health intervention previously and once the learning curve of the work teams in the surgical areas has been overcome.

We consider that more studies are needed to clarify the effect of the use of agile methodologies to improve the results of the implementation and local development of the ERAS protocols. Finally, we must analyse the possible causes of the lack of assimilation of these scalable protocols among professionals in the surgical areas of our environment, with the aim of knowing the limitations of this implementation.

REFERENCES

[1] Weiser T. G., Regenbogen S. E., Thompson K. D., Haynes A. B., Lipsitz S. R., Berry W. R., et al., An estimation of the global volume of surgery: a modelling strategy based on available data. *Lancet* 2008; 372: 139-44.

[2] Gómez-Ríos M. A., Abad-Gurumeta A., Casans-Francés R., Calvo-Vecino J. M. Claves para optimizar la eficiencia de un bloque quirúrgico. *Rev Esp Anestesiol Reanim* 2019; 66(2):104-112.

[3] Ferlay J., Soerjomataram I., Dikshit R., et al., Cancer incidence and mortality worldwide: sources, methods and major patterns in GLOBOCAN 2012. *Int J Cancer* 2015; 136:E359-86.

[4] 2019 Global health care sector outlook. *Deloitte.* [cited 2019 Jul 29]. Available online: https://www2.deloitte.com/global/en/pages/life-sciences-and-healthcare/articles/global-health-care-sector-outlook.html.

[5] Lee D., Haynes C., Deans G., Cook G. Implementing enhanced recovery after surgery in a district general hospital: implications of a pilot study. *J Eval Clin Pract* 2011; 17(06):1243-1245.

[6] United Nations. DESA/Population Division. *World Population Prospects 2019: Highlights.* Available online: https://population.un.org/wpp/Publications/ (Accessed 04/05/2021).

[7] Ashrafian H. Bariatric surgery: can we afford to do it or deny doing it? *Frontline Gastroenterol.* 2011; 2:82-89.

[8] Sammour T., Zargar-Shoshtari K., Bhat A., et al., A programme of Enhanced Recovery After Surgery (ERAS)is a cost-effective intervention in elective colonic surgery. *N Z Med J* 2010; 123:61-70.

[9] Torbe E., Louden K. an enhanced recovery programme for women undergoing hysterectomy. *Int J Gynecol Obstet* 2012; 119:S690.

[10] Mahesh B. P., Soragaon B., Annigeri A. R. Reduction of Patient Wait Time at a Multi-Specialty Hospital Using DMAIC Methodology and Factor Analysis. *Int. J. Eng. Technol.* 2018; 7:309-312.

[11] RCOG, Enhanced Recovery in Gynaecology, *scientific impact papers* no. 36 https://www.rcog.org.uk/globalassets/documents/guidelines/scientific-impact-papers/sip_36.pdf.

[12] Gustafsson U. O., Scott M. J., Schwenk W., et al., Enhanced Recovery After Surgery Society. Guidelines for perioperative care in elective colonic surgery: Enhanced Recovery After Surgery (ERAS®) Society recommendations. *Clin Nutr* 2012; 31(06):783-800.

[13] Dogan K., Kraaij L., Aarts E. O., et al., Fast-track bariatric surgery improves perioperative care and logistics compared to conventional care. *Obes Surg.* 2015; 25:28-35.

[14] Wilmore D. W., Kehlet H. Management of patients in fast track surgery. *BJM.* 2001; 322:473-476.

[15] Kalogera E., Bakkum-Gamez J. N., Jankowski C. J., et al., Enhanced recovery in gynecologic surgery. *Obstet Gynecol* 2013; 122:319-28.

[16] Birkmeyer J. D., Gust C., Dimick J. B., Birkmeyer N. J., Skinner J. S. Hospital quality and the cost of inpatient surgery in the United States. *Ann Surg* 2012; 255(01):1-5.

[17] Lee L., Li C., Landry T., et al., A systematic review of economic evaluations of enhanced recovery pathways for colorectal surgery. *Ann Surg* 2014; 259:670-6.

[18] Lemanu D. P., Singh P. P., Stowers M. D., et al., A systematic review to assess cost effectiveness of enhanced recovery after surgery programmes in colorectal surgery. *Colorectal Dis* 2014; 16:338-46.

[19] Feng F., Li XH., Shi H., et al., Fast-track surgery combined with laparoscopy could improve postoperative recovery of low-risk rectal cancer patients: a randomised controlled clinical trial. *J Dig Dis* 2014; 15:306-13.

[20] Lee L., Mata J., Ghitulescu G. A., et al., Cost-effectiveness of Enhanced Recovery Versus Conventional Perioperative Management for Colorectal Surgery. *Ann Surg* 2015; 262:1026-33.

[21] Keenan J. E., Speicher P. J., Nussbaum D. P., et al., Improving outcomes in colorectal surgery by sequential implementation of multiple standardised care programs. *J Am Coll Surg* 2015; 221(02):404-14.e1.

[22] Thiele R. H., Rea K. M., Turrentine F. E., et al., Standardisation of care: impact of an enhanced recovery protocol on length of stay,

complications, and direct costs after colorectal surgery. *J Am Coll Surg* 2015; 220(04):430-443.

[23] Nelson G., Kiyang L. N., Chuck A., et al., Cost impact analysis of Enhanced Recovery After Surgery program implementation in Alberta colon cancer patients. *Curr Oncol* 2016; 23:e221-7.I.

[24] Lau C. S., Chamberlain R. S. Enhanced Recovery After Surgery programs improve patient outcomes and recovery: a meta-analysis. *World J Surg* 2017; 41(04):899-913.

[25] Najjar P. A., Fields A. C., Maldonado L. J., Ward A., Bleday R. Differential Index-Hospitalization Cost Center Impact of Enhanced Recovery After Surgery Program Implementation. *Dis Colon Rectum.* 2020 Jun;63(6):837-841. doi: https://10.1097/DCR.0000000000001662. PMID: 32168094.

[26] Joliat G. R., Labgaa I., Petermann D., et al., Cost-benefit analysis of an enhanced recovery protocol for pancreaticoduodenectomy. *Br J Surg* 2015; 102:1676-83.

[27] Jing X., Zhang B., Xing S., et al., Cost-benefit analysis of enhanced recovery after hepatectomy in Chinese Han population. *Medicine* (Baltimore) 2018; 97:e11957.

[28] Nabhani J., Ahmadi H., Schuckman A. K., et al., Cost Analysis of the Enhanced Recovery After Surgery Protocol in Patients Undergoing Radical Cystectomy for Bladder Cancer. *Eur Urol Focus* 2016; 2:92-6.

[29] Relph S., Bell A., Sivashanmugarajan V., et al., Cost effectiveness of enhanced recovery after surgery programme for vaginal hysterectomy: a comparison of pre and post-implementation expenditures. *Int J Health Plann Manage* 2014; 29:399-406.

[30] Yoong W., Sivashanmugarajan V., Relph S., et al., Can enhanced recovery pathways improve outcomes of vaginal hysterectomy? Cohort control study. *J Minim Invasive Gynecol* 2014;21:83-9.

[31] Pache B., Joliat G. R., Hübner M., et al., Cost-analysis of Enhanced Recovery After Surgery (ERAS) program in gynecologic surgery. *Gynecol Oncol* 2019;154:388-93.

[32] Tatsuishi W., Kohri T., Kodera K., et al., Usefulness of an enhanced recovery after surgery protocol for perioperative management following open repair of an abdominal aortic aneurysm. *Surg Today* 2012; 42:1195-200.

[33] Petersen, J., Kloth, B., Konertz, J. et al., Economic impact of enhanced recovery after surgery protocol in minimally invasive cardiac surgery. *BMC Health Serv Res* 2021; 21: 254.
[34] Gani F., Makary M. A., Wick E. C., et al., Bundled payments for surgical colectomy among Medicare enrollees: potential savings vs the need for further reform. *JAMA Surg* 2016; 151(05):e160202.
[35] Wick E. C., Galante D. J., Hobson D. B., et al., Organisational culturechanges result in improvement in patient-centered outcomes: implementation of an integrated recovery pathway for surgical patients. *J Am Coll Surg* 2015; 221(03):669-677, quiz 785-786.
[36] McLeod R. S., Aarts M. A., Chung F., et al., Development of an Enhanced Recovery After Surgery guideline and implementation strategy based on the knowledge-to-action cycle. *Ann Surg* 2015; 262(06):1016-1025.
[37] McEvoy M. D., Wanderer J. P., King A. B., et al., A perioperative consult service results in reduction in cost and length of stay for colorectal surgical patients: evidence from a healthcare redesign project. *Perioper Med* (Lond) 2016; 5:3.
[38] Stone A. B., Grant M. C., Pio Roda C., et al., Implementation costs of an Enhanced Recovery After Surgery Program in the United States: a financial model and sensitivity analysis based on experiences at a quaternary academic medical center. *J Am Coll Surg* 2016; 222 (03):219-225.
[39] Ljungqvist O., Scott M., Fearon K. C. Enhanced recovery after surgery: a review. *JAMA Surg* 2017;152(03):292-298.
[40] MacFie J. Enhanced recovery after surgery is obsolete. *Dis Colon Rectum* 2016; 59(10):1002-1003.
[41] Pędziwiatr M., Kisialeuski M., Wierdak M., et al., Early implementation of Enhanced Recovery After Surgery (ERAS®) protocol compliance improves outcomes: a prospective cohort study. *Int J Surg* 2015; 21:75-81.
[42] Adamina M., Senagore A. J., Delaney C. P., Kehlet H. A systematic review of economic evaluations of enhanced recovery pathways for colorectal surgery. *Ann Surg* 2015; 261(05):e138.

[43] Morrison B., Kelliher L., Jones C. The economic benefits of enhanced recovery after surgery programmes. *Dig Med Res* 2019; 2:20.

About the Editor

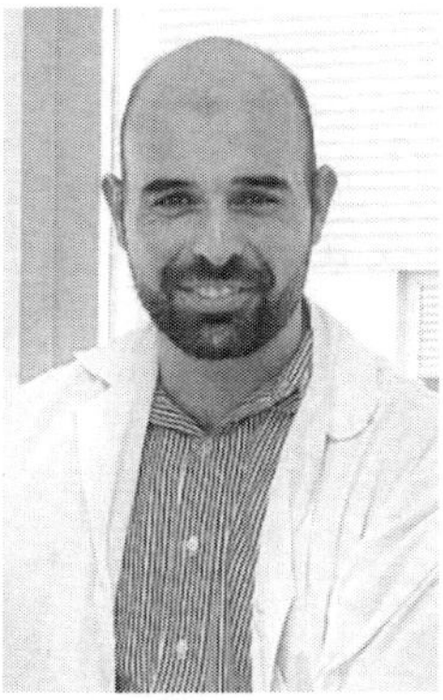

Jaime Ruiz-Tovar, MD, PhD

Professor of Surgery, Universidad Rey Juan Carlos.

Madrid, Spain

Email: jruiztovar@gmail.com

Jaime Ruiz-Tovar, MD, PhD, is General and Digestive Surgeon at Garcilaso Clinic (Madrid-Spain), where he is specialized in bariatric surgery. Professor of Surgery at Universidad Rey Juan Carlos. Head of the Bariatric Surgery section of the ERAS-Spain group (Enhanced Recovery After Surgery). He actually leads several investigational projects focused on bariatric surgery and surgical infections.

INDEX

A

B

C

D

E

S

T

U

W